'In our world today, where we struggle with the dissolution of community and trust in each other, with only the contractual communicative dimensions of political correctness as the tether to the social, what can we make of the underlying role of humour, comedy, and jokes, so often the source of offence and resentment? In *Race, Racism and Political Correctness in Comedy*, Jack Black shows us that the only way to achieve a proper universality under these conditions is through the subversive dimensions of comedy, itself. Drawing on the influential work of Lacanian theorists, such as Alenka Zupančič and Slavoj Žižek, Black teaches us about the politically subversive potentials of comedy, and how humour, more so than political correctness, is the only real way to go on the attack against social ills, like racism. Joining other leading Lacanian scholars, such as Zupančič and Todd McGowan, Black's book is sure to be a welcomed addition to the growing field of Lacanian studies of comedy.'

Matthew Flisfeder, author of *Algorithmic Desire: Toward a New Structuralist Theory of Social Media*

'This book provides a much-needed corrective to the asinine managerialist mindset that promotes the politically correct banality of safe spaces over the unpredictable challenges of critical thinking. Jack Black expertly demonstrates how the path to true seriousness is strewn with jokes. He puts the open-minded reader genuinely concerned about racism on the psychoanalyst's couch and reveals the various ways in which comedy is a highly resilient antidote to dominant ideological stupidities. University apparatchiks will not like this book – which is why I cannot recommend it highly enough.'

Paul Taylor, University of Leeds

RACE, RACISM AND POLITICAL CORRECTNESS IN COMEDY

In what ways is comedy subversive? This vital new book critically considers the importance of comedy in challenging and redefining our relations to race and racism through the lens of political correctness.

By viewing comedy as both a constitutive feature of social interaction and as a necessary requirement in the appraisal of what is often deemed to be 'politically correct', this book provides an innovative and multidisciplinary approach to the study of comedy and popular culture. In doing so, it engages with the social and cultural tensions inherent to our understandings of political correctness, arguing that comedy can subversively redefine our approach to 'PC debates', contestations surrounding free speech and the popular portrayal of political correctness in the media and society. Aided by the work of both Slavoj Žižek and Alenka Zupančič, this unique analysis adopts a psychoanalytic/philosophical framework to explore issues of race, racism and political correctness in the widely acclaimed BBC 'mockumentary', *The Office* (UK), as well as a variety of television comedies.

Drawing from psychoanalysis, social psychology and philosophy, this book will be highly relevant for postgraduate students and academic researchers studying comedy, race/racism, multiculturalism, political correctness and television/film.

Jack Black is a Senior Lecturer at Sheffield Hallam University. After completing his postgraduate studies at Loughborough University, his research has continued to explore the interrelationships between sociology, media and communications and cultural studies. Drawing upon 'traditional' media forms (newspaper analysis) as well as television and film studies, Jack's published work provides an interdisciplinary approach to the study of ideology, politics and power in both the media and popular culture.

RACE, RACISM AND POLITICAL CORRECTNESS IN COMEDY

A Psychoanalytic Exploration

Jack Black

Routledge
Taylor & Francis Group
LONDON AND NEW YORK

First published 2021
by Routledge
2 Park Square, Milton Park, Abingdon, Oxon OX14 4RN

and by Routledge
52 Vanderbilt Avenue, New York, NY 10017

Routledge is an imprint of the Taylor & Francis Group, an informa business

British Library Cataloguing-in-Publication Data
A catalogue record for this book is available from the British Library

Library of Congress Cataloging-in-Publication Data
A catalog record has been requested for this book

ISBN: 978-0-367-50895-1 (hbk)
ISBN: 978-0-367-50893-7 (pbk)
ISBN: 978-1-003-05169-5 (ebk)

Typeset in Bembo
by Taylor & Francis Books

For Alex

CONTENTS

ACKNOWLEDGMENTS

I would like to thank Tom Fletcher, Adam White and Stuart Whigham for inviting me to present early drafts of this work at their respective universities. I would also like to thank Tony Blackshaw for reading the first draft, and for encouraging me to continue. As always, I thank Alex – for all that need not be said.

INTRODUCTION

Comedy, political correctness and the case of Konstantin Kisin

In December 2018, Russian-born comedian Konstantin Kisin was asked to play a benefit gig for a UNICEF society at the School of African and Oriental Studies (SOAS) in London, UK (United Kingdom). The banality of this request would have gone largely unnoticed, if not for the outcry that Kisin's invitation created. Indeed, before performing his stand-up routine, Kisin was asked to sign a 'behavioural agreement', with the intention that the agreement would 'ensure' that Kisin's set would refrain from telling jokes on 'racism, sexism, classism, ageism, ableism, homophobia, biphobia, transphobia, xenophobia and Islamophobia or anti-religion or anti-atheism' (BBC, 2018). Kisin declined to perform.

In the days following Kisin's decline (which he subsequently made public), a variety of media reports and appearances – involving journalists, television personalities, fellow comedians and Kisin himself – sought to clarify the strange predicament that the comedian had found himself in (Bennett, 2018; Jefferies, 2019; Kisin, 2018; Malik, 2018). As evident in Kisin's (2018) account of the incident, the story quickly turned into a debate on 'political correctness' and the significance of comedy as a forum for discussing, challenging and critiquing common assumptions, values and beliefs.

Certainly, this type of 'story' is not a new one, with the relationship between comedy and political correctness proving a notable feature in contemporary debates on how comedy should approach issues relating to identity politics, taboo subjects and potentially offensive traditions. Nonetheless, for Kisin (2018), the relation between comedy and political correctness was one that reflected a growing trend across university campuses in the UK. Despite SOAS's declarations that the university and its students' union upheld the values of 'free speech', later emphasising that they did not require speakers to sign a 'behavioural agreement' (BBC, 2018), both the original contract and Kisin's (2018) frustrations were used to signify an apparent increase in the overbearing, oversensitive 'safe-spaces' that he believed were ubiquitously framing our everyday lives.

Indeed, it would seem that the 'over-sensitivity' of the contract is what proved particularly riling for Kisin, with him later stating that 'If someone writes a contract like that, the chances are that they will be hypersensitive, vigilant and trying to catch you out' (BBC, 2018). In a piece published in the UK newspaper the *Daily Mail,* Kisin stated that the contract's contents 'were as depressing as they were alarming' (Kisin, 2018). According to Kisin, 'There is a measure of cruelty at the heart of almost all comedy – even self-deprecating jokes have bite' (2018). Despite the ambiguity in Kisin's remarks (just how cruel can comedy be?), his comments resonate with a variety of comedians who have sought to draw upon taboo topics and subversive ideas in order to challenge (as well as propagate) traditional, conservative values regarding identity, sexuality, gender, racism, homophobia, disability, rape and pedophilia.

However, what was clear from both the media and public responses that Kisin received was the way in which these debates were ideologically framed around an apparent decline in liberal values of 'free speech'. In particular, while many protagonists of political correctness would advocate its proficiency in ensuring the rights and values of the individual's autonomy (Alibhai-Brown, 2018), both Kisin and his supporters saw the agreements' infringement as a reflection of an encroaching political correctness, bent on ensuring that the individual's capacity to share their opinion, whatever their political persuasion, remains beholden to a number of regulatory controls. Indeed, for Kisin, the list of 'inappropriate' topics was 'a laughable pastiche of today's politically correct times' (2018). Though the agreement was perceived as demonstrating 'the over-sensitivity of molly-coddled millennials, the so-called snowflake generation', as well as providing an example of the now well-recited refrain, 'political correctness gone mad', for Kisin, the agreement was 'more sinister than that' (2018). According to Kisin, the agreement reflected a form of 'Ideological oppression', similar to the Soviet Union, and one marked by the assertion that 'Britain's conviction in freedom of expression is waning' (2018).

Nonetheless, in the days following the incident, Kisin was asked to perform at a comedy event, where, as he later wrote:

> I read out the behavioural agreement form and got a few nice laughs. I then announced that I would be doing my normal set in the spirit of SOAS's rules to be 'respectful and kind'. 'Hello, my name is Konstantin Kisin,' I announced. 'Thank you very much – good night!' And walked off the stage to huge cheers.
> *(2018)*

While admonishing the UK's waning free speech and its over-reliance on 'safe-spaces', which were believed to unnecessarily curtail comic material, evidently Kisin did eventually find the exact space from which he was free to recite the agreement and incorporate it as part of his comic routine (this included his piece in the *Daily Mail*). In addition, the event became a formative theme in his proceeding stand-up tour. Nevertheless, both the incident and its ensuing debates offer a number of important and significant insights into the role of comedy and its ability to subversively challenge and critique social norms and values amidst a milieu of increasing awareness on the potentially harmful effects of stereotypes, typecasts and social and political 'labels' that are deemed inappropriate. What is noticeable is how these incidents continue to be framed in accordance with the actions, behaviours, routines and comic performances of a variety of well-known and widely celebrated comedians. In reflecting upon the Kisin incident, Stuart Jeffries remarked that:

> Comedy is in a period of extraordinary flux. The past two years have witnessed the reputations of revered comics, such as Louis CK and Aziz Ansari, implode in the wake of #MeToo allegations. Then there is the culture of unearthing old tweets, with standups being held to account for problematic 'jokes' they've made online (for Kevin Hart, it even cost him his most high-profile gig to date, hosting the Oscars).
>
> *(2019)*

Notably, the example of Louis CK exemplifies the ambiguity surrounding this flux. Before admitting to the allegations of sexual harassment that were directed towards him, Louis CK was widely promoted and heralded as a subversive comedian, 'poking fun at the inequalities of American society, while simultaneously acknowledging the ways they benefited him' (Jeffries, 2019). Though critics and commentators have since admonished Louis CK's behaviour, in many ways, these criticisms echo recent scholarship which has seen a turn away from comedy's subversive capacity towards discussions on the potential that comedy can provide in affording a 'radical' (but reactionary) (re)appraisal of contemporary issues and social problems (Fahs, 2019; Krefting, 2019).

For this book, the Kisin incident will serve as a prelude to exploring the subversive effects of comedy. Specifically, the following study and analysis will explore the various ways in which comedy *is* subversive. More importantly, this book will argue that it is through comedy's subversion that we can identify, expose and critique racist assumptions. The intention of this book is not to propose a clearly delineated list of 'good' comedy and 'bad' comedy, but rather to examine how and in what ways comedy can subversively challenge universal notions by seeking to establish a deliberate sense of uncomfortableness as fundamental to our relations with the other and ourselves. Key to this approach will be a considered examination of the hegemonic significance of political correctness as it is both promoted and disparaged in contemporary examples.

Central to this claim is the concern that in both promoting as well as denouncing political correctness, the relative significance of discourses *on* political correctness maintain a hegemonic universal function that both shapes and limits its own critique. Subsequently, by way of navigating this critique, this book will explore how such hegemony has become embroiled within discussions on multiculturalism, cultural diversity and 'race' relations, drawn primarily from a (neo)liberal ideological field. In doing so, the following chapters will seek to focus on the relationship between political correctness and examples of racism, paying particular attention to the ways in which political correctness seeks to manage and regulate human interaction. Here, a consideration of the subject's relation with the other, and how such dynamics are often presented in examples of race and racism, will be provided. However, before turning to these dynamics, the remainder of this introduction will seek to outline, define and introduce a number of key concepts and ideas that will serve to underpin the discussion that follows.

What is political correctness?

We can define political correctness as a form of avoidance that aims to curtail examples of offence that may be directed to a particular group (often a minority group). Before its re-appropriation by conservative critics in the 1990s, the term originated in the 1970s 'New Left' movement, serving as a form of self-parody against dogmatic forms of political assertion (Hall, 1994). For conservative critics, however, political correctness functions as a lynchpin for drawing together wider complaints against the erosion of 'traditional national cultures', with various opponents quick to denounce political correctness as a function of the 'nanny state'. Here, moral injustice and forms of inequality are frequently viewed as the fault of the individual – whatever their sex, race/ethnicity or physical capability. In part, this history points towards the term's ideological significance, one where the confusions which it creates can be used for alternative and opposing interests (Žižek, 2008a).

Indeed, some authors have questioned the hegemonic power of political correctness across both public and academic institutions, admonishing its ineffective approach to cultural tolerance and the regulations it imposes on social interaction (Alibhai-Brown, 2018; Esposito and Finley, 2019; Fry et al., 2018; Paglia, 2018; Schwartz, 2010, 2016, 2017; Žižek, 1997, 1998a, 1998b). This can be seen in appraisals of liberal multiculturalism, which, while aiming to ensure the rights of the individual (Balibar and Wallerstein, 1991; Kymlicka, 1996; Lentin and Titley, 2011), simply encourage a veneer of 'freedom', 'equality' and 'tolerance' (Žižek, 2002) that ultimately compels deeper antagonisms (Lentin and Titley, 2011). These antagonisms are marked by examples of fear, with proponents of multiculturalism seen as overly supporting the rights of minority groups. Certainly, while critics of political correctness have often conflated policies concerning inequality, with some suggesting that such policies remain guided by a 'Cultural Marxism' that seeks to profess and promote a hostility towards white, heterosexual men (Peterson, 2018), others have sought to connect the stand against political correctness as emanating from the fears and frustrations of a silent, predominantly white, working-class, majority (Kaufmann, 2018). In both cases, we see discussions on political correctness grounded in examples of fear: fear towards an increasingly hostile environment, limited in its ability to freely debate contentious issues, as well as a fear that, under a period of increased immigration, the history and culture of majority ethnic groups has been undermined and/or ignored. Occurring alongside criticisms regarding the 'success' of multiculturalism, immigration and cultural diversity, calculated attacks against political correctness remain a prominent feature in both public and political debates on 'free speech' and the autonomy of the individual (Paglia, 2018). Moreover, as evidenced in the election of US President Donald Trump in 2016, such attacks have also proven to be politically popular (Esposito and Finley, 2019).

Amidst these criticisms, it is apparent that the underlying aims and purposes of political correctness remain contested. Specifically, it is the ways in which these aims are administered and critiqued which serve to fuel its contestation. To this end, we can identify a number of contradictions within the term itself. First, while many critics of political correctness argue that it inhibits free speech, such calls often result in traditional forms of cultural orthodoxy that in fact limit the right to freely express novel ideas, philosophies and positions. Second, though advocates for political correctness seek to promote greater social equality, drawing upon gender, sexuality, ethnicity and disability, such forms of promotion can reify cultural experiences, resulting in regimented forms of interaction that ultimately undermines social interaction. Given these contradictions, political correctness serves a particular ideological function in obfuscating the subject's relations both to and with the other (Žižek, 2008a).

As evident in recent reviews on the impact of 'integration' within the UK, understandings of the other have become encompassed within various approaches which seek to manage the ways in which different cultures 'integrate' with one another (Cantle, 2001, 2008, 2012; Casey, 2016; Goodhart, 2013, 2017; Mathieu, 2017; Parekh Report, 2000). Such attempts to achieve some form of national unity are often grounded in an equivalence that prescribes 'an imaginary coherence … produced through the installation of an abstract universal horizon' (McMillan, 2013: 124). In the context of political correctness, it is through adopting this 'abstract universal horizon' that forms of human interaction are managed. In other words, political correctness remains dependent upon its own inherent 'boundaries' and forms of symbolic regulation. This approach seeks to deliberately align political correctness with ideological critique. Indeed, if we consider that 'the abstract universal is the point at which ideology creates a sense of universal applicability, of cohesion and of fullness: the generalised point of "common sense" by which we come to understand our shared social life' (McMillan, 2013: 155–156), then it is this point of 'common sense' which rallies those that seek to profess the importance of political correctness as something that should be upheld and maintained as well as those who seek to denounce political correctness as part of the 'nanny-state' – a position that is frequently projected via the announcement: 'political correctness gone mad!'

More importantly, these contrasting positions share a number of subtle similarities. That is, while attempts to critique political correctness, by their very nature, stand opposed to forms of political correctness, ultimately, this opposition remains grounded in a 'critical distance' that separates the anti-PC campaigner from the detrimental effects of a PC culture 'gone mad'. What is more, it is this same sense of 'critical distance' which is presented by those who profess to support the fundamental tenets of political correctness. As will be discussed in Chapter One, this is best reflected in late-night television chat shows and sketch performances where examples of irony, satire and cynicism are deliberately used to attack those who seek to openly denounce political correctness. Of greater concern, however, is that it is through examples of resistance, 'critical distance' and irony that the *ideological significance* of certain discourses is maintained. As Žižek notes when considering the success of the song 'Gangnam Style' by South Korean musician, Psy:

> 'Gangnam Style' is not ideology in spite of ironic distance, it is ideology because of it ... the self-mocking irony of 'Gangnam Style' makes palpable the stupid enjoyment of the rave music. Many listeners find the song disgustingly attractive, i.e., they 'love to hate it,' or, rather, they enjoy the very fact of finding it disgusting so they repeatedly play it to prolong their disgust.
>
> *(2014: 116)*

With regard to PC/anti-PC proponents, we can observe a shared sense of 'repeated disgust' from those who like to bemoan political correctness as well as those 'PC' individuals who just as easily denounce the bemoaners' frustrations. It is in this regard that arguments both for and against political correctness work to maintain its ideological significance.

To this extent, it is when one believes that the forms of subversion they are enacting are in some way criticising or undermining political correctness that 'such subversions ... serve as a way of preserving the very dynamism of that [PC] order' (Daly, 2010: 21). It is here that we get a proliferation of subversions – both supporting and challenging political correctness – that ultimately work to obfuscate or ignore our relations to/with the other (Daly, 2010). Over the course of this book, these contradictions will be drawn upon and used in order to examine the effectiveness of comedy's subversive potential. Key to this approach will be the assertion that 'Comedy adeptly lends itself to a kind of spectral analysis of the workings of power, fueled by its own power as comedy' (Zupančič, 2016: 219). Accordingly, it is through comedy, humour and the telling of 'risky' jokes that one can 'bypass the censorship of political correctness to be truly political' (Gherovici and Steinkoler, 2016: 13). Guiding such a political path, this book will be grounded in the Lacanian influences of both Alenka Zupančič and Slavoj Žižek. Drawing upon Lacan's dialectical approach to the subject, the work of both Zupančič and Žižek will be used to establish a path of comic subversion. While key terms drawn from Lacan's work will be discussed below, for now, a brief and introductory consideration of comedy's subversive potential will be provided.

Comedy's subversive ambiguity: Providing 'a distinct perception of reality'

There is, as Kamm and Neumann (2016) assert, no simple nor single definition of comedy. Instead, it presents a number of characteristics that 'temporarily suspend the rigid regimes of normality with performances, behaviour patterns, practices, dialogues and images of surreal absurdity, grotesque exaggeration and drastic vehemence' (Kamm and Neumann, 2016: 3). It is this temporal suspense of 'rigid regimes' which, for Berger, prescribes 'the experience of the comic … a very distinctive place' (2014: xvii). He elaborates:

> On the one hand, it is ubiquitous. Everyday life is full of comic interludes, of occasions for humor, of little jokes as well as more elaborate ones. What is more, the experience of the comic is universal. While its expression differs greatly from one culture to another, there is no human culture without it. On the other hand, the experience of the comic is highly fragile, fugitive, sometimes hard to remember. What seems funny in one moment may suddenly take on a tragic quality in the next moment, a joke may be so subtle that it barely reaches the level of full attention, and this is why only a short time later it may be difficult to recall just why something evoked amusement.
>
> *(Berger, 2014: xvii)*

This sense of universal fragility bears a certain apprehension when analysing the effects of comedy – that is, when one deliberately seeks to take comedy 'seriously' (Lockyer and Pickering, 2008). Indeed, to 'explain' a joke is to reduce its comedy to some form of analytical explanation that is so often conceived as not funny.

In contrast, for McGowan 'The failure to take comedy seriously is the most damaging attitude to take toward it' (2017: 179); equally, according to Lockyer and Pickering 'humour is far from trivial' (2008: 809). Instead:

> It is integral to social relationships and social interaction. It may be taken in certain contexts as light-hearted banter, but in other contexts, it can injure people's social standing, or cut deeply into relationships and interaction between people within and across different social groups.
>
> *(Lockyer and Pickering, 2008: 809)*

It is in this regard that 'comedy can be understood as an inherent element in the cultural–political discourse of society' (Brassett and Sutton, 2017: 248). Certainly, many theorists of comedy have examined the potential for comedy to be used as a form of resistance that challenges and opposes hegemonic groups/individuals (Collinson, 2002). Yet, in order to use comedy as a way of 'subversively broach[ing] serious political questions' (Gherovici and Steinkoler, 2016: 11), it is important that one considers the logics of subversion that such a path entails. As will be discussed further in Chapter Two, theorists of comedy, such as Henri Bergson (2008) and

Sigmund Freud (2003), have viewed comedy as maintaining a certain subversion of reality, affording a different outlook on reality itself. Thus, it is through challenging common sense, reason and arbitrary forms of human contact that comedy can subversively challenge established norms.

But what happens when comic subversion is itself incorporated as part of the established order? Here, Daly contends that 'the logics of subversion are essentially ambiguous' (2010: 6). Accordingly:

> What appears, on the surface, as contestation and challenge against a social totality may in reality become caught up in the latter and actually serve to reinforce and stabilise it: e.g. democratic subversion as an outlet for protest and good conscience but which implicitly accepts, and legitimises, the rules/grammar of political encounter. In order to reach the dimension of politics proper, the more radical question is whether forms of subversion can be developed that are capable of subverting the very logics of existing subversion.
>
> *(Daly, 2010: 6)*

It is under this logic that examples of inherent transgression, fetishistic disavowal and superego enjoyment prevail. The significance of this will be considered in Chapters Two and Four.

For now, it is important to emphasise that this brief introduction to the subversive potential of comedy is underscored by the contention that comedy 'is not just a physiological or psychological process, but also involves a distinct perception of reality' (Berger, 2014: 23). Drawing upon the work of Bergson, Berger elaborates:

> The comic experience provides a distinctive diagnosis of the world. It sees through the facades of ideational and social order, and discloses other realities lurking behind the superficial ones. The image of the jack-in-the-box, evoked by Bergson, says more than he proposed. One first sees an ordinary box, familiar and unthreatening. Then, suddenly, something or someone not ordinary at all pops out of the box. But it then becomes clear at once that this other something or someone was present in the box all along. The jack-in-the box reveals that things are not what they seem.
>
> *(2014: 34)*

Importantly, such revelation should not be viewed as offering some fundamental transformation of the subject, but rather reveal a sense of surprise – a comic surprise – that acknowledges and draws attention to what was there, but which was previously unacknowledged. Moreover, it is through such revelation that comedy's ability to approach the 'taboo' can be considered in conjunction with the fears, anxieties and frustrations which prove integral to examples of political correctness. Specifically, the argument presented in this book will be grounded in the consideration that these fears, anxieties and frustrations can be played with, approached and, more importantly, made fun of. It is on this basis that examples of political correctness and racism can be critiqued through the comic form.

Laughing at racism: Anti-racist racism and contextual determination

An important aspect of comedy and humour is that it allows for a number of tabooed topics to be approached and dissected. In the case of racist jokes 'humour [can] provid[e] a licence to be offensive', with Lockyer and Pickering pointing out that:

> 'only joking' is the classic let-out clause when a racist joke falls on unreceptive ears or when a gag with racist implications seriously backfires. The excuse assumes that a joke is just a joke and cannot be taken seriously. This is exactly the rhetorical effectiveness upon which offensive comic discourse relies. The consequence is our difficulty in objecting when humour is regarded as overstepping the mark and causing offence.
>
> *(2008: 812)*

To this extent, Billig has drawn attention to the importance of analysing the context where certain jokes are made, noting that:

> It is hard to make the argument that such joking is not racist when the jokes are being transmitted in an explicitly racist context. The sites in question specifically promote the jokes as racist humour and the continual use of the word 'nigger' in this context unambiguously links the jokes to a racist perspective.
>
> *(2005: 36)*

Notably, Billig's comments are drawn from his study of racist jokes found on far-right racist websites, such as that of the Ku Klux Klan. However, as Billig notes:

> These are not jokes that happen to be told by Ku Klux Klan supporters. The joke-tellers, in sending their jokes to the Website, have specifically wished to see these jokes portrayed as racist jokes in a context that supports the Ku Klux Klan. In transmitting these jokes the tellers are demonstrating their political loyalties and their racist hatred. If this joke-telling is not racist, then it would be hard to know what would qualify for that label.
>
> *(2005: 36)*

While not disagreeing with Billig's contention that such jokes are racist, it would seem that Billig's analysis falls short of the contextual importance he seeks to expose. Where would one find racist jokes, if not on a far-right racist website where racist jokes can be shared? Additionally, one can assume that the existence of such a website is used specifically by those who enjoy reading as well as uploading racist jokes (as well as laughing at them). Of greater concern, therefore, is the extent to which analyses of any racist 'context' can reassert 'racist'/'not-racist' distinctions and, as a consequence, work to maintain the racist assertions that such an analysis would wish to dissolve. Instead, what is ignored in Billig's account is the extent to which racism can ambiguously occupy the space of comedy.

With regards to the latter, it is in examples of an 'anti-racist racism' that comedy and race have frequently been considered. Indeed, many have critiqued the ways in which attempts to promote anti-racism *through* racism can work to normalise racist assertions (Hall, 1994). In such instances, critics have asserted that the effect of such comedy is that 'Bigots appreciate the rantings of the bigoted characters as the truth, whereas non-bigots see them as bigotry' (Howitt and Owusu-Bempah, 2005: 61). This is especially apparent in television comedies such as the BBC sitcom *Till Death Us Do Part* (1965–1975). Again, Billig highlights how:

> the portrayal of fictional characters uttering racist remarks or jokes can be humorous, because the audience is laughing at such characters. That was the justification for the racist remarks made by characters such as Alf Garnett in the BBC sitcom *Till Death Us Do Part* or Archie Bunker in the US sitcom *All in the Family*. Again, the reproduction of racist terminology for comedic purposes is deeply problematic. The context of reproduction is all important.
>
> *(2005: 27)*

The effects of contextual overdetermination will be further considered in Chapter Three. What is apparent in Billig's approach, however, is the extent to which such a contextual understanding serves to reinforce a form of relativism, whereby the joke's content is determined by the 'context' in which it is said. Accordingly, such approaches can work to disavow negative stereotypes and racist assertions by locating and fixing the racist remark or gesture to the cultural and historical context in which it is delivered. What remains ignored is the resort to racism in the first place and, more importantly, its recurrence across varying socio-historical contexts. While the 'context of reproduction' works to maintain a racist/not-racist binary distinction, of greater importance is the need to change these distinctions. For this to occur, it is argued that a turn to comedy's form can prove significant.

For example, if we believe that we can, however simplistically, delineate between 'good' (all 'Asians' are intelligent) and 'bad' (all Jews have big noses) stereotypes, then it is not necessarily the 'content' of the stereotype that is important, but its formal structure: namely, the 'framework' that allows for the stereotype to be used in order to support a lie or distortion of the 'truth' for ideological purposes. With regard to the use of stereotypes in comedy, what is required is an approach to comedy that seeks to explore the dialectical relation between comedy's 'content' and 'form'.

Content, form and psychoanalysis

Much of the discussion and analysis which has considered the various ways in which ethnic stereotypes are performed and contested within comedy remains grounded in the 'content' of these stereotypes – that is, 'what' is said, performed and enacted, rather than the formal, structural significances which underpin comedy's practice. Notably, Weaver (2010) has outlined how examples of 'reverse racism' seek to use comedy in order to re-structure the direction of the stereotype, with the underlying premise that the stereotype can be comically used by the racialised other in order to re-appropriate the racism that is directed at them. While such forms rely upon 'the sign-systems of earlier racism', so that 'earlier meanings have the potential to re-emerge, gain purchase and act rhetorically, Weaver contends that 'Any evaluation of a reverse discourse should, … be rephrased as a consideration of how the images in humour both *simultaneously* "play on" and "play off" the long-established stereotypes' (2010: 33). Crucially:

> We should begin with an acceptance of the poly-semic structure of the discourse and remove any overemphasis on the intentionality of the speaker, thus beginning from the position of the discourse as having a simultaneous, and paradoxical, racist and anti-racist potential.
>
> *(Weaver, 2010: 33)*

Certainly, Weaver's (2010) contentions should not be viewed as an attempt to simply reassert the contextual analysis that Billig's (2005) previous insights afford, but rather should be read with an explicitly dialectical accent. That is, it is through this 'poly-semic structure' (Weaver, 2010) that one can, paradoxically, present both a racist and anti-racist assertion.

This has a particular importance when analysing the significance of racist comedy. Indeed, when defining a joke based upon whether its content is racist or non-racist, we ultimately submit ourselves to a level of demarcation that, as evidenced in the previous critique of Billig, enforces a certain clear-cut distinction *between* what is allowed and what is not allowed. These distinctions remain tied to the content and the context where such content is shared. While certain racist remarks can be conceived as the result of a malignant, internal 'racism' within the individual's psychology (see Chapter Three), attempts to 'contextualise' racism, by way of simply examining the socio-historical context where such racism occurs, prove just as susceptible to forms of reductionism that merely re-apply individual and societal dichotomies.

By way of navigating this dichotomy, we can turn to Žižek's (2008a; 2012c) account of Freud's analysis of dreams, whereby it is revealed that 'if we seek the "secret of the dream" in the latent content hidden by the manifest text, we are doomed to disappointment: all we find is some entirely "normal" – albeit usually unpleasant – thought' (Žižek, 2012c: 297). What remains central to this use of Freud in Žižek's critique is the formal logic that maintains such content, a formal logic which bears a particular significance to psychoanalytic critiques of culture and the subject. Here, Dolar asserts:

> [Psychoanalytic] interpretation tries to circumscribe the point where interpretation fails, where no 'more faithful' translation can be made. It tries to

> pinpoint the dimension of the object in that tiny crack before different meanings get hold of it and saturate it with sense, the point that can never be successfully recuperated by the signifying chain. In other words, psychoanalysis differs from other interpretations by its insistence on the *formal level* of the uncanny rather than on its content.
>
> *(1991: 19–20 [italics added])*

It is this formal level that Zupančič (2008) applies to her analysis of comedy.

In clarifying this approach, Zupančič (2008) outlines the following comedy sequence: a presumptuous baron slips on a banana peel and, in falling to the ground, reveals himself to be a human subject, beholden to the laws of gravity, just like everyone else. What is significant in this example is the extent to which a figure of authority (the baron) is brought 'down to earth' through a moment of comedy (Bonic, 2011). From this, Zupančič (2008) emphasises the importance of form. Here she explains:

> It is not a question of what (which content) is subjected to comical treatment – Mother Teresa, Lenin, machismo, feminism, the institution of the family, or the life of a homosexual couple – it is a question of the mode of the comic processing itself.
>
> *(Zupančič, 2008: 30)*

Specifically, it is not the baron *slipping* which is comic, but the presumptuous way that the baron stands up and continues to *believe* himself to be a 'baron', which helps to draw our attention to the formal structure of the comic mode. This will be considered further in Chapter Two; for now, however, it is important to highlight how Zupančič's (2008) attention to 'the mode of the comic processing itself' echoes psychoanalytic accounts of popular culture, where, in examples ranging from Mary Shelley's *Frankenstein* – from which 'The monster can stand for everything that our culture has to repress – the proletariat, sexuality, other cultures, alternative ways of living, heterogeneity, the Other' (Dolar, 1991: 19) – to Steven Spielberg's *Jaws* (1975) – where 'the killer shark … may signify anything from repressed sexuality to unbridled capitalism or the threat of the Third World to America' (Žižek, 2008c: 158) – we observe how it is the 'form' itself (i.e. 'the shark') which is arbitrarily filled with various (ideological) 'content'. Instead, rather than determining which content is 'true' or 'false' one can draw attention to the underlying form that lends shape to this content. Primarily, this requires going 'beyond' the content in order to examine that formal aspect whose excessive significance proves integral to *this* content.[1] It is in this way that an understanding of 'true comedy' can be forged. Central to this approach, however, is achieving the short circuit that such a path requires.

Comedy's short circuit

As is clear from the argument presented thus far, this book will undertake an analysis of comedy that draws specifically from Lacanian psychoanalysis, as used in the work of Zupančič and Žižek, as well as a range of other academics who have applied Lacan's work to culture, race/racism and comedy. Though this approach will give specific attention to the ways in which the study of comedy can be subversively aided by Zupančič's concrete universal and Žižek's parallax view, it will also be noted how a psychoanalytic approach can prove adept at exploring the subject, the other and, more importantly, the subject's relations to/with this other.

In fact, these terms will prove integral to the arguments developed in Chapter Four and to the analysis of *The Office* in Chapter Five. For the moment, it is important that both terms are seen as synonymous with comedy's ability to induce a short circuit; a short circuit that bears a semblance with Berger's (2014) assertion that comedy can present a different perspective on reality. While Zupančič's (2008) *The Odd One In: On Comedy* was released under Žižek's 'Short Circuit' series (published by MIT Press) – with Žižek's (2006) *The Parallax View* the first title to be released in the series – there remains a certain affinity in each author's approach to comedy and, in particular, to the significance of a Hegelian approach to comedy and subversion.

In studies on comedy, this subversive significance is frequently overlooked, as McGowan points out:

> Most of the time, we view comedy as a kind of moral holiday, a time-out that releases us from the seriousness that governs everyday life. It has a palliative role that enables us to overlook or at least tolerate the contradictions of everyday life.
>
> *(2017: 179)*

It is through performing and enacting such contradictions that comedy can 'establis[h] a different type of social link, making explicit our imbrication in the signifying order' (Gherovici and Steinkoler, 2016: 10). Much like the futility of uncovering a certain 'meaning' behind a particular 'content', such uncovering proves integral to the inherent limits of knowledge itself and the 'impasse of epistemology' – an impasse that can tell us 'something about the ontological status of reality itself' (Kunkle, 2018: 9). For both Zupančič and Žižek (following Lacan), it is 'our ontology itself [... which is] configured as something incomplete and inconsistent, and this in turn is how ... a short-circuit between epistemology and ontology' can be achieved (Kunkle, 2018: 9). More to the point, it is the formal logic of this process which proves integral to comedy's subversive significance and to identifying how a Lacanian approach to ontology, the subject and the comic can present 'a practice aimed at invoking the disavowed foundations of the existing universal order' (McMillan, 2013: 94).

By way of exploring this disavowal and in order to offer some initial clarification, the following sections will briefly introduce a number of key concepts that will prove essential to the analysis that follows. While many of these terms have been drawn from the work of Lacan, they have formed a significant role in psychoanalytic approaches to culture, society and philosophy. Accordingly, whereas the following sections will consider these terms individually, their significance stems primarily from their integrated application, as the remainder of this book shall demonstrate.

Mind the 'gap'

As noted in the above section, a central tenet of Žižek's (1991, 2012a) philosophy has involved extending Lacan's ideas through the ontological contention that reality exists in its own incompleteness. That is, the constitution of reality is founded on the 'gaps' and inconsistencies which structure this reality. Much of this is drawn from Žižek's (2006) use of quantum physics and his adoption of Hegelian dialectics, or what he refers to as 'the classic Hegelian reversal' (Žižek, 2015: 108). Simply put:

> what at first appears as an impotence of limitation in our knowledge, as the impossibility of our grasping the wealth of natural phenomena conceptually, is turned into an impotence in nature itself. And, indeed, do we not find exactly the same constellation in quantum mechanics, where indeterminacy (complementarity) points towards a 'weakness of nature,' in its inability to fully determine itself?
>
> *(Žižek, 2015: 108–109)*

This has been extended in the work of Zupančič (2017), who highlights how 'any objectivized reality ... is a reality that is necessarily not directly accessible' (Kunkle, 2018: 15). As a result, 'Reality, like the subject, is always in excess of itself and inherently incomplete (split from within)' (Kunkle, 2018: 15).

Consequently, a key aspect of Žižek and Zupančič's work is to encourage us to accept and manoeuvre ourselves in relation to the inherent inconsistencies, contingencies and antagonisms that structure our reality. Moreover, it is an incomplete reality that ensures the centrality of ideology and phantasmatic formations which help bring coherence and stability to a chaotic world (Žižek, 2008a, 2008b). If we consider that such coherence and stability can be used to paper over (or redirect) the divisions, inconsistencies and instability which structure this reality, then we can begin to examine how a key part of comedy relies upon the sense of surprise – the shift in perspective – that it affords (Zupančič, 2008). It is this 'shift', explored in Chapter Two's discussion of the parallax view, which will prove central to outlining a form of subversion that deliberately draws upon such instability as integral to our human interactions.

The symbolic, the imaginary and the Real

The relation between the symbolic, the imaginary and the Real remains central to Lacanian understandings of the subject, society and the other. For Lacan, it is these three entwined registers which locate and define the subject's being. For example, it is the symbolic order which refers to what can be conceived as, or what is perceived to be, 'reality'. It refers to language and the customs that manage and give meaning to our social relations. In particular, our entry into the symbolic order is achieved through language, insofar that our existence, our sense of being, is always negotiated and managed through language's signifying system.

While the symbolic order is what structures our experience of reality, the imaginary constitutes the individual's 'lived' experience. Grounded in appearance (*how things appear to us*) and the importance of the image, it is here that the individual achieves a sense of coherence, a cohesive body, formed when we recognise and use certain 'images' to constitute our sense of 'self'. Drawn from Lacan's 'mirror stage', what is important is that the imaginary order pays tribute to a body that *was* perceived to be fragmented. It is this sense of fragmentation – of an inherent sense of lack – that avails the imaginary a certain projection from which fantasies of loss and completion are transposed onto an Other: the big Other and the other (discussed below). Wun elaborates:

> The fixation on a nostalgic wholeness and the accompanying anxieties from primordial lack are projected onto the subject's sense of self and relationship to counterparts. These images inform her ego and enable the subject to imagine herself as coherent and whole. In linguistic terms, her subjectivity attaches to signifiers for comprehension. However, this illusion of coherence wrapped around the ego obviates a fundamental recognition that the subject is not whole. Her identity and existence are related to other signifiers; moreover, she is also a screen for projections.
>
> *(2014: 465)*

Therefore, if the symbolic refers to what is commonly considered to be 'reality' – the language, social practices and forms of behaviour that constitute 'reality' – and if the imaginary is what confers an appearance of 'wholeness' for the subject, then what remains inherent to both these orders is what Lacan refers to as the Real.

For Lacan, the Real 'is neither a substance nor a process. Rather, it is something that interrupts a process, something closer to a stumbling block; it is an impossibility in the structure of the field of reality' (Zupančič, 2008: 160). As noted in the above description of the symbolic and the imaginary, any signifying order or sense of self is never determined nor fixed, but always marked by a sense of variability that results in the symbolic and imaginary orders being both fragile and incomplete (Moolenaar, 2004). Dean neatly captures this fragility and its effects on the subject when she notes that:

> Because one is never sure how one is seen, one is never certain of one's place in the symbolic order. How, exactly, are we being looked at? One never really knows who one is – despite all the cameras, files, media, and databases. … Who one is in the socio-symbolic order is uncertain – and ever-changing.
>
> *(2010: 57)*

Consequently, rather than being separate to both the symbolic and imaginary orders, it is the Real, in its capacity to 'interrupt', which constitutes the inherent inconsistency and instability of the symbolic order. This is most noticeable in experiences of guilt, shame, violence and anger and in the failure of language to properly and effectively 'make sense' of both the subject and their experiences (Carew, 2014; Kingsbury, 2017; Noys, 2010). It is in this sense that 'the [R]eal is detectable only in its effects, in symptoms and unsatisfied desire, in distortions and deformations of the symbolic order, in the tendency at the heart of all rational systems to deviate from their intended course' (Wilcox, 2005: 344–345).

This, undoubtedly, prescribes a certain level of ambiguity to the Real (Žižek, 1998a). As Žižek notes, 'the Real designates a substantial hard kernel that precedes and resists symbolization and, simultaneously, it designates the left-over, which is posited or "produced" by symbolization itself' (Žižek, 1998a: 36). It is, in short, 'impossible'; it is 'something which can neither be directly experienced nor symbolized – like a traumatic encounter of extreme violence which destabilizes our entire universe of meaning' (Žižek, 2014: 106). This is given further clarification in the following example, drawn from Lacan's reference to the 'smile' of the Cheshire Cat in Lewis Carroll's *Alice in Wonderland*:

> The persistent grin of Alice's Cheshire cat, the 'grin without a cat,' shows that even when the body dissolves, something indestructible is left as a remainder. This grinning grimace reveals the Lacanian Real, a beyond speech and understanding that uncannily insists.
>
> *(Gherovici and Steinkoler, 2016: 17)*

It is this uncanny insistence which has a significant impact and, as the following chapters will demonstrate, provides a certain affordance in producing a theoretical analysis which can prove adept at identifying those inconsistencies and instabilities that structure and frame human interaction.

As should now be clear, each of these three orders are deeply entwined, with the Real proving coterminous with the inconsistency that structures both the imaginary and the symbolic (Noys, 2010). In fact, Lacan would often present this entwinement via the 'Borromean Knot', whereby if any one of the intertwined circles were cut, all three would disintegrate. As a result, it is through the interdependence afforded to the symbolic, imaginary and Real that reality remains constituted through its inherent failure. It is not that each order works together to form some sense of integrated 'wholeness', but that what each order reveals is a certain failure in itself and the other orders. Instead, each order is constituted and maintained through its own failure so that neither order can exist on its own, but, instead, remains effectively tied to the other in its constitution.

Absence, parallax and spectre

For Lacan and his followers, a key aspect of identifying or acknowledging the Real is in exploring 'the effects of absence' (McMillan, 2013: 119). Accordingly, while the Real '"does not exist" within the positive contours of reality', McMillan emphasises how 'it produces a range of effects that identifies its presence' (2013: 119). It is here that the Real bears a particular significance to Žižek's parallax view, as Wood notes:

> certain ambiguities or paradoxes are ineradicable, so that sometimes all that we can do is to maintain a 'parallax view,' by holding open both of the two inconsistent perspectives. This fundamental antagonism or paradox of the Real proves to be the only 'sameness' that always recurs.
>
> *(2012: 17)*

It is this 'sameness' which Zupančič (2019) locates in relation to comedy. Here, 'the Real is the register of repetition as coincidence, rupture, surprise (one could also say: of sameness as novelty)' (Zupančič, 2008: 163). What is important, however, and what will prove integral to examining comedy's subversive significance, is the extent to which we can 'use the Real to reconfigure our symbolic order' (Kunkle, 2014: 5). It is in this way that comedy can help 'radicalise' societal norms and values through confronting the Real and 'traversing' the fantasies that structure and frame our social interactions.

The importance of absence is continued in Žižek's (2012a, 2017b) assertions that reality is never 'complete' but constituted in the failure of its symbolisation; in the failure to ever eradicate, cover or mask the Real. To this end, there is no clear separation between 'reality' and 'illusion', but, instead, just various ways in which we can, through analyses of fantasy and forms of ideological critique, identify how our reality is sustained through a certain foreclosure that obscures reality's incompleteness. It is this foreclosure which underscores Lacan's contention 'that there is no reality without the spectre, that the circle of reality can be closed only by means of an uncanny spectral supplement' (Žižek, 2012b: 21). It is these spectral supplements which bear an affinity to the Real and which confer that 'reality is never directly "itself"' (Žižek, 2012b: 21). Instead, reality:

> presents itself only via its incomplete-failed symbolization, and spectral apparitions emerge in this very gap that forever separates reality from the real, and on account of which reality has the character of a (symbolic) fiction: the spectre gives body to that which escapes (the symbolically structured) reality.
>
> *(Žižek, 2012b: 21)*

The importance of this 'spectral apparition' is that it gives 'presence' to that constitutive absence which maintains society and social relations. Thus, it is in the act of acknowledging, identifying or confronting – all of which prove integral to Žižek's assertions that we should 'look awry' at reality – this 'absent presence' as the Real which is forever obscured in our socio-symbolic constructions. While the importance of this 'absent presence' will be considered in Chapter Three, we can, for now, locate Lacan's symbolic, imaginary and Real orders in relation to Žižek's (2012a, 2015) ontological contentions in order to emphasise the importance of fantasy and its significance for both the subject and society.

Objet petit a

According to Lacan, the *objet petit a* is a central feature in analyses of the subject. In Lacanian parlance, the *objet petit a* (*objet a*) refers to the object cause of desire. That is, it is not the object that the subject desires, but rather that which causes this desire in the first place. Importantly, it 'sets our desire in motion' by affording 'the formal frame which confers consistency on our desire' (Žižek, 2008b: 53). Paradoxically, therefore, the *objet a* is an immaterial 'object' which bears a certain material significance. Indeed, if we remember that due to the Real, any 'imaginary' (imaginary order) representation that one holds of oneself can be breached, thwarted and undermined, then the *objet a* is that 'object' – that stumbling block – which announces the subject (Verhaeghe, 2018). To this extent, the *objet a* 'stands for the unknown X, for what is "in you more than yourself"' (Žižek, 2017b: 54). In other words, it is what represents the subject's inscription in 'objective' reality.

Notice how this description prescribes a dialectical inflection to traditional object-subject dichotomies (Žižek, 2015). It is the *objet a* which signals that aspect of an object which posits 'its unreachable core', yet, it is precisely because of this designation that 'the very point of the inscription of subjectivity into the object' is achieved (Žižek, 2017: 54). To help clarify this term, Žižek frequently draws upon the example of love:

> what causes love is some elusive *je ne sais quoi* in the beloved, some X that cannot be pinned down to any perceptible particular feature of the beloved; but this X does not exist in itself, it is the inscription of my desire into the object (which is why, as they say, a human being appears sublime only to the gaze of the subject in love with him/her).
>
> *(Žižek, 2017: 54)*

For comedy, the 'object *a* is a material sensitive point of a system, a point that comedy plays with abundantly' (Zupančič, 2008: 101). It is through such 'play' that the significance of the *objet a* can help draw attention to the importance of (self-) division and repetition in comedy as well as allowing us to identify the limits that underscore the subject and Other's incongruity (McGowan, 2017).

Fantasy and ideology

For Lacan, fantasy provides a constitutive role in an individual's subjectivity (Sharpe and Turner, 2018). More importantly, according to Žižek (2008b), our conceptions of fantasy should not stand separate to 'reality' – fantasy does not mask or cover up a 'real' reality, as described in Marx's false consciousness – instead, fantasy is what conceals the Real for the subject, it is what regulates the subject's desire. Accordingly, if we remember that the subject's entry into the symbolic order rests upon a certain separation of the subject from their bodily experience, then, as McMillan notes, 'We humans, unlike our fellow animals, cannot purely react upon instinct or enjoy our bodies. Instead, upon entry into the symbolic order, the subject loses access to total materiality' (2013: 48). It is this loss, this sense of some repression beyond the entry into the language, which results in a recourse to fantasy that seeks to afford the subject a certain level of self-consistency. Fantasy is what allows us to manage our inherent alienation and the basic impasse (the lack) in both the subject and society.[2]

In sum, fantasy permits us to manage our sense of self and our relations with the other/Other. Ideological critique, therefore, is what encourages us to examine in what ways certain fantasy formations conceal the Real. So often throughout history, societies have used ideological formations, grounded in fantasy, to make sense of and/or obscure those inherent antagonisms that structure social relations, and it is in this way that ideological critique is not a process that can be 'escaped' from, but rather something that requires a radical de-centralisation, a certain de-subjectivisation, which reveals to the subject the 'gap' in reality. It is this acknowledgment that, again, lays bare the constitutive role of ideology and fantasy in underscoring reality's inconsistency and which, as Chapter Four will detail, can prove subversively effective.

The big Other and the other

Avoiding any biological or psychological reductionism, Lacan adopted a dialectical approach to the subject and 'the other'. For the latter, Lacan distinguished between two forms of other: 1) the big Other; and, 2) the other.[3] First, the big Other is what refers to society itself. Working in correspondence with the symbolic order, it is the locus that is always presupposed and whose immateriality maintains and structures our social interactions through its virtuality. The significance of the big Other is that it occupies that 'third' location which upholds and maintains a conversation between two individuals. It is that which acknowledges the polite greetings which mark an introduction ('Good morning', 'Did you have a good weekend?'), and which ensures the consistency of the conversation. Accordingly, 'As the big Other is the (presup)position of an immaterial and ideal order, its (libidinal) function is to guarantee the ultimate meaning and consistency of the subject's experience' (Garcia and Sanchez, 2008). To this extent, the existence of the big Other works off of a certain reification, yet it is:

> This reification [which] acknowledges our capacity for detaching the concept of the Other from any specific person and even from any physical entities such as rivers and trees and stones. Lacan further thinks that it is by this abstraction of the concept of Otherness that we generate a concept of God. When Lacan declares that 'it is impossible not to believe in God', he is

> pointing to the inevitable generation of some such avatar of the Other in the structure of our minds.
>
> *(Benson, 2018)*

In fact, this reference to God proves integral to Lacan's assertion that, paradoxically, 'the big Other does not exist'. That is, it 'exists' only on the basis that subjects act 'as if' it exists. Indeed, as will be detailed in Chapter Four, the significance of this 'as if' realisation echoes the inconsistency of the symbolic order and 'the fact that the big Other is [not] just a retroactive illusion masking the radical contingency of the real', so that 'we can simply suspend this "illusion" and "see things as they really are"', but that it is this '"illusion" [that] structures our (social) reality itself: its disintegration leads to a "loss of reality"' (Žižek, 1991: 71). One should now begin to see the interconnections between the subject and the social that psychoanalysis can provide. Much like the fantasies that structure the subject's being, the inconsistency of reality is itself constituted and held together through those spectral supplements and ideological formations that help maintain reality's consistency, and which underscores the consistency of meaning and experience that is afforded to the big Other.

Accordingly, while in our everyday routines we act on behalf of the big Other, at the same time we also spend the majority of our lives with 'other' subjects, and it is through this relation with the other that our sense of self is dialectically marked. The importance of the other will be discussed further in Chapters Two and Three; for now, it is essential to note that it is through this dialectic that our social relations are always marked by an inherent limit and a fundamental difference. Though as subjects we remain both separate from but also linked to the other, it is these 'imaginary limits' which will prove integral to developing a conception of the other that does not resort to fake forms of sentimental attachment or examples of racist fantasy (Zupančič, 2019).

The Master-Signifier

The purpose of the Lacanian Master-Signifier is that it provides a quilting point to the signifying system. That is, it represents a nodal point from which the endless deferral of signifiers is stalled and fixed to a certain 'Master-Signifier' which prevents any further deferral. Importantly, while Master-Signifiers attempt to fix meaning, they are not necessarily stable. With regard to political correctness, Penhallurick notes how:

> some of the enterprises rather unthinkingly characterized under the umbrella term 'political correctness' can be seen as attempts to abolish or replace or taboo harmful master-signifiers. Another response to negative, imposed master-signifiers is to seize them, accept them but turn them positive.
>
> *(2010: 204)*

Accordingly, while for some, politics reflects the struggle to present one's Master-Signifier (Laclau, 2000), such signifiers are inherently 'empty'. That is, in most cases the exact feature that underscores a particular Master-Signifier may not necessarily be known to the individual or group adopting that Master-Signifier. In short, there is no 'essence'.

Nonetheless, it is the imposition of a Master-Signifier which endows a certain thing with an unknowable aspect that underpins the significance of *that* feature. For example, in the case of nationality, such as 'British', or in the case of a particular political persuasion, such as 'Communist', what we often see amongst their adherents, is a reference to some mysterious feature which emanates from the failure of language to fully distinguish what this feature is (Žižek, 2015). This excess of language is only curtailed, managed or bounded by the imposition of the Master-Signifier which affords some form of closure.

This use of the Master-Signifier bears a certain affinity with the function of *objet a*. As Vogt notes, 'The *objet a* is thus something like the master signifier of the master signifier (which a merely discursive ideology critique misses)' (2007: 63). Certainly, the significance of the Master-Signifier is not to reify that 'impossible object' which it seeks to uphold, but rather to tease, critique and pull apart the 'excessive instability or impossibility that, when traversed, can generate the experience that there is no Other of the Other' (Vogt, 2007: 63). If we consider the case of anti-Semitism, then, despite the 'Jew' functioning as that Master-Signifier whose possession of a certain object (*objet a*) provides the antagonistic attribute that prevents society's smooth functioning, it is the 'recognition that the "Jew" does not possess what anti-Semitism confers on him – *objet a* – [which] entails … identification with the symptom' (Vogt, 2007: 63). It is this surplus attribute which draws attention to the excesses of the social system itself, allowing us to perceive – or traverse – the fantasy formations that both obscure and obstruct such recognition in the first place.

'There is no…' and ex-sistence

It is here that we can begin to draw together a number of important threads in the above introductions. It is these threads which can be pulled together through Lacan's notion of the Real, the virtual existence of the big Other and the fundamental asymmetry which marks both the subject and the other. Certainly, this is not intended to present human relations as being tied to an inevitable sense of animosity and disagreement. Instead, it is to draw attention to those fantasy formations which structure our relations with the other and vice versa.

One notable area where such fantasies play a pivotal role in our relations with the other is in Lacan's declaration that 'There is no sexual relation'. Certainly, such an assertion does not declare that all sexual relations are marked by animosity and failure, but that any sexual relation – and here we can expand his ideas to human relations in general – are marked by a certain antagonism or dialectical understanding. Here, 'the amorous relation is not a relationship, but a struggle between two opposites, each in an asymmetrical position vis-à-vis the other' (Roudinesco, 2014: 83), and it is this asymmetry which is played out in our discussions on 'gender'. Notably, these debates have resulted in what can often seem like a proliferation of gender identities, reflected in the ever-expanding LGBTQIA+ title. This will be discussed further in Chapter One's account of identity politics; for now, Kunkle notes how this expanding list is 'an attempt to overcome binaries of normative heterosexuality' (2018: 13); an attempt that reveals how a level of negativity is 'intrinsic to sex' (Kunkle, 2018: 5), and, by extension, how this sense of negativity is reflected in Lacan's non-relationship.

This is not a simple fetishisation of negativity or lack, but a decisive account of how such absence can be positively asserted and used as a formative feature of our human relations. More to the point, it is to draw attention to the fact that the 'reality' of any relationship is one marked by a certain excess which is grounded in reality's incompleteness (the 'gap'/'split' within reality, see above). This excess is demonstrably performed when, if one was to ask you to describe that feature of your partner which you love the most, the ability to concentrate such a task on one specific feature would prove particularly difficult, almost impossible. The question itself would at least require a certain dexterity as you make sure to identify the 'correct' feature (imagine the reply: you identify that particular feature only for the response to be: you only like that 'bit' about me?). What this reveals, however, is the inherent impasses which always frame our relations with the other and, more importantly, ourselves. For Žižek:

> Therein resides the key feature of the properly Hegelian dialectic of the subject-object. The couple subject-object is never a simple duality, since one of its terms (subject) is structurally split into two: subject as opposed to object, the subject in the common sense, the agency which mediates, dominates, forms the object; and subject, insofar as it emerges in the domain of objectivity itself, as the void of negativity, as the radical frustration of all endeavour to attain objective existence. I am effectively a subject when I fail to find any 'objective correlative', any objective content in which I can fully recognise myself, apropos of which I can say: 'that's me!' Hysteria is the name for this frustration, for the question 'Is that really ME?' which arises apropos of every identification.
>
> *(2001b: 108 [emphasis in original])*

Here, being is always 'non-all'; there is always a certain excess that remains intimately tied to the lack at the heart of being. Again, this notion of a 'non-all' refers explicitly to a certain positivisation of negativity. Indeed, 'Lacan associates the non-all both with the register of the symbolic (the field of language) and with the register of the real', so that 'the marker "all" relates to the imaginary closure of being into One' (Tomšič, 2018: 109). In doing so, any wholeness or closure to the One is itself predicated on a certain 'ex-sistence' which marks our ontological incompleteness (Tomšič, 2018). It is in this regard that we can explore how our relations with the other are marked by the *possibility* of failure (going too far in your desire to be polite, offending someone for not being polite enough). It is, in short, to draw attention to the Real that ex-sists in any social relationship or field of representation: an ex-sistence that is not only separate from, but also fundamental to, our symbolic and imaginary orders, as evident in its missed opportunities, its failures and its shadowy, spectral supplements (Moolenaar, 2004). The significance of this ex-sistence is reflected upon in the following remarks from Žižek:

> Something that doesn't exist can be efficient, it can leave traces in (symbolic) reality. God doesn't exist, but its inexistence leaves traces in our reality. More precisely, God *qua* Cause is a retroactive effect of its own traces-effects, in the same way that a political cause only exists in the series of its effect: communism only exists insofar as there are individuals fighting for it (or attacking it), motivated by it in their activity.
>
> *(2016: 348)*

It is these 'traces' which comedy performs, and which, more importantly, can be used to subvert the inherent inconsistencies in our abstract universal assumptions via the 'gap' that comedy ex-poses. Indeed, it is these traces which blur as well as structure our relations with the other. Corresponding with Lacan's 'non-relationship', we can consider how any form of intimacy with the other – be this a husband or wife, a long-term partner, a close friend, or even a work colleague who you see on a daily basis – is marked by a certain 'extimacy'.[4] It is this sense of extimacy with the other that will be examined in relation to comedy, with specific attention given to how our 'non-relationships' can be rethought in the context of comedy.

Chapter outlines

In Chapter One, attention is given to examining how a central theoretical and, indeed, aesthetic component of the UK's post-war comedy history is the entwined development of a decidedly postmodern account of 'subversion' supplemented with a 'politically correct' and culturally driven identity politics. In order to examine this development, the emergence and success of Alternative Comedy during the late 1970s, will be used to identify a number of key themes, evident in both the relative dominance of postmodern critiques of ideology as well as the level of subversion that has typically been appropriated to Alternative Comedy. Moreover, this critique will go beyond the emergence of political correctness in the 1970/1980s in order to consider how the impact of 1960s counter-cultural movements signalled a diversion away from class struggle towards an emphasis on identity politics. The resonance of this period is one that continues to be identified in popular commercial culture and in the prevalence for forms of irony, satire and cynicism in comedy. Indeed, while offering the *potential* for subversion, such comic forms are criticised for providing a supplementary role in supporting the development of neoliberalism (grounded in the autonomy of the individual under free market capitalism) as well as programmes of cultural diversity (steered by a liberal multicultural perspective). As a result, it is highlighted that examples of liberal multiculturalism have introduced new forms of regulation as well as a greater sense of guilt and anxiety in discourses on political correctness and 'politically correct' behaviour. Rather than directly opposing this hegemony, this chapter emphasises how one can draw attention to the inherent *excesses* of the system itself and, as a consequence, present opportunities for subversive resistance. It is this type of subversive resistance that lays visible the inherent failures that characterise the abstract universality of political correctness.

Chapter Two begins with a critical discussion of the importance of incongruity in studies on comedy, humour and jokes. Early philosophical accounts, including the work of Immanuel Kant (2007) and Henri Bergson (2008), are outlined in order to distinguish the various ways in which comedy can reveal as well as induce a sense of incongruity for the subject. Of greater significance, however, is that this work will be used to introduce a closer analysis on the effects of incongruity, as discussed in both Simon Critchley's (2002) and Agnes Heller's (2005) analyses of comedy. Notably, both authors are employed in order to expand upon the relative importance of comedy's incongruity, before turning to a materialist critique of comedy and its subversive potential. In view of both Critchley (2002) and Heller (2005), this critique will be grounded in Zupančič's (2008) adoption of the Hegelian concrete universal, elucidating how comedy can provide a short circuit between the universal and particular; a form of reflexivity whereby the universal is performed through its own 'exception'. Indeed, it is through this constituted exception that comedy obtains a subversive significance. Importantly, this consideration is supplemented with two additional approaches: Todd McGowan's (2017) analysis of comedy as dialectically predicated on lack and excess and Žižek's (2006) notion of parallax. These additional considerations draw attention to the formal structure of comedy and, specifically, its material implications. In contrast to comedy studies, which focus predominantly on the 'content' of comedy, this chapter will conclude this 'formal' importance with a discussion on the differences between the joke and comedy sequence as well as the performative significance of the 'comedy character'.

In developing the critique laid out in Chapter Two, Chapter Three serves to examine how our conceptions of race bear an imaginary and symbolic consequence that remains grounded in the 'intricate complexion … of racism' (Mitchell, 2012: 37). Notably, this chapter develops upon the arguments presented in Chapters One and Two by detailing how such 'complexion' is ignored, obfuscated or overlooked in examples of political correctness. In particular, this will detail how forms of racial tolerance are pervasively grounded in forms of intolerance, and that by obfuscating the significance of race, through private regulation (tolerating the other's difference, but maintaining a distance to such difference), the hegemonic power of liberal multiculturalism and political correctness locates the other as both 'traumatic' and 'excessive'. Central to this approach are the distinctions Hsiao (2010) draws between the spectre and spectacle of race. Specifically, Hsiao's (2010) distinctions will be used to examine how the effects of race and racism can have both a material and immaterial significance, so that any racialised depiction – any 'spectacle' – is shadowed and haunted by the spectre of race. Thus, it is argued that, in accordance with Lacanian approaches to race, racism and the Real (Hook, 2004, 2008; Mitchell, 2012), Hsiao's (2010) race as spectre can explore those instances of human (mis)communication, whereby comedy's Real subversion is used to redefine our relations with political correctness and the other.

Chapter Four provides a final precis on the significance of comedy. This argument is predicated on two underlying contentions: first, that our approach to comedy should not refrain from those excessive elements which allow us to aver the Real; and, second, that we cannot approach the other without being aware of the reflexive short circuit that is required when encountering the Real of *their* as well as *our* otherness. Moreover, it is asserted that it is in the failure of political correctness to effectively curtail racism that the spectral presence of race, as well as the inherent inconsistencies of the symbolic/big Other and universal, can be identified. In fact, this 'failure' will be used to outline a comic space from which what cannot be said can at least be approached via a form of comic interaction grounded in an acknowledgment of absence and (possible) exclusion. Here, we can turn to those moments of comedy where the performance of a politically correct situation is rendered 'comical' by identifying the fundamental lack which destabilises its universal authority. In part, this requires turning to comedy's capacity to perform those inherent excesses that posit a fundamental lack in the universal. It is through approaching this excess that comedy can perform, in exaggerated ways, the inherent contradictions *in* political correctness.

Chapter Five affords a critical analysis of an example of racism drawn from the UK sitcom *The Office* (2001–2003). Specifically, attention is given to examining the performance of a racist joke from episode one, series two, 'Merger'. While a synopsis of the episode is provided, critical attention will then be given to examining four notable scenes. These four scenes have been selected for consideration due to their performance of a 'black man's cock' joke by the show's lead character, David Brent (Ricky Gervais). Although it is acknowledged that the reference to a 'black man's cock' is embedded in racial fantasies, this analysis considers the *ways* in which David's attempts to build morale amongst his colleagues clashes with his politically (in)correct intentions. Indeed, the purpose here is not to expose the joke as racist, but rather to examine how this racial exchange can subversively be used to challenge examples of political correctness. This is achieved by drawing attention to the following characteristics: the spectacle and spectre of race; the comic significance of the Real other; lack and self-estrangement in the comic character (David Brent); and the presumptuous authority of political correctness.

In conclusion, final consideration is given to outlining how examples of political correctness, though being supported in theory, are, in practice, detrimental to tackling racism. Drawing upon and summarising the analysis of *The Office* provided in Chapter Five, it is argued that the ineffectiveness of political correctness can be comically subverted in analyses of popular culture. The role of comedy in this culture will now be considered.

Notes

1 Žižek elaborates: 'take a well-known elementary example from the analysis of melodramas: the emotional excess that cannot express itself directly in the narrative line finds its outlet in the ridiculously sentimental musical accompaniment or in other formal features' (2001a: 59).
2 This is what Lacan refers to as 'symbolic castration'; the virtual castration that one feels when language can never fully articulate the body's materiality.
3 For clarity, this book will distinguish between the two 'others' via the 'big Other's' capital 'O' and 'the other's' lowercase 'o'.
4 Zupančič refers to such 'extimacy' as denoting 'an excluded interiority or an included exteriority' (2019: 90).

References

Alibhai-Brown, Y. 2018. *In Defence of Political Correctness*. London: Biteback Publishing.

Balibar, E. and Wallerstein, I. 1991. *Race, Nation, Class: Ambiguous Identities*. London: Verso.

BBC. 2018. Comedian refused to sign 'behavioural agreement' before gig [online]. Available from: www.bbc.co.uk/news/newsbeat-46541002 [Accessed 1 March 2019].

Bennett, S. 2018. A 'safe space' contract for comedians is a bit silly… but the backlash is just as ludicrous [online]. *Chortle*. Available from: www.chortle.co.uk/correspondents/2018/12/14/41910/a_safe_space_contract_for_comedians_is_a_bit_silly…_but_the_backlash_is_just_as_ludicrous [Accessed 21 December 2018].

Benson, P. 2018. The concept of the Other from Kant to Lacan. *Philosophy Now*. Available from: https://philosophynow.org/issues/127/The_Concept_of_the_Other_from_Kant_to_Lacan [Accessed 30November 2020].

Berger, P. L. 2014. *Redeeming Laughter: The Comic Dimension of Human Experience*, 2nd edn. Berlin, Germany: De Gruyter.

Bergson, H. L. 2008. *Laughter: An Essay on the Meaning of the Comic*. Rockville, MD: Wildside Press.

Billig, M. 2005. Comic racism and violence. In: S. Lockyer and M. Pickering, eds. *Beyond a Joke: The Limits of Humour*. Basingstoke: Palgrave Macmillan, 25–44.

Bonic, N. 2011. Psychoanalysis and comedy: The (im)possibility of changing the socio-symbolic order. *S: Journal of the Jan Van Eyck Circle for Lacanian Ideology Critique*, 4, 91–108.

Brassett, J., and Sutton, A. 2017. British satire, everyday politics: Chris Morris, Armando Iannucci and Charlie Brooker. *British Journal of Politics and International Relations*, 19 (2), 245–262.

Cantle, T. 2001. *Community Cohesion: Report of the Independent Review Team – The 'Cantle Report'*. London: Home Office.

Cantle, T. 2008. *Community Cohesion: A New Framework for Race and Diversity*. Basingstoke: Palgrave Macmillan.

Cantle, T. 2012. *Interculturalism: The New Era of Cohesion and Diversity*. Basingstoke: Palgrave Macmillan.

Carew, J. 2014. 'Why is there nothing rather than something': Less than nothing's new metaphysics. *International Journal of Žižek Studies*, 8 (1), 1–16.

Casey, L. 2016. *The Casey Review: A Review into Opportunity and Integration*. London: Department for Communities and Local Government.
Collinson, D. L. 2002. Managing humour. *Journal of Management Studies*, 39 (3), 269–288.
Critchley, S. 2002. *On Humour*. London: Routledge.
Daly, G. 2010. Causes for concern: Žižek's politics of loving terror. *The International Journal of Žižek Studies*, 4 (2), 1–23.
Dean, J. 2010. *Blog Theory: Feedback and Capture in the Circuits of Drive*. Cambridge: Polity.
Dolar, M. 1991. 'I shall be with you on your wedding-night': Lacan and the uncanny. *October*, 58, 5–23.
Esposito, L. and Finley, L., eds. 2019. *Political Correctness in the Era of Trump*. Newcastle-Upon-Tyne: Cambridge Scholars Publishing.
Fahs, B. 2019. Reinvigorating the traditions of second-wave radical feminism: Humor and satire as political work. *Women's Reproductive Health*, 6 (3), 157–160.
Freud, S. 2003. *The Joke and its Relation to the Unconscious*, trans. Joyce Crick. London: Penguin.
Fry, S., Peterson, J., Dyson, M. E. and Goldberg, M. 2018. *Political Correctness Gone Mad?* London: Oneworld Publications.
Garcia, G. I. and Sanchez, C. G. A. 2008. Psychoanalysis and politics: The theory of ideology in Slavoj Žižek. *The International Journal of Žižek Studies*, 2 (3). Available from: https://zizekstudies.org/index.php/IJZS/issue/view/9 [Accessed 30 November 2020].
Gherovici, P. and Steinkoler, M. 2016. Introduction. In: P. Gherovici and M. Steinkoler, eds. *Lacan, Psychoanalysis, and Comedy*. New York, NY: Cambridge University Press, 1–22.
Goodhart, D. 2013. *The British Dream: Successes and Failures of Post-War Immigration*. London: Atlantic Books.
Goodhart, D. 2017. *The Road to Somewhere: The Populist Revolt and the Future of Politics*. London: Hurst & Company.
Hall, S. 1994. Some 'politically incorrect' pathways through PC. In: S. Dunant, ed. *The War of the Words: The Political Correctness Debate*. London: Virago Press, 164–184.
Heller, A. 2005. *Immortal Comedy: The Comic Phenomenon in Art, Literature, and Life*. Lanham, MD: Lexington Books.
Hook, D. 2004. Racism as abjection: A psychoanalytic conceptualisation for a post-apartheid South Africa. *South African Journal of Psychology*, 34 (4), 672–703.
Hook, D. 2008. The 'Real' of racializing embodiment. *Journal of Community & Applied Social Psychology*, 18, 140–152.
Howitt, D. and Owusu-Bempah, K. 2005. Race and ethnicity in popular humour. In: S. Lockyer and M. Pickering, eds. *Beyond a Joke: The Limits of Humour*. Basingstoke: Palgrave Macmillan, 45–62.
Hsiao, L.-C. 2010. Color (un)conscious: Psychoanalysis, resistance, and the specter/spectacle of race. *Concentric: Literary and Cultural Studies*, 36 (1), 159–187.
Jaws, 1975. Film. Universal Pictures.
Jeffries, S. 2019. Is standup comedy doomed? The future of funny post-Kevin Hart, Louis CK and Nanette [online]. *The Guardian*. Available from: www.theguardian.com/culture/2019/jan/19/is-standup-comedy-doomed-future-of-funny-kevin-hart-louis-ck-nanette [Accessed 29 January 2019].
Kamm, J. and Neumann, B. 2016. Introduction: The aesthetics and politics of British TV comedy. In: J. Kamm and B. Neumann, eds. *British TV Comedies: Cultural Concepts, Contexts and Controversies*. Basingstoke: Palgrave Macmillan, 1–22.
Kant, I. 2007. *Critique of Judgement*. New York, NY: Cosimo.
Kaufmann, E. 2018. *White Shift: Populism, Immigration and the Future of White Majorities*. London: Penguin.

Kingsbury, P. 2017. Uneasiness in culture, or negotiating the sublime distances towards the big Other. *Geography Compass*, 11 (6), 1–11.

Kisin, K. 2018. What a joke! His dissident grandfather fled Russia for the freedoms of Britain. Now comedian Konstantin Kisin has faced ludicrous censorship by snowflake students here. His withering response? [online]. *Daily Mail.* Available from: www.dailymail.co.uk/news/article-6493921/Comedian-signed-behaviour-agreement-reveals-family-fled-censorship-Soviet-Russia.html [Accessed 21 December 2018].

Krefting, R. 2019. Hannah Gadsby stands down: Feminist comedy studies. *JCMS: Journal of Cinema and Media Studies*, 58 (3), 165–170.

Kunkle, S. 2014. Act. In: R. Butler, ed. *The Žižek Dictionary*. London: Routledge.

Kunkle, S. 2018. The formalization of impasse. *Continental Thought & Theory: A Journal of Intellectual Freedom*, 2 (2), 3–17.

Kymlicka, W. 1996. *Multicultural Citizenship: A Liberal Theory of Minority Rights*. Oxford: Clarendon Press.

Laclau, E. 2000. Identity and hegemony: The role of universality in the constitution of political logics. In: J. Butler, E. Laclau and S. Žižek, eds. *Contingency, Hegemony, Universality: Contemporary Dialogues on the Left*. London: Verso, 44–89.

Lentin, A. and Titley, G. 2011. *The Crisis of Multiculturalism: Racism in a Neoliberal Age*. London: Zed Books.

Lockyer, S. and Pickering, M. 2008. You must be joking: The sociological critique of humour and comic media. *Sociology Compass*, 2/3, 808–820.

Malik, K. 2018. We could all do with being a little less sure of ourselves [online]. *The Guardian*. Available from: www.theguardian.com/commentisfree/2018/dec/16/we-could-all-do-with-being-a-little-less-sure-of-ourselves [Accessed 21 December 2018].

Mathieu, F. 2017. The failure of state multiculturalism in the UK? An analysis of the UK's multicultural policy for 2000–2015. *Ethnicities*, 18 (1), 43–69.

McGowan, T. 2017. *Only a Joke Can Save Us: A Theory of Comedy*. Evanston, IL: Northwestern University Press.

McMillan, C. 2013. *Žižek and Communist Strategy: On the Disavowed Foundations of Global Capitalism*. Edinburgh: Edinburgh University Press.

Mitchell, W. J. T. 2012. *Seeing Through Race*. Cambridge, MA: Harvard University Press.

Moolenaar, R. 2004. Slavoj Žižek and the real subject of politics. *Studies in Eastern European Thought*, 56, 259–297.

Noys, B. 2010. The horror of the Real: Žižek's modern gothic. *The International Journal of Žižek Studies*, 4 (4). Available from: http://zizekstudies.org/index.php/IJZS/issue/view/20 [Accessed 30 November 2020].

Paglia, C. 2018. *Provocations: Collected Essays*. New York, NY: Knopf Doubleday.

Parekh, B. 2000. *The Future of Multi-Ethnic Britain: The Parekh Report*. London: Profile Books.

Penhallurick, R. 2010. *Studying the English Language*. Basingstoke: Palgrave Macmillan.

Peterson, J. B. 2018. *12 Rules for Life: An Antidote to Chaos*. London: Penguin.

Roudinesco, E. 2014. *Lacan: In Spite of Everything*. London: Verso.

Schwartz, H. S. 2010. *Society Against Itself: Political Correctness and Organizational Self-Destruction*. London: Karnac.

Schwartz, H. S. 2016. *Political Correctness and the Destruction of Social Order*. Berlin, Germany: Springer.

Schwartz, H. S. 2017. *The Revolt of the Primitive: An Inquiry into the Roots of Political Correctness*. New York, NY: Routledge.

Sharpe, M. and Turner, K. 2018. Fantasy. In: Y. Stavrakakis, ed. *Routledge Handbook of Psychoanalytic Political Theory*. London: Routledge, 187–198.

The Office. 2001–2003. TV Series. BBC Two/One.

Till Death Us Do Part. 1965–1975. TV Series. BBC One.
Tomšič, S. 2018. Toward a materialist ontology. *Continental Thought & Theory: A Journal of Intellectual Freedom*, 2 (2), 82–117.
Verhaeghe, P. 2018. Lacan's answer to alienation: Separation. *Crisis and Critique*, 6 (1), 365–388.
Vogt, E. 2007. Exception in Žižek's thought. *Diacritics*, 37 (2–3), 61–77.
Weaver, S. 2010. The 'Other' laughs back: Humour and resistance in anti-racist comedy. *Sociology*, 44 (1), 31–48.
Wilcox, L. 2005. Don DeLillo's Libra: History as text, history as trauma. *Rethinking History*, 9 (2–3), 337–353.
Wood, K. 2012. *Žižek: A Reader's Guide*. Chichester: Wiley-Blackwell.
Wun, C. 2014. The anti-black order of no child left behind: Using Lacanian psychoanalysis and critical race theory to examine NCLB. *Educational Philosophy and Theory*, 46 (5), 462–474.
Žižek, S. 1991. *Looking Awry: An Introduction to Jacques Lacan through Popular Culture*. Cambridge, MA: MIT Press.
Žižek, S. 1997. Multiculturalism, or, the cultural logic of multinational capitalism. *New Left Review*, 1 (225), 28–51.
Žižek, S. 1998a. *Tarrying with the Negative: Kant, Hegel, and the Critique of Ideology*. Durham, NC: Duke University Press.
Žižek, S. 1998b. Love thy neighbour? No, thanks! In: C. Lane, ed. *The Psychoanalysis of Race*. New York, NY: Columbia University Press, 154–175.
Žižek, S. 2001a. *The Fright of Real Tears: Krzysztof Kieslowski between Theory and Post-Theory*. London: British Film Institute.
Žižek, S. 2001b. The feminine excess: Can women who hear divine voices find a new social link? *Millennium Journal of International Studies*, 30 (1), 93–109.
Žižek, S. 2002. The only good neighbor is a dead neighbor. *Identities: Journal for Politics, Gender and Culture*, 2 (2), 9–31.
Žižek, S. 2006. *The Parallax View*. Cambridge, MA: MIT Press.
Žižek, S. 2008a. *The Sublime Object of Ideology*. London: Verso.
Žižek, S. 2008b. *The Plague of Fantasies*. London: Verso.
Žižek, S. 2008c. *Enjoy Your Symptom!: Jacques Lacan in Hollywood and Out*. New York, NY: Routledge.
Žižek, S. 2012a. *Less Than Nothing: Hegel and the Shadow of Dialectical Materialism*. London: Verso.
Žižek, S. 2012b. Introduction: The spectre of ideology. In: S. Žižek, ed. *Mapping Ideology*. London: Verso, 1–33.
Žižek, S. 2012c. How did Marx invent the symptom. In: S. Žižek, ed. *Mapping Ideology*. London: Verso, 296–331.
Žižek, S. 2014. *Event: A Philosophical Journey Though a Concept*. Brooklyn, NY: Melville House.
Žižek, S. 2015. *Absolute Recoil: Towards a New Foundation of Dialectical Materialism*. London: Verso.
Žižek, S. 2016. *Disparities*. London: Bloomsbury.
Žižek, S. 2017. *Incontinence of the Void: Economico-Philosophical Spandrels*. Cambridge, MA: MIT Press.
Zupančič, A. 2008. *The Odd One In: On Comedy*. Cambridge, MA: MIT Press.
Zupančič, A. 2016. Power in the closet (and its coming out). In: P. Gherovici and M. Steinkoler, eds. *Lacan, Psychoanalysis, and Comedy*. New York, NY: Cambridge University Press, 219–234.
Zupančič, A. 2017. *What is Sex?* Cambridge, MA: MIT Press.
Zupančič, A. 2019. Love thy neighbor as thyself?! *Problemi International*, 3 (3), 89–108.

1

POLITICAL CORRECTNESS AND COMEDY

Political correctness and the 'postmodern turn': Comedy, humour and the problem of subversion

In the introduction chapter a brief attempt was made to offer some form of definition to the term 'political correctness' (PC). While various definitions abound, what has remained constant throughout its usage and history is its ability to be a contentious but also vague term that is grounded in predominantly negative and disparaging descriptions (Penhallurick, 2010). For this reason, Penhallurick argues that political correctness has often been conceived as:

> an extremist movement dedicated particularly to the removal of all offensive and even potentially offensive expressions from the English language. People assume that it is an assault on their freedom of expression, and that the day will soon come when we are forced into not uttering words like *short* or *fat* or *old*. In fact, it's already come. Political correctness gone mad!
>
> *(2010: 165)*

Penhallurick's reference to 'freedom of expression' bears a particular frustration towards those rallying against the dogmatism of political correctness. Consequently, though many have tied its emergence to the political left – originally the term was meant to refer to an excessive political gesture (Hall, 1994) – today it is often viewed, both positively and negatively, as a means for promoting one's moral superiority as well as an advocation of one's right to free expression (Thakkar, 2019).

However, while the term 'politically correct' has gained wider usage in the latter half of the twentieth century, 'The tension between the right to speak freely and the right to live in a society where offensive communication is monitored and regulated has longstanding roots within the philosophical study of pragmatics and morality'

(Das and Graefer, 2017: 6). In particular, the management of 'offensive communication' bears a historical relation to the performance of comedy, with Kamm and Neumann highlighting how 'As early as 1625, Francis Bacon in his essay "Of Discourse" admonished writers that certain subject matters should not be exposed to ridicule' (2016: 12). Equally, Stourton notes how sixteenth century religious tensions between Protestants and Catholics could, today, be re-interpreted alongside contemporary debates on the restrictions that political correctness poses. In accordance with the concern that contemporary PC advocates are promoting a repressive 'PC culture', Stourton details how, in 1569, the performance of the York Mystery Plays[1] was 'suppressed by the Elizabethan authorities for being too Catholic' (2008: 7). Stourton argues that 'Since Protestantism was the "politically correct" religion of the day it is reasonable to say that the plays were, in fact, victims of sixteenth-century Political Correctness' (2008: 7). Consequently, while any single definition of political correctness can offer 'only a partial understanding of a complex territory' (Das and Graefer, 2017: 6), the management of offence and the suppression of that which is deemed to offend – be it a certain subject matter or an expression of one's beliefs – suggests that 'the idea of ideological "correctness"' (Stourton, 2008: 8) posits a long and significant history within the marginalisation of certain 'minority' groups and in the management of forms of insult.

In fact, despite its varied history, debates on political correctness have continued to persist and, since the end of the Second World War, have become embroiled in a number of significant political and cultural confrontations, ranging from an over-zealous liberal bias in academic institutions to serving as a form of cultural Marxism bent on imposing its own moral agenda. Though the term remains tied to certain political agendas and conspiracy theories, its usage continues to bear an accusatory significance. Dunant notes that, 'To call someone PC is less a description than an insult, carrying with it accusations of everything from Stalinism/McCarthyism to (even worse?) having no sense of humour' (1994: vii). While political correctness is geared towards preventing 'offence', it has, in the case of right-wing politicians, been used as a way of emphasising the detrimental impact of forms of censorship on political actions that are frequently deemed to be in the interests of a 'political elite'. Drawing upon the linguist Anna Szilagyi (2017), Quirk highlights how far-right politicians often 'lin[k] "political correctness" to negative connotations', including 'the subordination of "ordinary people" by an intellectual elite', the over-zealous promotion of forms of 'censorship', which seeks to manage what can and can't be said, and an open disregard for 'important issues [which] go damagingly unaddressed by politicians who fear that they will cause offence' (Quirk, 2018: 59). It is against this backdrop that examples of political correctness draw together both politics and culture under a climate of fear, anxiety and frustration, with the hysterical nature of political correctness contriving to redefine any story, insinuation or representation into a debate on the *correct* type of label, description or language to use.

Indeed, although these debates have proved to be politically divisive, the significance of political correctness – both positive and negative – has remained central to post-war debates regarding one's individual autonomy and one's location in an increasingly globalised economy set within a varying cultural milieux. Accordingly, while, for some, political correctness continues to maintain a political importance, through its aversion to social hierarchies, culturally, examples of political correctness have heralded a cultural eclecticism, whereby the intermingling of high and low culture has taken shape within a commercially orientated cultural apex where the relationship between culture and capital is now inseparable (Adorno, 2003). This has seen political arguments increasingly steered by one's cultural location, with social mobility being orchestrated by an ability to increase one's 'cultural capital'.

This change has proven particularly significant following the emergence of the post-war welfare state and the subsequent broadening of social democracy in the UK and Western Europe. As evident in the fight for civil rights in the US, the 1960s were notable for delivering a number of critical movements tied to issues of postcolonialism, anti-war and nuclear disarmament, gay rights and 'second-wave' feminism, where, for many, the 'personal' was now political. This diffusion of politics dispelled political action across a variety of fronts; a process that was echoed in critical theory's shift from Marxism's economic reductionism towards the importance of culture as an ideological tool (McMillan, 2013). Notably, the move towards 'culture' served to decentre 'class struggle', with the significance of 'class' giving way to debates on one's gender, sexuality and race/ethnicity, as well as the various ways in which these were (and are) discursively produced both on, and through, the subject (McHoul and Grace, 2015).

As a consequence, these 'New Social Movements' resulted in a political picture that was largely 'post-political' (Habermas, 1981). That is, such movements were not just concerned with political change, but with a wider social and cultural redefinition of how one could achieve and discover their self-realisation through a shift in one's cultural outlook and through a potential array of available lifestyles. In principle, such redefining steered clear of any top-down centralisation. Instead, a 'protest from below' was enacted by deconstructing privileged interpretations through forms of radical plurality (Derrida, 1997). Working 'outside' the 'normal' and emboldened by a new focus on affect and a decentred politics grounded in one's cultural well-being (and not just one's material well-being), these movements would increasingly be perceived as 'postmodern' (Agger, 1994; Flisfeder, 2019).

Sharing in the subversive zeitgeist, which had been established across Europe and the US in the 1960s (Eagleton, 2003), the emergence of postmodernism provided 'a reaction to modern narratives of history, including liberal and Enlightenment narratives of progress, and dialectical models of change and transformation, particularly Marxist historical materialism' (Flisfeder, 2017: 149). Positioning itself in stark contrast to the 'grand narratives' which had sought to explain and even predict the decline of capitalism (Jameson, 1991; Lyotard, 1984), postmodernism redirected attention to the importance of language as an act of power.

Specifically, the act of naming would be conceived as a decree of power, with postmodern politics focusing on the significance of discourse in both shaping and understanding cultural and historical texts as well art, language and aesthetics. The emergence of a postmodern approach to culture and politics closely followed broader changes in critical theory and Western philosophy, most notably in what would become known as the 'discursive/linguistic turn'. By directing attention to the ontological significance of language (McMillan, 2013), and through extending the ideas of Ferdinand de Saussure, academic disciplines such as philosophy, literary studies, Marxism and psychoanalysis would find themselves paying closer attention to the relationship between power and language via new forms of critical inquiry that reconsidered the human condition and the study of reality. In part, this focus on language placed greater emphasis on the indeterminacy of meaning and power, with various political movements seeking to assert their own interpretations and understandings of society (Laclau and Mouffe, 1985). Importantly, the 'discursive turn' provided a renewed focus on culture and its impact on politics and identity. By reconsidering the use of 'labels' in approaching issues of human rights and free speech, debates on feminism and multiculturalism sought to trace the discursive effects of power relations on the subject, subjectivity and 'human nature' (Chomsky and Foucault, 2006; Foucault, 2002).

Significantly, these debates considered the position of the subject in relation to ideological discourses, which both constituted and 'subjected' the subject to established identity formations and social relations. Alongside commercial culture, greater emphasis was placed on the individual – both as a source of contention and as an aesthetic form of artistic creation (Jameson, 1991). This focus on the individual, grounded in forms of self-reflexivity and self-conscious understanding, underscored postmodernism's critique of meta-narratives and fuelled its subversion of traditional forms of authority, with greater attention now paid to the ambivalences that permeated conceptions of the 'self'. In short, the ambivalence, uncertainty and ambiguity which characterised the postmodern condition would be reflected in examples of 'postmodern humour', whereupon self-reflective modes of cultural expression were enacted in comical forms that conferred a wry commentary on popular culture as well as humorously critiquing the boundaries that inhibited and curtailed conventional social roles.

Notably, postmodernism's conflation with a humorous aesthetic was not necessarily tied to any specific 'content' but rather served to reveal a certain 'attitude', that was perpetuated in 'a readiness to go beyond conventional ways of looking at the world' (Vasantkumar, 1998: 213). In doing so, conventional forms of understanding the social, the individual and their interdependence were played with, redefined and recreated in postmodern texts that were marked by a multiplicity in their construction and interpretation (Weaver, 2011). Specifically, 'postmodern humour' would draw upon irony, satire, pastiche, paradox, montage, polysemy and ambiguity in order to blur and distort traditional genre conventions. By mixing comic genres, examples of 'postmodern humour' subversively dislodged and critically undermined the pomposity of power and its positions of authority, with the authorial intention of the postmodern text becoming, in some instances, difficult to conceive (Olsen, 1990). What became apparent in the 'interpenetration' of post-modernism with humour was the extent to which its self-reflexivity deliberately blurred the boundaries between the 'object' of humour and the very 'style' in which this humour was employed (Vasantkumar, 1998: 213). Whereas not every postmodern formation could be conceived as comical, the sense of ambivalence that postmodern humour relied upon would ultimately result in postmodernism itself being perceived as a joke (Vasantkumar, 1998).

Outside of comedy, such 'ambivalence' worked to bolster critics of post-modernism, who sought to decry the pursuit of infinite, non-hierarchical interpretations as undermining an academic pursuit for objective truth and rational understanding. Such criticisms bear just as many inaccuracies as they do detractors (Jordan Peterson is notable, in this instance, for conflating criticisms of both post-modernism and political correctness), but what is evident in such contentions – and postmodern humour in general – is an underlying connection, or rather tension, between postmodernism's ability to subvert established discourses *and* its use of enlightenment principles, grounded in modernism's recognition of the individual and the other's difference. Flisfeder notes:

> Although modernism, … was concerned with the dislodging of authority, we might say that postmodernism is what emerges when the challenge to authority *becomes* the norm. When the subversion of authority itself seemingly becomes the authoritative position. This puts postmodern criticism in a difficult position, and is one reason why it is often charged with being overly relativistic.
>
> *(2017: 65)*

In fact, for Flisfeder, the apparent 'success' of postmodern criticism has resulted in the normalisation of subversive forms of resistance that 'makes it difficult to conceive the truly radical potentials of postmodernism' (2017: 26). Here, the paradoxes of postmodernism are reflected by the fact that while it 'has had the advantage of bringing greater attention to the critique of cultural stereotypes in modern texts, … it has also drained the desire for social and political transformation' (Flisfeder, 2017: 84).[2] As a result, postmodernism remains indebted to its own inherent limitations and to a sense of plurality, which seeks to conform to a variety of cultural tastes. With regard to these limitations, postmodernism's inability to present the 'new' means that it ends up 'rel[ying] on ironic modes of presentation' that 'becom[e] part of the aesthetic of postmodern irony and parody' (Flisfeder, 2017: 75). Indeed, 'Because everything has already been said, novelty and originality prove difficult' (Flisfeder, 2017: 75).

To this end, the subversive potential of postmodern humour was one that remained tied to an aesthetic formation grounded in plurality and unending cultural eclecticism (Flisfeder, 2017). This eclectic plurality has served to encourage forms of hyper-liberalism which remain indebted to a symbolic play of differences that simply encourages the individual to tolerate difference – different identities etc. – without ever making the *commitment* that acknowledging this difference requires. This underscores postmodernism's transformation from a radical form of critical inquiry into an arm of late capitalism, exacerbating capitalism's own inherent contradictions through the promotion of various forms of 'cultural identity'. Arguably, it is postmodernism's 'loosening' of conceptual boundaries and its understanding of the subject as constituted by a plurality of discourses which has proven adept at securing dominant forms of cultural commodification (Adorno and Horkheimer, 1997; Flisfeder, 2017, 2019). Drawing from the work of Frederic Jameson (1991, 1996), McMillan argues that Jameson can help shed light on these contradictions, noting how:

> the burgeoning development of social identities that came with the birth of postmodernism became a seamless cure for the ills of overproduction, as, along with the financialisation of capital, new social identities were ideal for the development of new products and new markets. These markets were generated by the 'new social movements' and cultural identifications that developed alongside the turn to language and emphasis upon cultural differentiation amongst Leftists.
>
> *(2013: 35)*

It is in this regard that such 'movements have provided the impetus for the liberation of very real limitations upon subjective expression' and, as a result, 'they cannot be considered to be subversive' (McMillan, 2013: 35). This emphasises the difficulties in producing real forms of subversion, especially when such challenges are now the 'norm'. In part, this has helped to buttress the inherent paradoxes that underscore political correctness, most notable in the extent to which political correctness can often be used and critiqued by both the political left and right.

To this extent, the emergence of political correctness can be attributed to a post-ideological predicament, whereby the potential to resort to post-ideological assertions amongst the liberal left remained grounded in a politicisation of identity, from which structural forms of inequality went largely unchallenged. Under a logic of promoting greater inclusivity and social equality, and with 'overtones of enforcing tolerance and prescribing behaviour' (Dunant, 1994: viii–ix), political correctness would eventually be embroiled in campus debates that would seek to manage and curtail any form of 'offensive behaviour' (Hall, 1994). Dunant notes:

> it was perhaps inevitable that PC should lead to such absurdities as the Antioch College code of sexual behaviour which insisted on verbal agreement before any and every stage of sexual courtship, and to accusations that Andrew Marvell's ode 'To His Coy Mistress' was simply a sophisticated piece of sexual harassment.
>
> *(1994: ix)*

Accordingly, whether one was proclaiming for, in the above instance, greater diversity in educational curriculums, or criticising the overbearing tendency of political correctness to both regulate and manage human behaviour, 'What seemed most characteristic of the PC issue was the way it cut across the traditional left/right divide, and divided some sections of the left from others' (Hall, 1994: 166). Closer consideration of this division reveals an underlying concern not only in the *ways* in which political correctness has come to catalyse recent and ongoing political predicaments, but also alludes to far deeper changes within Western society since the end of the Second World War. In fact, over the course of the 1970s, these changes would take shape within a social context of tumultuous political and economic change, with postmodernism seeking to subvert the political regimes and social values that had previously been tied to European colonialism and patriotic nationalism as well as rigid class structures, racial hierarchies and patriarchal control. This new 'revolutionary' zeal in social, cultural and political terms would buttress a growing capitalist framework, underpinned by an increasing number of transnational corporations and an increasingly integrated international market predicated on the economic expansion of debt (Žižek, 1999).

As a result, new opportunities for the autonomy of the free individual were increasingly steered by a burgeoning capitalist reality (Fisher, 2009). Here, a growing focus on the desire and needs of the self-made individual, set against a steep decline in national industries and a political instability that would see a turn away from post-war social democracy towards the hegemonic control of a New Right grounded in a decidedly neoliberal agenda, would come to characterise the 1970s. In the UK, this steer towards the right was directed by the continued electoral success of Margaret Thatcher and her Conservative governments. Instilling 'a long-term, historic transformation of British society' (Hall, 1994: 169), Hall elaborates on how this 'New Right':

> Use[d] [its] political power in order to 'wind up' one whole historical era – the welfare-state, Keynesian, full-employment, comprehensive education-era on which the postwar settlement was constructed – and its replacement by another entirely new type of social order. Its outlook penetrated deep into social, moral, sexual and family life. It … more or less comprehensively transformed all our public institutions – forcing them, through the application of new principles of enterprise management, either to directly obey or indirectly to 'mimic' the market. It has a philosophy, a recipe for everything: for remodeling not only how we behave as citizens and voters, but as mothers, fathers, children, teachers, doctors and lovers.
>
> *(1994: 170)*

Yet, this new social order would be subject to a number of popular cultural counter-movements, with a key trend emerging in comic performances whose offbeat style and unique take on contemporary cultural debates would specifically draw from a politically correct oeuvre that was directed at challenging old orders and established hierarchies. Here, the emergence of Alternative Comedy would serve as a radical and reactionary genre, geared towards exposing and exploring the inconsistencies of popular culture through new forms of comic performance.

Out with the old, in with the new: Alternative Comedy and political correctness

Emerging from the Comedy Store venue, situated in Soho, London, comedians and scholars have noted how the rise of Alternative Comedy during the 1980s (Friedman, 2014; Lee, 2010; Quirk, 2018) marked a decidedly political turn in British comedy. While 'remembered as the moment when comedy grew a political conscience rooted in egalitarianism, specifically addressing the areas of class and marginalized identities and seeking new forms which were innovative and experimental' (Quirk, 2018: 8), it was in the stand-up routines and comic cabarets of a variety of British comedians that the importance of social values pertaining to sexism, class, homophobia and racism were presented (Friedman, 2014; Norris, 2014). In contrast to the stand-up comedians who had graced TV schedules during the 1970s, Alternative Comedy forged itself in reaction to 'the offensive comedy rife in working men's clubs and similar entertainment milieux [which] had filtered through in diluted form to television and radio', and which was, as noted by Lockyer and Pickering, 'replete with racist and sexist stereotypes' (2008: 810). Instead, for Alternative Comedy, 'Packaged gags and tired catchphrases were swept away by comic onslaughts against Thatcherism, middle-class foibles and male hypocrisies' (Lockyer and Pickering, 2008: 810). In fact, the anti-Thatcher motifs of Alternative Comedians proved a reoccurring theme, with 'the overt adoption of a left-wing political stance … commonly discussed as a reaction to the specific historical circumstances of Thatcherism' forming a constitutive feature of comic routines (Quirk, 2018: 51–52).

From stand-up to the alternative cabarets, the success of Alterative Comedy led to television work that would make household names of Ade Edmondson, Rik Mayall, Nigel Planer, Dawn French and Jennifer Saunders. Performing as 'The Comic Strip', their success was rewarded in television productions such as the pioneering series, *The Comic Strip Presents…* (1980–2016). Following this success, *The Young Ones* (1982–1984) would later draw upon the traditional sitcom genre in order to portray, parody and comment upon political and social issues of the time.

Consequently, while a key tenant of Alternative Comedy's success can be seen in its ability to critically 'introduc[e] political correctness as a best practice … turn[ing] the frequent recourse to racist, sexist, and homophobic stereotype, which had previously been a staple of popular comedy, into a taboo' (Quirk, 2018: 5), its comic exposition of cultural identities would bear a notable resemblance to postmodernism's self-reflexive irony and its penchant for parody and imitation (Jameson, 2009). Over the course of the 1990s, the political significance of Alternative Comedy would become increasingly ambiguous, with a tendency towards pretentiousness, shock and 'ironic incorrectness' (Hunt, 2013).

Matched by a period of neoliberal ascendance (Fukuyama, 2006), the inherent tensions in the political significance of Alternative Comedy would be exposed, with Brassett asserting that while 'Alternative comedy was about equality between races and sexes, freedom of expression, modernity and progress in a critical liberal vein. … [I]ts success was also arguably a failure' (2015: 178). Here, 'The opposition between "alternative comedy" and "white racist stand-up" was gradually deconstructed into a social compromise of political correctness' (Brassett, 2015: 178), with the political hegemony of neoliberalism finding itself embroiled in a cultural tension torn between PC's 'multicultural' diversity and a reactionary new-laddism (Brassett, 2015). Although remaining 'outside' the mainstream politically, 'Alternative comedy expounded the values of a newly emergent liberal class: educated, cosmopolitan, travelled' (Brassett, 2015: 178).

Instead, 90s television comedies, such as *Men Behaving Badly* (1992–2014) and *Knowing Me, Knowing You with Alan Partridge* (1994), would help to reinvent the 'male fool' as a historical comedy trope (Norris, 2014), developing upon that which had previously been seen in character's such as Anthony Aloysius Hancock (Tony Hancock), in *Hancock's Half Hour* (1956–1960) and *Hancock* (1961), as well as Basil Fawlty (John Cleese) in *Fawlty Towers* (1975–1979). While echoes of Alternative Comedy would continue in the success of Vic Reeves and Bob Mortimer's *Shooting Stars* (1993–2011), for many 'The narratives surrounding politically correct humour became seen … as a restrictive, institutionalised mechanism' (Norris, 2014: 173). For Norris (2014) this resulted in the emergence of a 'post-political correctness', with various comedians ignoring or openly mocking politically correct rhetoric. Here, comedians such as Chris Morris, and his widely acclaimed *Brass Eye* (1997–2001), self-knowingly criticised political correctness by comically performing its 'reactionary' tendencies and not its progressive intentions (Norris, 2014).

Furthermore, with the election of Tony Blair's New Labour government, discussions on and attitudes towards political correctness were marked by a growing individualism within British society (Fisher, 2009). Though, on the one hand, successive New Labour governments sought to promote minority interests, typically associated with the left (such as homosexuality, race, etc.), on the other hand, these interests would frequently be promoted via a consumer-led focus on the individual (Hewison, 2014; Pitcher, 2009). Accordingly, under 'third-way neoliberalism … the ideological antagonisms of the 1970s and 1980s were downplayed and difference was emphasised through the articulation of discourses such as multiculturalism' (Salter, 2016: 120). In fact, 'While multiculturalism undoubtedly had its merits, the possibility of political change that may challenge the dominant hegemony became increasingly distant, as the practices of neoliberalism became normative and institutionalized' (Salter, 2016: 120). The impact of these political and social changes would continue into the new millennium, with debates on political correctness, especially in comedy, taking on an added significance.

During the first decade of the new millennium, the politicisation of identity remained a contentious topic in television comedies and stand-up routines, with arguments both for and against political correctness taking centre-stage (Kamm and Neumann, 2016). Admired television comedians, such as David Jason and Rowan Atkinson, openly criticised the encroachment of political correctness in contemporary comedy, with others denouncing the restrictions it seemed to place on the importance of 'free speech' (Kamm and Neumann, 2016). In particular, British comedian Ricky Gervais would come to draw upon 'politically incorrect' themes in both his stand-up and sitcoms (alongside his collaborator, Stephen Merchant). Though often perceived to be 'pushing' the boundaries of political correctness, 'Liberal popular comedians such as Ricky Gervais or Jimmy Carr' continue to be both lauded and admonished for 'build[ing] jokes or comedy routines around race, ethnicity or even incest or paedophilia arguing that free speech is a pillar of western democracy' (Das and Graefer, 2017: 3). Central here is the 'liberal' framing of these comedians and their promulgation of a 'free speech' that remains predicated on one's political autonomy to incite challenging views, ideas and/or beliefs. While it would seem that the objectives of political correctness are now widely derided by those comedians who frequently frame their comic routines under the rubric of 'free speech', what is of greater significance is the extent to which these arguments seek to achieve a sense of liberal autonomy that bears a striking resemblance to politically correct attempts to challenge traditional power structures. It is amidst these contradictions that assertions of liberalism occupy a position both for and against political correctness.

Therefore, what has remained a central theoretical and, indeed, aesthetic component of the UK's post-war comedy history is the corresponding relation between postmodernism's subversive aims and a political rhetoric which has sought to challenge established hierarchies by drawing upon a 'politically correct' and culturally driven identity politics. In part, one can assert that it is perhaps the success of postmodernism which has encouraged the turn to a centrist politics grounded in a neoliberal economic agenda. Indeed, for Flisfeder, it is postmodernism's subversive resistance which has ensured that, under late capitalism, the 'alternative' is now a fundamental 'part of the mainstream' (2017: 26):

> As the commodity has taken precedence over daily life, it has become increasingly difficult to discern any concrete figure antagonistic to the project of emancipation. Under the reign of the commodity, even the bourgeoisie as a primarily cultural (as opposed to economic) category has lost its clout. Even the Right, today, is largely antibourgeois, preferring to combine populist rhetoric with the uninhibited logic of the market (figures like Donald Trump and Sarah Palin, and the former mayor of Toronto, Rob Ford are exemplary here). … Our situation today presents us with the paradox of a class struggle on the Right, where the latter appears to be more capable of interpellating the working class, by presenting the postmodern Left – tied rhetorically to the validation of political correctness – as the ruling class.
>
> *(Flisfeder, 2017: 150)*

In view of this history, the following sections will seek to identify a number of key themes drawn from postmodern critiques which, in accordance with examples from comedy, have resided themselves to forms of irony, satire and cynicism. While offering the *potential* for subversion, it will be argued that such comic forms work to support and maintain a decidedly non-subversive approach.

The failure of postmodern subversion: Irony, satire and cynicism

In his work on British comedy, Brassett (2009, 2015) has examined how irony and satire have proved a staple feature of British comedians. Indeed, in accordance with the post-imperial decline of Britain, Ward (2001) contests that the use of irony helped Britain manage the loss of empire, locating the UK within a new military and economic hegemony orchestrated by the US and Soviet Union. Through the use of irony, Britain's geopolitical position could be poked at, played with and made fun of (Brassett, 2009; Ward, 2001). More importantly, such an ironic stance in British comedy would reveal a certain ambiguity that, while directed towards examples of self-depreciation, could be used to assert a frustrated and reactionary form of political significance. To this extent, examples of irony would serve to permit a form of self-detachment; a space from which the self and society could be viewed from a critical distance.

According to Berger, 'The word *irony* comes from the Greek for dissembling' (2014: 26). Here, 'The ironist plays a game of pretending with his audience. He always means something else than what he says – more than he says, or less so, or at any rate something different' (Berger, 2014: 26). In doing so, examples of irony can frequently result in difficulties assessing the political motivations and underlying meanings of certain 'ironic' performances. This is especially apparent in the case of racist jokes, where the distance afforded by irony can allow the comedian to 'hide behind' a shield of their own self-distance, often reflected in the reply: 'I was being ironic'. Moreover, such forms of irony are not necessarily tied to the UK context. As Detweiler's comments on the use of irony in the popular US comedy *Seinfeld* (1989–1998) highlight, the show's ironic stance would often serve 'as a means of distancing itself from and relieving itself of responsibility for the earnest moral and political issues of the world' (Detweiler, 2012: 729). Brassett's contentions follow a contrary path, with him asserting that such 'distancing' does not have to centre on 'relieving oneself of responsibility', but rather, in accordance with Richard Rorty's work on irony, can 'suggest a *reflective distance* in discussions of global ethics' (Brassett, 2009: 236 [italics added]). Here, Brassett details how examples of British irony have allowed the UK to 'realise that recognising our contingency can be both playful and tragic' (2009: 240). What remains important in these cases, however, is the way in which we recognise and perform such contingency, with the tragic itself providing a certain transgressive relief that can be comically realised, recognised and played with.

In this regard, Brassett (2015) has commended the work of Ricky Gervais and Stephen Merchant, with Gervais's performances providing their own 'ironic turn'. In fact, according to Brassett:

> Gervais's more personal deprecation nurtured a form of social pain, partly a social pain of being British, and partly the pain of surviving a post-industrial Britain. If the economy was the centre of politics, then *The Office* was the appropriate stage for examining the tensions of social life.
>
> *(2015: 179)*

Such tensions, however, are not just reflected in examples of irony, but have also featured in forms of satire. Whereas, historically, 'Select Greeks and Romans used satirical comedy at symposia to demonstrate the elite's supposed superiority over the masses' (Hughey and Muradi, 2009: 227), in the post-war period, satire has often functioned as a way of making fun of and even ridiculing important political figures and their policies (Colletta, 2009). To this end, 'satire is the deliberate use of the comic for purposes of attack' (Berger, 2014: 146), and, as Berger (2014) elaborates, has become a constitutive feature of almost all forms of comic expression. Central here is the way in which it draws attention to the expectant ideal and its subsequent frustrations (Davis, 1993).

In fact, these frustrations would frequently find themselves directed towards examples of satire that, in the UK, would coalesce with the social realism genre, lending political satire a decidedly popular appeal. Here, the 'satire boom' in British comedy would mimic examples of 'British' irony, providing 'a mechanism of public critique and questioning of the establishment: a particular(ly) British mood of self-deprecation [that] reflected an uncertain position in the world and doubts over the excess of empire' (Brassett, 2015: 177). This was most notable in the British sitcom *Till Death Us Do Part* ('*Till Death*') (1965–1975), whose 'anti-liberal messages' were 'presented as laughable satire' (Bebber, 2014: 254). Bebber highlights how the aims of the series' writer, Johnny Speight, were reflected in 'Speight's intentional use of vulgar, racist and sexist language ... born of his sensitivity to any form of censorship', and used 'to undermine bourgeois liberalizing discourses' so as to 'reveal working-class life intimately and accurately' (2014: 260). However, such portrayals would ultimately rely upon a certain ambiguity of intent. As a result, Speight's depiction of 'working-class men as rough' and his desire to undermine the views and values 'of more "respectable" liberals in 1960s society' (Bebber, 2014: 259) meant that it could often be very difficult to determine whether the 'jokes', performed as part of the racist ramblings of the show's protagonist, Alf Garnett (Warren Mitchell), were steered towards Alf's own presumptuousness or were instead directed at his naive 'liberal' son-in-law and daughter. To this extent, examples of satire were, in accordance with the 1960s counter-culture, predicated on a form of 'punching up'; a critique that would continue into the 1980s with *Spitting Image* (1984–1996).

Nonetheless, though many have commented upon the apparent decline in British satire, Brassett notes how:

> An interesting facet of the austerity period in mainstream British politics has been the rise (or return) to prominence of an apparently radical set of satirists.

> Comedians like Russell Brand, Charlie Brooker and Stewart Lee have consolidated already strong careers with a new tranche of material that meets a widespread public mood of disdain for the failure and excess of 'global capitalism'.
>
> *(2015: 168–169)*

Echoed in comedies such as *The Thick of It* (2005–2012), the satirical comedy of Brand, Brooker and Lee has frequently 'engag[ed] in a satirical critique of sound-bite culture, personality and gesture politics' (Brassett and Sutton, 2017: 249). The problem, however, is that this often runs the 'risk that satire will confirm what "we already know"' (Brassett and Sutton, 2017: 249). For Brassett and Sutton, 'This appears to be a political dilemma of comedy', with examples of satire and irony offering 'a tranquilising effect …, whereby things may be terrible, but "hey at least we can laugh"' (2017: 249). Consequently, although examples of irony and satire are undoubtedly funny, of greater concern is that these examples never go beyond the performance of a hyper-farcity that often steers towards the ridiculousness (Hughey and Muradi, 2009). Instead, such 'open-ended' performances merely present social and political critiques that fall short of enacting any considered form of political resistance that can challenge the established orders which they seek to ridicule. As a result, they maintain a rather cynical approach.

Accordingly, whereas the above discussion has sought to draw upon examples of irony and satire, it is argued that one of the prevailing features of British comedy – and here one can trace a line beginning with the emergence of Alternative Comedy to the present – is a prevalence for cynical forms of comic depiction. Here, British comedy frequently resorts to examples of trivialisation, which, while remaining critical of certain political figures, movements and broader social and cultural changes, has, nevertheless, only served to maintain a paradoxical position in popular (postmodern) culture. Moreover, such cynicism corresponds with a neoliberal agenda and the right of the individual to critically dismiss the cultural, political and social consensus. Reflecting a 'post-politically correct' attitude in British comedy, Norris notes how examples such as the animated sketch comedy *Monkey Dust* (2003–2005) traded in a post-Cool Britannia melancholy which was 'reinforced by the complicit nature of each protagonist within the sketches, locked in the confines of their own fractured narratives and blocked by a contemporary existence that was defined by apathy' (Norris, 2014: 99).

In other instances, such apathy and cynicism were performed through absurdity. Drawing upon the comedy series *Brass Eye*, Brassett and Sutton highlight how 'the absurdity of *Brass Eye* not only satirises the limited nature of British political discourse but also *deliberately performs it*' (2017: 254). What is problematic is that it performs it in a farcical manner grounded in a cynical distance. While Morris's work may engender ambiguity and uncertainty in its political direction (if there is one), his comedy remains grounded in a distance between the onscreen farcity and the reality it seeks to critique. It remains cynical, rather than subversive.

To this end, we can consider how comedy's reliance on examples of irony, satire and cynicism ultimately provide it 'an ambiguous ethical position' that 'is as dependent upon the contingencies that it mocks as it is critical of them' (Brassett, 2015: 187). In fact, Hughey and Muradi (2009) refer to our current predicament in comedy as working off a form of 'hyper-irony' and 'manic-satire'. Drawing specifically on *South Park* (1997–present) and *Family Guy* (1999–present), they note how:

> acts of irreverant parody are goals in and of themselves. It matters little as to the target of caricature – whether it is censorship, religion, the media, or the mainstream populace – in so long as the process of spoof, ridicule, and lampoon is engaged.
>
> *(Hughey and Muradi, 2009: 226)*

Indeed, this has also been noted in other examples of animated comedy, including the previously mentioned *Monkey Dust* (Norris, 2014) and *The Simpsons* (1989–present). In his comparison of *South Park* and *The Simpsons*, Jansen (2003) notes how both shows have sought to critically satirise our liberal capitalist democracy, while at the same time remaining embedded within this model as part of its functioning. This is perhaps best reflected in *South Park's* criticism of the commercialisation of Christmas and their inclusion of the character, 'Mr. Hanky – the Christmas poo'. In fact, as Jansen highlights, 'The harsh satiric gesture involved in creating a Christmas icon from fecal matter hardly needs to be stressed, but perhaps the most ironic twist in this case is that Mr. Hankey has become a Christmas commodity in our world' (2003: 34). Jansen adds:

> The same question could be asked of *The Simpsons* since, not only has it introduced phrases like 'Don't have a cow, man,' and 'Cowabunga, dude' into the cultural lexicon, it has also sold countless t-shirts featuring Bart's image underneath such captions.
>
> *(2003: 34)*

As a result, shows such as *South Park, Family Guy* and *The Simpsons* often serve to 'promote dominant and conservative viewpoints while simultaneously targeting and ridiculing them' (Hughey and Muradi, 2009: 220). This contradiction, it is argued, has become a formative feature of comedy's postmodern condition, so that, 'Through parody, irony, and self-reflexivity, postmodernism is able to both legitimize and subvert culture (both high culture and mass culture) at the same time' (Flisfeder, 2017: 73–74).

What the above discussion has sought to imply, therefore, is that when certain jokes or comedy performances seek to employ irony, satire and cynicism, they frequently succumb to a liberal position that privileges the individual's ability to admonish those in power as well as wider social and cultural movements (Lee, 2010). To this end, if one is to suggest that 'liberalism' is particularly adept at using comedy to satirise or ironically portray figures of authority, as argued by Dagnes (2012), then it is more often the case that such comedy relies upon a sense of cynicism that both creates as well as supports a distance and/or detachment between the comic performance and the social context in which this comedy is performed. Although examples of irony, satire and cynicism are indeed funny and, as a consequence, constitute an important part of any comic arsenal, these forms of comedy fail to offer a substantiated subversive critique. Instead, such comic expressions work from an enforced distance *between* the comic performance and the subject of comedy (what Lacan refers to as the subject of enunciation (the comic-subject) and the subject of the enunciated (the subject of comedy)). Here, 'satire and irony … blur the line between the representation of hegemony and counter-hegemony' to the extent that in the case of racist, sexist or anti-Semitic jokes, 'irony and satire can simultaneously reaffirm racist ideologies, while also presenting alternative and antiracist narratives' (Hughey and Muradi, 2009: 212). In other words, the cynical, satirical and ironic comic who 'reaffirms racist ideologies' can always maintain a distance between themselves (enunciation) and the content of the joke (enunciated). In fact, these contradictions go some way to exposing the functioning of ideology as it pertains to examples of irony and cynicism.

As noted in Žižek's (2008a) critique of ideology, it is in accordance with examples of 'ironic distance' (or, 'radical' critique) that dominant ideologies maintain their power (Žižek, 2008a). Here, ideology:

> appears precisely as its opposite, as a radical critique of ideological utopias. The predominant ideology today is not a positive vision of some utopian future but a cynical resignation, an acceptance of how 'the world really is,' accompanied by a warning that if we want to change it (too much), only a totalitarian horror can ensue. Every vision of another world is thereby dismissed.
>
> *(Žižek, 2019a: 20)*

In short, our cynicism works to support hegemonic ideologies, by allowing us to dis-identify with ideological power. This cynicism is underscored by what Žižek refers to as an example of fetishistic disavowal, depicted in the attitude: 'I know very well, but nevertheless…'. To this end, while one can maintain a cynical attitude – a distance from the hopelessness of the situation – one, nevertheless, continues to remain embedded in the situation and its ideological parameters. Key here is that any actual change to the situation goes amiss. As a result, Contu refers to forms of cynicism, especially in comedy and humour, as a 'decaf resistance':

> Decaf resistance, just as decaf coffee, makes it possible for us to enjoy without the costs and risks involved. We can have the thing (coffee) without actually having it. I am suggesting that what are construed as new forms of resistance – the unofficial transgressions in the underground of neoliberal working life (i.e., skepticism, humor, cynicism, etc.) – consist of an edulcorated resistance.
>
> *(2008: 374)*

More importantly, we can begin to see how such forms of 'decaf resistance' serve to embody liberalism's own inherent transgressions (Contu, 2008). Although his comments refer to examples of satire, Bogel captures how this inherent transgression often revolves around false forms of difference, arguing that 'Satire … is a rhetorical means to the production of difference in the face of a potentially compromising similarity, not the articulation of differences already securely in place' (Bogel, 2001: 42). We can tie this 'production of difference' to postmodernism's focus on culture and its politicisation of identity politics via forms of political discussion that deliberately steer away from actual political action. More to the point, whereas postmodernism undoubtedly encourages an experiment with the self that can challenge as well as promote new forms of identity, such processes are counterbalanced by a more insidious form of subjection – an unrelenting need to perform oneself in 'new ways' (Žižek, 1999).

Ultimately, what we are left with in today's comedy landscape is a cynical scepticism whose radical and subversive alternatives remain embedded within the formal limits of a postmodern cultural practice that maintains the dominant ideological field. Accordingly, we can begin to locate these contradictions in the 1960s counter-culture and, in the case of comedy, in underlying contradictions that emerged in the Alternative Comedy movement. In fact, drawing upon the comments of British comedian Stewart Lee, Quirk notes that Alternative Comedy 'was a business model that exploited individual talent, competition, and self-motivated labour' (2018: 5). Echoing the normalisation of postmodernism's cultural critique, Quirk demonstrates how 'Alternative Comedy itself came, in some ways, to constitute a new form of artistic hegemony' (2018: 6), a hegemony which has resonated in the failures associated with postmodernism's subversive potential (Flisfeder, 2017).

To this extent, we can trace the prevalence of cynicism within certain comic performances alongside wider social and cultural contradictions which have come to permeate contemporary society. More importantly, delineating this path leaves us with a central question: how can comedy be subversive? Indeed, this question remains a pertinent one, especially when we consider how discussions on the 'failure' of postmodern subversion seek to frame this failure as emanating from the universalisation of liberal democracy under late capitalism. In outlining this critique, the remainder of this chapter will seek to explore how examples of liberal multiculturalism have come to structure our relation to cultural tolerance, identity politics and multicultural understandings of difference.

Liberal multiculturalism

In discussions on the emergence of political correctness, and in accordance with the previous discussion on comedy, Hall (1994) elaborates upon the idea that political correctness is often perceived through a liberal lens that focuses on the individualisation of personal rights. Alongside postmodernism's deconstruction of identity, liberal assertions of the autonomous individual (or 'Self') have developed upon postmodernism's capacity to question established conceptual boundaries by defending the individual's self-recognition. In fact, although postmodernism sought to position itself against liberalism's attempts to conceive the Self as both rational and centred, liberal discourses on cultural and ethnic integration have served to emphasise those values associated with Enlightenment principles, including secularism, individualism and freedom of expression. As a consequence, 'Individuals embedded within this [liberal/neoliberal] ideology focus upon themselves as their primary asset and the enhancement of the self as a pro-social – an inherently "good" and "correct" – behaviour' (Quirk, 2018: 65). Moreover, this contemporary ideological constellation is one that is marked by a neoconservative populism and liberal multiculturalism that is itself closely imbricated with a focus on the other, and, specifically, *their* enjoyment (Žižek, 1998). It is this infatuation with the other which forms part of a postmodern episteme that regularly returns to the promotion of cultural, racial and ethnic differences under an overarching sense of 'shared ethical substance' (Žižek, 2008c: 24).

The promulgation of a 'shared ethical substance', untainted by cultural antagonisms, is reflected in the work of Will Kymlicka, a key proponent of the liberal multiculturalist approach. Drawing upon the liberal framework, Kymlicka's (1996) creation of a shared *civic identity* is one that is grounded in cultural differences and, in particular, the integration of minority groups. To this end, Kymlicka (1996) believes that 'majority' and 'minority' tensions do not necessarily need to result in violence, but instead the autonomy and value of the individual can work alongside forms of cultural membership (Boulden and Kymlicka, 2015; Kymlicka, 1996). Key here is Kymlicka's (1996) ability to highlight that it is liberalism's principles of equality and individual autonomy which can promote as well as protect minority cultures through positive accommodations and special protections. Indeed, 'The central claim of the theory is that minority groups ought to have state protections in place so as not to be wrongfully disadvantaged due to their cultural status' (Maciel, 2014: 383). In doing so, the freedom to express oneself and to freely associate with a variety of collectives is pluralistically encouraged and it is in this way that a shared civic identity can help populate cultural diversity (Kymlicka, 2017).

What remains significant in Kymlicka's approach, however, is the extent to which his liberalism binds him to a form of cultural tolerance that, while remaining open to the diversity of majority and minority cultures (and, specifically, indigenous cultures), works off a liberal/illiberal dynamic that undermines such tolerance. That is, whereas Kymlicka is indebted to the promotion of cultural equality, his liberalism is one that remains posited on an inherent limit that reveals its own contradictions. This is exemplified in an approach that, on the one hand, respects the autonomy of the individual (and, by extension, their specific culture), but which, on the other, seeks to condemn 'illiberal' cultures and practices that undermine such autonomy. Under these circumstances, Kymlicka's (1996) argument falls upon the assertion that illiberal cultures should be 'liberalised'; an assertion which suggests that cultures which stem from 'a non-liberal provenance' are inevitably viewed as handicapped in some from (Van Oenen, 2010: 297). As Van Oenen asserts: 'Having a non-liberal provenance, for Kymlicka, is basically a handicap that can be compensated for through amendments (or provisos)' (2010: 298). Indeed, 'Such a framework implicitly presupposes the background of dominant, liberal culture, and consequently conceives of recourse to minority culture as merely a measure to fill a "lack"' (Van Oenen, 2010: 298). To this extent, Kymlicka's 'liberal thought strategically invokes multicultural thought to safeguard white political authority during episodes of crisis' (Baldwin, 2009: 532).

It is in view of such assertions that we can begin to draw contentions between Kymlicka's use of liberalism to promote cultural *tolerance* and Žižek's (1998, 2006a, 2006b, 2006c, 2008c) fundamental concern that liberal multiculturalism results in a pervasive homogenisation of culture that is controlled through fear, arrogance and apathy. In fact, with regards to the issue of cultural tolerance, Bunting notes how:

> Tolerance has become something of a founding mythology for western developed nations: our tolerance is regarded as a mark of our superiority over many less tolerant, less developed nations around the world. Our tolerance – in contrast to the intolerance of many of our ancestors – is evidence of the concept of historical progress.
>
> *(2011)*

Echoing Bunting's assertions, Žižek's critique is grounded in the consideration that examples of liberal tolerance circulate around two ways of relating to the other: 1) a respect for the other's culture; and, 2) an underlying fear of being 'too close' to the other – conceived in examples of harassment and the often-cited need *to be* culturally tolerant and, thus, tolerated (Bunting, 2011). Malik asserts that:

> The irony of multiculturalism as a political process is that it undermines much of what is valuable about diversity as lived experience. When we talk about diversity, what we mean is that the world is a messy place, full of clashes and conflicts. That's all for the good, for such clashes and conflicts are the stuff of political and cultural engagement.
>
> *(2010)*

These 'lived experiences' of a 'messy' world 'full of clashes and conflicts' is fundamentally undermined by an overriding desire, on behalf of those advocates of tolerance, to manage and minimise the potential effects of these 'clashes and conflicts'. In fact, 'They seek to minimise such conflicts by parcelling people up into neat ethnic boxes, and policing the boundaries of those boxes in the name of tolerance and respect' (Malik, 2010). Certainly, this is not to suggest that a successful form of multiculturalism should be grounded in violent clashes that simply place ethnicity against ethnicity. Instead, it is to consider how such management is underscored by a pervasive sense of anxiety, which is often ignored, but demonstrably reflected when we consider where our efforts to be 'tolerant' start and finish. Indeed, after donating our money to a homeless charity, after contributing to our local food banks, after sharing the concern that our nation should be accepting more refugees… is all this enough? What we often find with arguments grounded on tolerance is that such forms of tolerance can excessively imbue the individual with feelings of guilt (am I doing enough?). It is here that we can begin to observe how such pervasive forms of tolerance 'perfectly reproduce the paradox of the superego: the more you obey what the pseudo-moral agency demands of you, the more guilty you are' (Žižek, 2017: 21).

To this end, examples of liberal multiculturalism have introduced new forms of regulation that have resulted in greater feelings of guilt and anxiety (Dean, 2006). Insofar as being reminded 'that we are not enjoying properly' and that we 'are not doing anything right', we ultimately remain tied to a 'malevolent superego, empowering it to torment us all the more' (Dean, 2006: 38, 39). This failure to perform the correct type of politically correct behaviour, the regulated ways in which our work lives are organised and managed around the fear of harassment (Westwood and Johnston, 2011), and the constant questioning as to whether our tolerance is 'enough' (Radcliffe, 2012), all serve to underscore the universal hegemony of liberal multiculturalism.

The universality of liberal multiculturalism

As a universal form, liberal multiculturalism seeks to maintain a 'neutral' position in debates on cultural and ethnic relations. To help clarify the particular ways in which this 'universal position' achieves its sense of neutrality, we can turn to an example from film, and, in particular, Manoharan's account of Marvel Studios' *Avengers: Endgame* (2019):

> In the climax of Endgame, Ironman wields magical infinity stones and eliminates all those on Thanos' side, making him a more ruthless killer than Thanos who only killed half of the earth[/Universe]. Yet, Ironman will never be seen as a war criminal because he was restoring that which always was and should be – the liberal order. The bottom line of the entire Avengers film franchise seemed to be one single point, that a superrich superhero like Tony Stark/Ironman, who made his fortune through manufacturing weapons, would sacrifice his life for the sake of humanity. Throughout the MCU [Marvel Comic Universe] series, we were exposed to a defense of the American military-industrial complex, foreign interventionism, mass surveillance, targeted assassinations, and the stockpiling of weapons of mass destruction. Endgame was a justification for all that and more. The left-leaning *The Guardian*, however, felt a greater need to celebrate the diversity component of the movie. One does feel compelled to conclude that liberal multiculturalism is, indeed, the hegemony of our times!
>
> *(2019)*

As evident in Manoharan's reference to *The Guardian*, it is possible to identify how, under (neo)liberalism, there has been an equivalence of difference, which serves to depoliticise 'previously dispersed political demands' (Salter, 2016: 121) under a widely accepted and largely unchallenged narrative of 'inclusivity'. In doing so, liberal multiculturalism becomes its own universal, grounded in the disavowal or obfuscation of its own limitations and, as seen in *Endgame*, in an ideological justification of the liberal order itself.

In fact, it is amidst such liberal hegemony that examples of liberal multiculturalism can work to maintain a Eurocentric and, indeed, patronising, position (Žižek, 1998). Accordingly, while multiculturalism '"respects" the Other's identity' it does so by 'conceiving of the Other as a self-enclosed "authentic" community towards which he, the multiculturalist, maintains a distance rendered possible by his privileged universal position' (Žižek, 1997: 44). It is under such circumstances that 'the multiculturalist respect for the Other's specificity *is* the very form of asserting one's own superiority' (Žižek, 1997: 44 [italics added]). This superiority is maintained in 'a disavowed, inverted, self-referential form of racism, a "racism with a distance"' (Žižek, 1997, 44) and can be seen in examples of political correctness which coalesce with a 'liberal attitude that perceives itself as surpassing the limitations of its ethnic identity (as a "citizen of the world" without anchors in any particular ethnic community)' (Žižek, 1997, 47). Indeed, for multi-billionaires such as Bill Gates and Richard Branson, the claim to be a 'global citizen', devoid of any ethnic hindrance, underscores a desire to remove the state, to dissolve borders and, in view of capitalist development, ensure the unhindered expansion of capital into new 'emerging' markets. Ironically, it is these same individuals that our governments now deal with in order to 'solve' our ecological and humanitarian problems (Vidal, 2012). It is here that the politically correct desire to rid oneself of one's ethnic identity hegemonically functions to maintain a clear delineation between the multicultural/cosmopolitan subject and the 'ethnically driven' other. It is this function which allows liberal multiculturalism to serve as an 'empty universal' (Žižek, 1997).

This universality is accentuated when we consider how examples of liberal multiculturalism work off a desire to 'liberalise' or patronisingly aid the subject in their relations with the other. In each instance, we see narratives grounded in 'affect' and steered towards examples of 'victimisation' (Zupančič, 2003), which, rather than a more modest change in the social situations that embody such antagonisms, find themselves mistakenly drawn to identifying those external enemies ('the other') who are, in some way or another, deemed culpable for these antagonisms. While Žižek (1997) considers these features as being central to relations with the other under late-capitalism (an argument that will be returned to in his discussion of the 'decaffeinated other'), it remains important to highlight how these characteristics circulate around a cultural anxiety to/with the other that can result in: 1) open forms of racism and xenophobia (far right fascism, national populism); and 2) a hyper-liberal politics that undermines and/or obscures interactions with the other (identity politics).

It is with regards to the latter that examples of 'politically correct multiculturalism and their distortion of a certain type of alliance politics' have, according to Žižek, resulted in 'chains of equivalence between a widening set of differential struggles' (Žižek and Daly, 2004: 14). It is this 'widening chain' of difference which inhibits Real political action. Žižek elaborates:

> While there is nothing wrong in principle with establishing such forms of solidarity, the problem arises where this type of politics begins to assume, in a commonsense way, a basic levelling of the political terrain where all groups are taken to suffer equally ('we are all victims of the state/global capitalism/ repressive forces ...'). In other words, there is a danger that equivalent politics becomes so distorted that it becomes a way of disguising the position of those who are truly abject: those who suffer endemic poverty, destitution and repressive violence in our world system.
>
> *(Žižek and Daly, 2004: 14)*

In short, such equivalence serves the function of a fantasy by working to obscure Real engagement with those victims that stand outside the liberal-capitalist order; or, when considering this order itself, engaging in fundamental changes that would redefine the very order from which these problems arise (Dean, 2006). Instead, the 'levelling of the political terrain' (Žižek and Daly, 2004: 14) becomes incorporated in examples of identity politics, which, according to Gandesha (2018), have become overly focused on narratives of separated equality which undermine political protests against racial oppression. For Gandesha:

> identity politics is based on a particular ... account of experience as expressed in the statement 'You wouldn't understand because it's a black, Asian or queer, thing.' It is a staking out of a proprietary relation to an experience understood not as a process and a social relation but as a thing. This then leads not to a juridical discourse but a moralistic one based on the claiming of special victim status based on such reified experience.
>
> *(2018)*

Gandesha's comments bear a semblance to Žižek's critiques of identity politics (1997, 1998, 2018): both critically denounce the 'reified' importance of promoting politics grounded in 'majority-minority' experiences. Here, Žižek adds:

> Identity politics reaches its peak (or, rather, its lowest point) when it refers to the unique experience of a particular group identity as the ultimate fact which cannot be dissolved in any universality: 'only a woman/lesbian/trans/Black/ Chinese knows what is it to be a woman/lesbian/trans/Black/Chinese.' While this is true in a certain trivial sense, one should thoroughly deny any political relevance to it and shamelessly stick to the old Enlightenment axiom: all cultures and identities can be understood, provided that one makes an effort to

> get it. *The secret of identity politics is that, in it, the white/male/hetero position remains a universal standard; everyone understands it and knows what it means, which is why it is the blind spot of identity politics, the one identity it is prohibited to assert.*
>
> (2018: 175 [italics added])

Notably, Žižek's argument is not to reassert 'the white/male/hetero position' but instead draw attention to the fact that it is exactly this identity which has found itself reinvigorated in the rise of far-right and populist politics. More importantly, the emergence of identity politics is characteristically performed in assertions of political correctness, which seek to embed collective disadvantages in one's individual identity (Hall, 1994). The problem here is that 'It reflects the spread of "the political" from the public to the private arena' (Hall, 1994: 167).

Certainly, this critique is in no way intending to paint liberal multiculturalism as a straw man, beholden to the wide range of issues that underscore the various criticisms which have been levelled at multiculturalism in general. Indeed, Titley and Lentin make it clear that:

> Ironically, working through the idiom of multicultural failure is a form of political correctness; a way of talking about issues of migration, identity, power, belonging, legitimacy and socio-political anxiety while steering clear of a lexicon associated with the overt history of a shameful, racist past.
>
> (2011)

To this end, both the current and preceding critiques seek to work *within* the confines of political correctness in order to (re)approach those '*ways* of talking about' cultural diversity. It is approaching this cultural diversity through the lens of political correctness that the following discussion will now consider.

Political correctness: A Žižekian critique

The above discussion has sought to draw attention to the specific socio-political arrangements which have emerged in the wake of liberal multiculturalism; a multiculturalism that celebrates particular identities, while encouraging such celebration under closer forms of regulated control and social anxiety. It is in this sense that examples of political correctness have provided 'The ideological coordinates [… to] liberal multiculturalism' (Žižek, 2008c: 17). That is, by relying upon a reified ethnic particularity, examples of a politically correct superiority – a superiority that universally elevates the tolerant multiculturalist – are grounded in attempts to define the rules of social behaviour via forms of management that demarcate such behaviour along lines of harassment. In doing so, examples of politeness – what Žižek considers as those 'implicit unspoken regulations, … [and] questions of tact, … that [… are] part of our spontaneous sensitivity' (2015: 61) – are undermined by a regulated, even contractual, form of social interaction. Indeed, what becomes apparent in Žižek's approach is how human interaction relies upon an 'ambiguously imprecise domain' of what constitutes politeness (2015: 60). It is this ambiguity which is ignored in accounts of political correctness and which penalises and regulates intersubjective behaviour.

Therefore, by way of concentrating our critique of political correctness under the abstract neutrality that liberal multiculturalism prescribes, we can draw attention to the following characteristics: 1) a sense of guilt; 2) a latent cultural arrogance; 3) a denial of the other's agency; 4) a 'management' of the other; and 5) a presupposing of harassment.

1) A sense of guilt

While examples of political correctness can lead to the reassertion of a white, male, heterosexual identity, it is also the case that such assertions can result in feelings of 'white guilt'. As previously noted, this criticism is not intended to resolve this issue by arguing for the reaffirmation of such identities, nor does it suggest that any failure to assert this identity does not already speak to its hegemonic position (the need not to mention it). Instead, it is *this* hegemonic identity ('white/male/hetero') which is maintained in a sense of neutrality that, despite professing disgust at the intolerance of others, ensures that such neutrality is masked by examples of 'white guilt' that support such neutrality. Moreover, such guilt incurs a form of indulgence, whereby the politically correct subject can profess their cultural sensitivity, while not actually meeting the demands of engaging with cultural diversity. As Žižek notes:

> The problem with the self-denial of white identity is not that it goes too far but that it does not go far enough: while its enunciated content seems radical, its position of enunciation remains that of a privileged universality. So, yes, they declare themselves to be 'nothing,' but this very renunciation to a (particular) something is sustained by the surplus-enjoyment of their moral superiority.
>
> *(2019b)*

2) A latent cultural arrogance

Attempts to renunciate one's Eurocentric culture, masked in examples of political correctness, invariably promote a cultural arrogance that paradoxically works to maintain certain 'illiberal' practices (such as genital mutilation, polygamy and the wearing of religious attire). That is, while the advocation of a politically correct stance towards promoting various cultural idiosyncrasies can work to position the 'multicultural subject' as distinct to the less open, more xenophobic, 'lower' working class, at the same time, it is through a desire to promote the alterity and exoticness of the other's culture that liberalism's illiberal contradictions can be observed. These tensions can be identified in Kymlicka's (1996) desire to locate cultural diversity within the confines of a Western-European liberal paradigm. Here, 'the imposition of Western values as universal human rights, and the respect for different cultures independently of the horrors that can be part of these cultures', can work to:

> cove[r] up the antagonisms within each of these particular ways of life, justifying acts of brutality, sexism and racism as expressions of a particular culture that we have no right to judge by foreign 'Western values'.
>
> *(Žižek, 2017: 66)*

3) A denial of the other's agency

The third critique of political correctness is its patronising ability to romanticise the other, a feature that was clearly expressed during the 2015 refugee crisis. While Western-liberal celebrities sought to encourage residents of the UK to offer their spare rooms to refugees (Laville, 2015), such gestures masked a form of ideological interpellation that effectively de-humanised the other. Whereas these calls drew attention away from the underlying cause of the crisis (EU military interventions in Libya), they also inhibited any real form of criticism, instead portraying the refugees as helpless, dehumanised individuals, devoid of any personal agency.

4) A 'management' of the other

In its efforts to curtail the possibility of harassment and to promote tolerance, examples of political correctness permit greater forms of regulated control, which inevitably seek to manage social interactions by ensuring that those 'private' differences, which constitute the other, do not impact upon the public sphere. This is perhaps best reflected in large corporations whose workplaces are frequently subject to 'diversity training' and tolerance initiatives. Here, 'Modes of normative control can be seen as extending to notions of appropriate organizational behaviour and civility and judgements pertaining to these matters have come to incorporate behaviours labelled as harassment' (Westwood and Johnston, 2011: 789). Delineating such behaviours has resulted in the desire to manage and police those 'unspoken regulations' and forms of 'tact' that inevitably frame how we relate and behave with the other (Žižek, 2015: 61). However, in the wake of recent 'Hollywood scandals' surrounding Harvey Weinstein and the efforts of the #MeToo movement, there is the potential that such movements may indoctrinate new forms of 'violent' behaviour. Notably, 'In downplaying the complexity of sexual interactions, it not only blurs the line between lewd misconduct and criminal violence *but also masks invisible forms of extreme psychological violence as politeness and respect*' (Žižek, 2018: 151 [italics added]).

5) A presupposing of harassment

By modulating social interactions, it becomes apparent that examples of political correctness are marked by a level of presupposition. Here, the act of coordinating and managing certain forms of behaviour regarding how one should and should not behave is to presume the advent of harassment, before any harassment has actually taken place. Indeed, such forms of regulation bear a retroactive significance which, in a process akin to that of the 'precogs' (mutants who are able to foresee crime before it occurs) in Philip K. Dick's *Minority Report* (2002), seeks to catch politically incorrect behaviour before such behaviour has even occurred. As a result, one is left in a constant 'state of emergency' where the threat of harassment remains virtual and non-actualised. This is not to suggest that one deliberately ignores examples of harassment, but that the *threat* of harassment can lead to pre-emptive forms of regulation. This is perhaps best reflected in examples of seduction:

> there is no seduction which cannot at some point be construed as intrusion or harassment because there will always be a point when one has to expose oneself and 'make a pass'. But, of course, seduction doesn't involve incorrect harassment throughout. When you make a pass, you expose yourself to the Other (the potential partner), and her[/his] reaction will determine whether what you just did was harassment or a successful act of seduction.
>
> *(Žižek, 1999)*

While this, and the above criticisms, point to the paradoxes inherent within political correctness, we can see how such presupposed regulations serve to inhibit and limit human interaction.

Liberal multiculturalism and political correctness: Promoting race, ignoring racism

In the case of 'race' and racism, we can begin to see how examples of political correctness, often reflected in claims of 'colour-blindness', work to mask examples of racism and inequality. What these claims ignore is how:

> Race is built with the bodies of myths as well as myths about bodies, and it is constituted as a reality that cannot be erased by fiat. That is why we see and recognize racial identities and accompany them with statements and narratives, and why the notion that we can be 'color blind' is so problematic.
>
> *(Mitchell, 2012: 20–21)*

By attempting to achieve and promote toleration, examples of political correctness can repress 'racism' and eroticise 'race' (Žižek, 1998). Here, politically correct narratives rely upon implicit counter-narratives, which serve to maintain undisclosed and openly ignored forms of racism, despite their appeals to the contrary (Lentin and Titley, 2011; Titley and Lentin, 2011; Žižek, 1997, 1998). Accordingly, while political correctness aims to achieve a sense of 'correctness' by 'eliminat[ing] a genuine political space of disagreement' (Swyngedouw, 2015:

138), equally, 'the notion that western societies are post-race, whether this comes from a right-wing or a liberal perspective, is in fact a denial of the experience of the lived experience of racism' (Lentin, 2014: 1280). These 'post-race' assertions are frequently articulated in examples that seek to divert attention away from the significance of race as a political factor towards a refracted political space where the centrality of race is divested across a number of other cultural formations.

Certainly, this is not meant to reintroduce the importance of 'experience' as a reified form of exposing racial differences, but rather draw attention to how discussions on 'race', particularly in the West, are often framed as 'non-racist' discussions. Here, Lentin and Titley (2011) note how phrases such as 'playing the race card' work to deprive 'race' as a significant political attribute, providing a form of obfuscation that depoliticises accounts of racialisation.

To this extent, scholarly work has frequently highlighted the ways in which forms of 'neo-racism' work to both assert and deny racist effects through a focus on culture as opposed to biology (Balibar and Wallerstein, 1991). Gilroy warns: 'The habitual resort to culture as unbridgeable division needs to be interpreted with care', so that whereas 'The logics of nature and culture have converged, … it is above all the power of race that ensures they speak in the same deterministic tongue' (2004: 6). Accordingly, by referring to culture instead of race, 'racial' discussions are predicated on the assertion that one 'not be reminded of racism' (Lentin, 2018: 411).

Therefore, if one is to remain critical of the effects of political correctness as a form of critique that seeks 'To dispute racial common sense' (Gilroy, 2004: 10), then it is important that such critiques do not fall foul of the post-racism/not-racist allusion that 'race', as a social category, no longer holds prevalence in contemporary societies (Lentin, 2018). In fact, as evidenced in Žižek's (2008a) work on ideology, one way that ideology remains pertinent is via the paradoxical assertion that we are living in a post-ideological era. Rather, Žižek (2008a) contends that, in accordance with popular culture, post-ideological assertions derive their power by appearing as non-coercive. Post-race debates serve a similar function by denouncing the significance or ideological importance of race, while obfuscating underlying forms of racism.[3] As a result, Žižek contends that:

> Today's racism is strictly (post)modern; it is a reaction to the 'disenchantment' inflicted by the new phase of global capitalism. One of the commonplaces of the contemporary 'post-ideological' attitude is that today, we have more or less outgrown divisive political fictions (of class struggle, etc.) and reached political maturity, which enables us to focus on real problems (ecology, economic growth …) relieved of their ideological ballast – however, it is as if today, when the dominant attitude defined the terrain of the struggle as that of the Real ('real problems' versus 'ideological chimeras'), the very foreclosed political, as it were, *returns in the Real* – in the guise of racism, which grounds political differences in the (biological or social) Real of the race.
>
> *(2008b: 211)*

Žižek's reference to the 'Real of the race' will be returned to in Chapter Three, but for now, we can begin to see how attempts to assert a 'post-racial' society echo the postmodern, liberal multicultural transformation of political struggles into cultural (racial) struggles. Under such circumstances, it is possible to see how racism, instead of being conceived as 'an *effect* of exploitation', is instead portrayed through the assumption that racism is 'an *effect* of our intolerance of other cultures' (Žižek cited in Taylor, 2009: 157 [italics added]). In doing so, racism becomes obfuscated and perceived as an individual or group's inability to display the colour-blind, moral superiority of the liberal subject. Again, it is through such forms of 'colour-blindness' that a privileged universal position is maintained (McGowan, 2018), so that 'at the core of this disavowal of race, whiteness operates as the universal, unmarked signifier through its disavowal of embodiment itself' (Winnubst, 2004: 41). In such instances, it is our relation to race which becomes the focus of toleration, leaving the effects of racism largely unchallenged.

Nonetheless, despite these criticisms it is pertinent that one does not simply seek to undermine examples of political correctness by way of any reactionary critique. In part, such criticisms can serve to maintain the hegemonic status of political correctness, via examples of cynicism, which, as the above discussion on comedy has highlighted, are incorporated as part of the ideological field. Such critical deflection remains fundamental to the liberal order (Manoharan, 2019). What is important here is that rather than directly opposing these discourses, one can instead draw attention to the inherent *excesses* of the system itself and, as a consequence, can pose opportunities for subversive resistance. It is this type of subversion which can help to draw attention to the inherent failures that characterise universal notions, such as those seen in the above discussions on liberal multiculturalism and political correctness. Integral to this failure is the very way in which these universal notions rely upon forms of 'self-exclusion'. Here, McGowan elaborates on how:

> Society's self-exclusion ensures that no one really belongs, … in order to obscure this universal failure of belonging, societies have recourse to racism, xenophobia, and other form of exclusion. They exclude in order to hide the fact that everyone is always already excluded. Certain groups must embody non-belonging so that others can believe that they belong.
>
> *(2016: 613)*

Identifying those 'exceptions' that underscore the universal form is what proves integral to Žižek's (2008a) critique of ideology, and which can expose those 'points of exception' that highlight the fissures and falseness of the universal and its inherent negation.

In part, we see this same process followed in Žižek's (2012) subversive appropriation of certain terms that are usually associated with the political right. Notably, his use of the term *Leitkultur* (which translates to dominant culture) has also been adopted by the German right as a call to oppose further immigration (Sayeau,

2013). Instead, Žižek (2012) uses the term not to denounce cultural difference, but to argue that our own *Leitkultur* should be a common struggle in cultural difference. In this sense, Žižek is not deferring to the racist rhetoric of the political right, nor is he succumbing to the moral righteousness of the liberal left, but rather, he refocuses our attention on the failed efforts of an abstract, liberal multiculturalism and how, despite its efforts, racism continues to thrive.

In the case of comedy, these discussions take on an added significance. For Pérez:

> If color-blind racism tends to be concealed, racism in comedy is hidden in plain sight. The strategies that comics learn suggest another possible answer to the question of how racism is communicated in a society that disavows racist speech: racism is expressed in public and overtly, but its offensiveness is deflected, in part, by the use of strategies that make the performers seem 'not racist,' even as they say racist things.
>
> *(2013: 479)*

Therefore, while not denying the racist potential of certain comic strategies, both intentional and unintentional, what remains pertinent in Perez's account is the extent to which 'racism in comedy is hidden in plain sight'. Such 'hiding' does not necessarily have to follow a process of deflection, but rather can highlight how such deflection has become a formative part of the comic sequence – that is, its own inherent limitation, negation and exception. To this end, it is in the comic performance that a unique strategy in unveiling and re-approaching racism can be formed. As the following chapter will consider, it is in this way that we can begin to identify comedy's subversive potential.

Notes

1 The York Mystery Plays (York Corpus Christi Plays) were a series of plays celebrating the Festival of Corpus Christi that were performed by York's Craft Guilds. Drawing upon the Old and New Testaments, the plays were suppressed in the mid-sixteenth century.

2 This is perhaps best reflected in the case of art (Flisfeder, 2017, 2019; Paglia, 2015). Here, Paglia has noted that 'The end result of four decades of postmodernism permeating the art world is that there is very little interesting or important work being done right now in the fine arts. Irony was a bold and creative posture when Duchamp did it, but it is now an utterly banal, exhausted, and tedious strategy. Young artists have been taught to be "cool" and "hip" and thus painfully self-conscious. They are not encouraged to be enthusiastic, emotional, and visionary. They have been cut off from artistic tradition by the crippled skepticism about history that they have been taught by ignorant and solipsistic postmodernists. In short, the art world will never revive until postmodernism fades away. Postmodernism is a plague upon the mind and the heart' (2015).

3 This is echoed by Gilroy who notes that 'anyone who makes a fuss about racism, past or present' can be subject to the assertion that they are 'getting things out of proportion, engaging in witch-hunts, practicing empty moralism, or indulging in the immature outlooks of "loony leftism" and, above all, "political correctness"' (2004: 159).

References

Adorno, T. W. 2003. *The Culture Industry: Selected Essays on Mass Culture*. London: Routledge.

Adorno, T. W. and Horkheimer, M. 1997. *Dialectic of Enlightenment*. London: Verso.

Agger, B. 1994. Derrida for sociology? A comment on Fuchs and Ward. *American Sociological Review*, 59 (4), 501–505.

Avengers: Endgame. 2019. Film. Walt Disney Studios Motion Pictures.

Baldwin, A. 2009. The white geography of Lawren Stewart Harris: Whiteness and the performative coupling of wilderness and multiculturalism in Canada. *Environment and Planning A*, 41, 529–544.

Balibar, E. and Wallerstein, I. 1991. *Race, Nation, Class: Ambiguous Identities*. London: Verso.

Bebber, B. 2014. *Till Death Us Do Part*: Political satire and social realism in the 1960s and 1970s. *Historical Journal of Film, Radio and Television*, 34 (2), 253–274.

Berger, P. L. 2014. *Redeeming Laughter: The Comic Dimension of Human Experience*, 2nd edn. Berlin, Germany: De Gruyter.

Bogel, F. V. 2001. *The Difference Satire Makes: Rhetoric and Reading From Jonson to Byron*. Ithaca, NY: Cornell University Press.

Boulden, J. and Kymlicka, W. 2015. Introduction. In: J. Boulden and W. Kymlicka, eds. *International Approaches to Governing Diversity*. Oxford: Oxford University Press, 1–24.

Brass Eye. 1997–2001. TV Series. Channel 4.

Brassett, J. 2009. British irony, global justice: A pragmatic reading of Chris Brown, Banksy and Ricky Gervais. *Review of International Studies*, 35, 219–245.

Brassett, J. 2015. British comedy, global resistance: Russell Brand, Charlie Brooker and Stewart Lee. *European Journal of International Relations*, 22 (1), 168–191.

Brassett, J. and Sutton, A. 2017. British satire, everyday politics: Chris Morris, Armando Iannucci and Charlie Brooker. *British Journal of Politics and International Relations*, 19 (2), 245–262.

Bunting, M. 2011. The problem with tolerance [online]. *The Guardian*. Available from: www.theguardian.com/commentisfree/belief/2011/sep/05/tolerance-frank-furedi [Accessed 10 January 2019].

Chomsky, N. and Foucault, M. 2006. *The Chomsky-Foucault Debate: On Human Nature*. New York, NY: The New Press.

Colletta, L. 2009. Political satire and postmodern irony in the age of Stephen Colbert and Jon Stewart. *The Journal of Popular Culture*, 42 (5), 856–874.

Contu, A. 2008. Decaf resistance: On misbehavior, cynicism, and desire in liberal workplaces. *Management Communication Quarterly*, 21 (3), 364–379.

Dagnes, A. 2012. *A Conservative Walks into a Bar: The Politics of Political Humor*. New York, NY: Palgrave Macmillan.

Das, R. and Graefer, A. 2017. *Provocative Screens: Offended Audiences in Britain and Germany*. Gewerbestrasse, Switzerland: Palgrave Macmillan.

Davis, M. 1993. *What's So Funny?: The Comic Conception of Culture and Society*. Chicago, IL: University of Chicago Press.

Dean, J. 2006. *Žižek's Politics*. New York, NY: Routledge.

Derrida, J. 1997. *Of Grammatology*. Baltimore, MD: The John Hopkins University Press.

Detweiler, E. 2012. 'I was just doing a little joke there': Irony and the paradoxes of the sitcom in *The Office*. *The Journal of Popular Culture*, 45 (4), 727–748.

Dick, P. K. 2002. *Minority Report*. London: Gollancz.

Dunant, S. 1994. Introduction: What's in a word? In: S. Dunant, ed. *The War of the Words: The Political Correctness Debate*. London: Virago Press, vii–xv.

Eagleton, T. 2003. *After Theory*. London: Allen Lane.

Family Guy. 1999–present. TV Series. Fox.

Fawlty Towers. 1975–1979. TV Series. BBC Two.

Fisher, M. 2009. *Capitalism Realism: Is There No Alternative?* Ropley: O Books.

Flisfeder, M. 2017. *Postmodern Theory and Blade Runner*. New York, NY: Bloomsbury.

Flisfeder, M. 2019. Postmodern Marxism today: Jameson, Žižek, and the demise of symbolic efficiency. *The International Journal of Žižek Studies*, 13 (1), 23–56.

Foucault, M. 2002. *The Order of Things: An Archaeology of the Human Sciences*. London: Routledge.

Friedman, S. 2014. *Comedy and Distinction: The Cultural Currency of a 'Good' Sense of Humour*. Abingdon: Routledge.

Fukuyama, F. 2006. *End of History and the Last Man*. New York, NY: Free Press.

Gandesha, S. 2018. Not only the difference between identities but the differences within them [online]. openDemocracy. Available from: www.opendemocracy.net/en/not-only-difference-between-identities-but-differences-within-them/ [Accessed 20 November 2018].

Gilroy, P. 2004. *After Empire: Melancholia or Convivial Culture?* Abingdon: Routledge.

Habermas, J. 1981. New social movements. *Telos: Critical Theory of the Contemporary*, 49, 33–37.

Hall, S. 1994. Some 'politically incorrect' pathways through PC. In: S. Dunant, ed. *The War of the Words: The Political Correctness Debate*. London: Virago Press, 164–184.

Hancock. 1961. TV Series. BBC.

Hancock's Half Hour. 1954–1960. TV Series. BBC.

Hewison, R. 2014. *Cultural Capital: The Rise and Fall of Creative Britain*. London: Verso.

Hughey, M. W. and Muradi, S. 2009. Laughing matters: Economies of hyper-irony and manic-satire in South Park & Family Guy. *Humanity & Society*, 33, 206–237.

Hunt, L. 2013. *Cult British TV Comedy: From Reeves and Mortimer to Psychoville*. Manchester: Manchester University Press.

Jameson, F. 1991. *Postmodernism, or, The Cultural Logic of Late Capitalism*. Durham, NC: Duke University Press.

Jameson, F. 1996. Five theses on actually existing Marxism. *Monthly Review*, 47, 1–10.

Jameson, F. 2009. *The Cultural Turn: Selected Writings on the Postmodern, 1983–1998*. London: Verso.

Jansen, D. A. 2003. 'Time to lose faith in humanity': 'The Simpsons', South Park', and the satiric tradition. *Studies in Popular Culture*, 26 (1), 27–36.

Kamm, J. and Neumann, B. 2016. Introduction: The aesthetics and politics of British TV comedy. In: J. Kamm and B. Neumann, eds. *British TV Comedies: Cultural Concepts, Contexts and Controversies*. Basingstoke: Palgrave Macmillan, 1–22.

Knowing Me, Knowing You with Alan Partridge. 1994. TV Series. BBC Two.

Kymlicka, W. 1996. *Multicultural Citizenship: A Liberal Theory of Minority Rights*. Oxford: Clarendon Press.

Kymlicka, W. 2017. Liberal multiculturalism as a political theory of state-minority relations. *Political Theory*, 46 (1), 81–91.

Laclau, E. and Mouffe, C. 1985. *Hegemony and Socialist Strategy: Towards a Radical Democratic Politics*. London: Verso.

Laville, S. 2015. Bob Geldof offers to house four refugee families [online]. *The Guardian*. Available from: www.theguardian.com/uk-news/2015/sep/04/bob-geldof-jk-rowling-mary-portas-stan-collymore-refugees-welcome [Accessed 3 December 2018].

Lee, S. 2010. *How I Escaped My Certain Fate: The Life and Deaths of a Stand-Up Comedian*. London: Faber and Faber.

Lentin, A. 2014. Post-race, post politics: The paradoxical rise of culture after multiculturalism. *Ethnic and Racial Studies*, 37 (8), 1268–1285.

Lentin, A. 2018. Beyond denial: 'Not racism' as racist violence. *Continuum*, 32 (4), 400–414.
Lentin, A. and Titley, G. 2011. *The Crisis of Multiculturalism: Racism in a Neoliberal Age*. London: Zed Books.
Lockyer, S. and Pickering, M. 2008. You must be joking: The sociological critique of humour and comic media. *Sociology Compass*, 2/3, 808–820.
Lyotard, J.-F. 1984. *The Postmodern Condition*. Minneapolis, MN: University of Minnesota Press.
Maciel, R. 2014. The future of liberal multiculturalism. *Political Studies Review*, 12, 383–394.
Malik, K. 2010. Multiculturalism undermines diversity [online]. *The Guardian*. Available from: www.theguardian.com/commentisfree/2010/mar/17/multiculturalism-diversity-political-policy [Accessed 12 January 2019].
Manoharan, K. 2019. Avengers and the endgame of liberalism [online]. *The Philosophical Salon*. Available from: https://thephilosophicalsalon.com/avengers-and-the-endgame-of-liberalism/ [Accessed 7 May 2019].
McGowan, T. 2016. The location of silent comedy: Charlie Chaplin's outsider and Buster Keaton's insider. *Quarterly Review of Film and Video*, 33 (7), 602–619.
McGowan, T. 2018. The absent universal: From the Master Signifier to the missing signifier. *Problemi International*, 2 (2), 195–214.
McHoul, A. and Grace, W. 2015. *A Foucault Primer: Discourse, Power and the Subject*. London: Routledge.
McMillan, C. 2013. *Žižek and Communist Strategy: On the Disavowed Foundations of Global Capitalism*. Edinburgh: Edinburgh University Press.
Men Behaving Badly. 1992–2014. TV Series. ITV; BBC One; Channel 4.
Mitchell, W. J. T. 2012. *Seeing Through Race*. Cambridge, MA: Harvard University Press.
Monkey Dust. 2003–2005. TV Series. BBC Three.
Norris, V. 2014. *British Television Animation, 1997–2010: Drawing Comic Tradition*. Basingstoke: Palgrave Macmillan.
Olsen, L. 1990. *Circus of the Mind in Motion*. Detroit, MI: Wayne State University Press.
Paglia, C. 2015. Camille Paglia: 'Postmodernism is a plague upon the mind and the heart' [online]. *Fausto Mag*. Available from: https://faustomag.com/camille-paglia-postmodernism-is-a-plague-upon-the-mind-and-the-heart/ [Accessed 10 January 2019].
Penhallurick, R. 2010. *Studying the English Language*. Basingstoke: Palgrave Macmillan.
Pérez, R. 2013. Learning to make racism funny in the 'color-blind' era: Stand-up comedy students, performance strategies, and the (re)production of racist jokes in public. *Discourse & Society*, 24 (4), 478–503.
Pitcher, B. 2009. *The Politics of Multiculturalism: Race and Racism in Contemporary Britain*. Basingstoke: Palgrave Macmillan.
Quirk, S. 2018. *The Politics of British Stand-Up Comedy: The New Alternative*. Gewerbestrasse, Switzerland: Palgrave Macmillan.
Radcliffe, T. 2012. Tolerance is not enough to learn the art of living with others [online]. *The Guardian*. Available from: www.theguardian.com/profile/timothy-radcliffe [Accessed 16 February 2019].
Salter, L. 2016. Populism as a fantasmatic rupture in the post-political order: Integrating Laclau with Glynos and Stavrakakis, Kōtuitui. *New Zealand Journal of Social Sciences Online*, 11 (2), 116–132.
Sayeau, M. 2013. Enjoy his symptoms? [online]. *The White Review*. Available from: www.thewhitereview.org/feature/enjoy-his-symptoms/ [Accessed 3 March 2019].
Seinfeld. 1989–1998. TV Series. NBC.
Shooting Stars. 1993–2011. TV Series. BBC Two; BBC Choice.
South Park. 1997–present. TV Series. Comedy Central.

Spitting Image. 1984–1996. TV Series. ITV.
Stourton, E. 2008. *It's a PC World*. London: Hodder & Stoughton.
Swyngedouw, E. 2015. Depoliticized environments and the promises of the Anthropocene. In: R. L. Bryant, ed. *The International Handbook of Political Ecology*. Cheltenham: Edward Elgar Publishing, 131–148.
Szilagyi, A. 2017. A linguist explains how the far-right hijacked political correctness [online]. *Quartz*. Available from: https://qz.com/886552/a-linguist-explains-how-the-far-right-hijacked-political-correctness [Accessed 31 May 2019].
Taylor, A. 2009. *Examined Life: Excursions with Contemporary Thinkers*. New York, NY: The New York Press.
Thakkar, J. 2019. Putting the political back in politically correct [online]. *The Chronical of Higher Education*. Available from: www.chronicle.com/article/Putting-the-Political-Back-in/246476 [Accessed 2 March 2020].
The Comic Strip Presents...1982–2016. TV Series. Channel 4; BBC Two.
The Simpsons. 1989–present. TV Series. Fox.
The Thick of It. 2005–2012. TV Series. BBC Four; BBC Two.
The Young Ones. 1982–1984. TV Series. BBC Two.
Till Death Us Do Part. 1965. TV Series. BBC One.
Titley, G. and Lentin, A. 2011. The crises of multiculturalism [online]. *openDemocracy*. Available from: www.opendemocracy.net/en/opendemocracyuk/crises-of-multiculturalism/ [Accessed 10 March 2019].
Van Oenen, G. 2010. Three cultural turns: How multiculturalism, interactivity and interpassivity affect citizenship. *Citizenship Studies*, 14 (3), 293–306.
Vasantkumar, J. J. C. 1998. Postmodernism and jokes. In: A. A. Berger, ed. *The Postmodern Presence: Readings on Postmodernism in American Culture and Society*. London: Altamira Press, 212–238.
Vidal, J. 2012. Bill Gates backs climate scientists lobbying for large-scale geoengineering [online]. *The Guardian*. Available from: www.theguardian.com/environment/2012/feb/06/bill-gates-climate-scientists-geoengineering [Accessed 5 April 2019].
Ward, S. 2001. 'No nation could be broker': The satire boom and the demise of Britain's world role. In: S. Ward, ed. *British Culture and the End of Empire*. Manchester: Manchester University Press, 91–110.
Weaver, S. 2011. Liquid racism and the ambiguity of Ali G. *European Journal of Cultural Studies*, 14 (3), 249–264.
Westwood, R. and Johnston, A. 2011. Reclaiming authentic selves: Control, resistive humour and identity work in the office. *Organization*, 19 (6), 787–808.
Winnubst, S. 2004. Is the mirror racist? Interrogating the space of whiteness. *Philosophy & Social Criticism*, 30 (1), 25–50.
Žižek, S. 1997. Multiculturalism, or, the cultural logic of multinational capitalism. *New Left Review*, 1 (225), 28–51.
Žižek, S. 1998. *Tarrying with the Negative: Kant, Hegel, and the Critique of Ideology*. Durham, NC: Duke University Press.
Žižek, S. 1999. You may! [online]. *London Review of Books*. Available from: www.lrb.co.uk/v21/n06/slavoj-zizek/you-may [Accessed 10 January 2019].
Žižek, S. 2006a. Preface to the paperback edition: The big other between violence and civility. In: R. Butler and S. Stephens, eds. *Slavoj Zizek: The Universal Exception*. London: Continuum, vii–xxxii.
Žižek, S. 2006b. Why we all love to hate Haider. In: R. Butler and S. Stephens, eds. *Slavoj Zizek: The Universal Exception*. London: Continuum, 33–41.

Žižek, S. 2006c. A leftist plea for Eurocentricism. In: R. Butler and S. Stephens, eds. *Slavoj Zizek: The Universal Exception*. London: Continuum, 183–208.

Žižek, S. 2008a. *The Sublime Object of Ideology*. London: Verso.

Žižek, S. 2008b. *The Plague of Fantasies*. London: Verso.

Žižek, S. 2008c. The violence of the liberal utopia. *Distinktion: Scandinavian Journal of Social Theory*, 9 (2), 9–25.

Žižek, S. 2012. *The Year of Dreaming Dangerously*. London: Verso.

Žižek, S. 2015. *Absolute Recoil: Towards a New Foundation of Dialectical Materialism*. London: Verso.

Žižek, S. 2017. *In Defense of Lost Causes*. London: Verso.

Žižek, S. 2018. *Like a Thief in Broad Daylight: Power in the Era of Post-Humanity*. London: Allen Lane.

Žižek, S. 2019a. *The Relevance of the Communist Manifesto*. Cambridge: Polity.

Žižek, S. 2019b. They are both worse! [online]. *The Philosophical Salon*. Available from: https://thephilosophicalsalon.com/they-are-both-worse/ [Accessed 27 February 2019].

Žižek, S. and Daly, G. 2004. *Conversations with Žižek*. Cambridge: Polity Press.

Zupančič, A. 2003. *The Shortest Shadow: Nietzsche's Philosophy of the Two*. Cambridge, MA: MIT Press.

2

SUBVERSIVE COMEDY

Comedy's incongruity

Examples of comedy's ability to draw attention to what is incongruent, disparate and separated from the 'normal' has underscored scholarly work that has examined its theoretical significance and its subversive, even radical, potential (Giappone, 2018; McGowan, 2014, 2017; Zupančič, 2008). Here, McGowan highlights how comedy can often work to subversively 'disrup[t] the flow of everyday life' by 'call[ing] social authority into question' and by 'upset[ting] our usual way of thinking' – in fact, if it didn't 'it would fail to be funny' (2014: 201). Implicit in McGowan's (2014) account is the significance of an 'incongruity' within the comic experience. According to Berger, 'From its simplest to its most sophisticated expressions, the comic is experienced as incongruence' (2014: xiv). This incongruity is brought to bear in 'the professor lecturing on some profound topic while trying to hide his erection, [and] the politician whose fervent speech is interrupted by an unstoppable sneezing fit' (Berger, 2014: viii), each of which displays how it is the incongruity between these positions of authority and their various 'mishaps' which helps to induce a comic effect. In short, humour is caused by an incongruence between what *occurs* and what we *expect*.

Understanding the significance of comedy's incongruence has formed an important feature of a variety of studies which have examined the formal structure of comedy and humour (Critchley, 2002a; Freud, 2003; Heller, 2005, Zupančič, 2008). Indeed, drawing upon the work of Swabey (1961), Berger highlights 'that since about the eighteenth century … there have been different views as to how to define this incongruity …, and more importantly as to whether the incongruity is only perceived subjectively or has an objective referent' (2014: 32). Such thinking has aligned comedy's incongruence with wider discussions on both the purpose and function of philosophy (Nikulin, 2014), as well as the human condition (Berger, 2014; Critchley, 2002a; Heller, 2005; Zupančič, 2008). Subsequently, before delving into a more focused discussion on the significance of incongruity as it pertains to the work of Simon Critchley and Agnes Heller, it is important that we briefly acknowledge its relation to the work of both Immanuel Kant and Henri Bergson.

Kant and Bergson

It was in the work of Kant (2007) that comedy's incongruity was first considered. Specifically, Kant sought to trace how, during the telling of a joke, the listener is subject to an unreasonable suggestion that proves incongruous to their social setting or what is believed to be common sense. While this endows the joke with a critical incentive, by drawing attention to what is commonly believed to be convention, it is, more importantly, the expectation inherent to the joke's final resolution (its 'punchline') which results in laughter. As Heller notes, for Kant, 'laughter is an affect which occurs when a tense expectation suddenly empties itself into nothing' (Heller, 2005: 134). In doing so:

> The comedic situation sets up expectations which move in a destabilizing, even threatening direction relative to our mundane understandings, but then there is a resolution and we realize that there was *nothing* (threatening) there at all – it was just a joke.
>
> *(Westwood, 2004: 788–789)*

Accordingly, though detective novels dissolve the tension into 'something' (the final 'who done it'), in the case of comedy, its tension is dissolved into 'nothing', except laughter (Heller, 2005).

Continuing this line of inquiry, Henri Bergson (2008) considered how incongruity occurs when there is a displacement 'between mind and body, or between life and matter' (Berger, 2014: 29). Laughter results when an involuntary action occurs on behalf of a conscious individual. In this way, Bergson (2008) believed that laughter was a decidedly 'human phenomenon', with humans being the source of laughter (other 'animals' do not laugh) and with the act itself remaining a social activity specific to human beings. For Bergson (2008), it was this 'human source' which gives laughter and the comic mode its cause. Here, the displacement between 'life and matter', takes place when the 'human' begins to mimic, reflect or perform the mechanical. For example, when we consider *that* particular idiosyncrasy which constitutes a certain individual and mimic it, we get a mechanical reproduction which produces laughter. Equally, when we watch a comedic imitation of a well-known individual, or when a particular subject follows a social convention to the letter (like a machine), we get life reduced to the mechanical and it is this which subjects the human to the comic, presenting the subject as a 'thing' (Bergson, 2008). In the latter, we can think of Charlie Chaplin in *Modern Times* (1936) excessively reproducing the frenetic movement of the machine, or a more recent example from the television series *Little Britain* (2003–2006), where David Walliams's character mechanically replies: 'Computer says, no'. In these instances, it is the displacement of life and matter, towards the material thing, which produces the comic.

What remains central to both Kant and Bergson's incongruity, however, is the effect of the joke and its relation to the subject. According to Heller, 'as far as the technique and strategy of the body of the joke is concerned, incongruity theories best describe how jokes are constituted and how they work to take effect' (2005: 155). It is this contradictory aspect of the joke's narrative which underscores Kant's own solution that such contradiction, and its tense expectation, is what dissolves into nothing. This 'nothing' is what accompanies the experience of hearing a joke and its punchline. For Moreall, it is this expectation – or shock – which is indicative of the fact that 'We live in an orderly world where we have come to expect certain patterns', and, as a consequence, 'When we experience something that doesn't fit these patterns, that violates our expectations, we laugh' (Morreall, 1982: 244–245).

In what follows, further attention will be paid to examining the effects of comedy's incongruity in relation to the work of Simon Critchley and Agnes Heller. Clearly, by drawing upon these two thinkers I am not intending to provide an expansive list of philosophy's contributions to comedy and humour.[1] Instead, these two authors have been drawn upon due to the various ways in which their work builds upon the study of comedy (notably, Freud) as well as the combined importance that each can provide when examining comedy's 'subversive potential'. Moreover, in light of the previous chapter's discussion, the following question will be proposed: if comedy and humour can be used by those in power in order to maintain their authority, that is, if it is asserted that hegemonic ideologies are adept at including their own self-critique as part of their ideological message (Žižek, 2008a), then in what ways can comedy maintain a subversive edge? The following sections will offer some initial solutions to this question.

Simon Critchley

According to Critchley, comedy provides an anarchic function by incongruously interrupting what is 'normal' and everyday. Indeed: 'A true joke, ... suddenly and explosively lets us see the familiar defamiliarized, the ordinary made extraordinary and the real rendered surreal' (Critchley, 2002a: 10). It is in this way that comedy, humour and the delivering of 'a true joke' can help separate oneself from the immediacy of the social environment, forging an 'incongruity between what we expect to be the case and what actually takes place in the joke' (Critchley, 2002a: 3). Rather positively, Critchley (2002a) asserts that this incongruity can help provide a space for change, by drawing attention to those elements that were not expected or previously included. Such subversion emanates from the 'distance' which is obtained via comedy's ability to bring into focus a sharp distinction between the self (or audience) and our everyday, routine experiences. That is, 'humour is produced by a disjunction between the way things are and the way they are represented in the joke' (Critchley, 2002a: 1).

For Critchley, this 'disjunction' bears a phenomenological significance, with the effects of humour bringing us back to earth through a form of estrangement: 'It is a practice that gives us an alien perspective on our practices. It lets us view the world as if we had just landed from another planet' (2002a: 66). Such estrangement is a decidedly subversive move in that while one is left separated – and, therefore, distanced – from their surroundings, it is through humour's disjunctive form that one is shocked into learning something 'new' about themselves and their shared communities. As a result, the comedian bears a semblance with the philosopher – indeed, 'a family resemblance' whereby both professions 'as[k] us to look at the world askance, to imagine a topsy-turvy universe where horses and dogs talk and where lifeless objects become miraculously animated' (Critchley, 2002b: 103).

There is much that can be taken from Critchley's analysis, with such '*dissensus communis*' or 'uncommon sense' providing a 'momentary' jolt for the subject and defamiliarising what is often taken for granted (Critchley, 2002b: 111). Ethically and politically, Critchley argues that such experiences can prove conductive for achieving a radical non-self-coincidence of the ego; an ego that 'does not only become an object, [… but] becomes what we might call an *abject object*' (Critchley, 2002a: 97). While Critchley assumes that there is a 'self' to begin with, it is in acknowledging the self/ego as an abject object that a more modest and limited conception of the human condition can be achieved through the laughter that comedy induces.

However, what remains pertinent to Critchley's approach to comedy is how the effects of humour can leave the subject estranged from their immediate social and cultural context. In other words, through a sense of distance, comedy is able to separate the subject from what they consider to be 'normal' and 'taken-for-granted' and, in doing so, can reveal moments of subversion and political resistance. However, the problem with such distance is that it relies upon a form of fantasy from which the subject is suddenly separated and removed from the actions around them. The effect of this subversion is that it encourages a form of cynical detachment – or distance – from the social setting. This is acknowledged by Critchley (2002a) when he recounts a group of employees, whom he observes participating in an organisational team bonding exercise. In speaking with the employees, Critchley (2002a) notes that, whereas the employees were aware of the ridiculous activities that they were required to partake in, they nevertheless sought moments of comedy as a way of cynically subverting the various activities which had been organised. Here, Critchley notes how 'such fun is always capable of being ridiculed by informal, unofficial relations amongst employees, by backchat and salacious gossip' (2002a: 14), and it is in this way that the employees were able to achieve a cynical distance.

Critchley's empowered sense of cynicism is one that is undermined when considered in accordance with Žižek's (2008a) critique of ideology. As noted in Chapter One, hegemonic ideologies maintain their authority via the precondition that one can achieve a cynical distance and ironic detachment from ideology (Žižek, 2008a). That is, it is through encouraging its own self-critique that ideology continues to maintain a significance in our – supposedly – post-ideological age.

Moreover, we can see how, in the above example, such temporary cynical resistance bears a notable resemblance to Bakhtin's (1984) carnivalesque.[2]

In his study of Rabelais, 'a time of comedy in which festival and laughter displace everyday life' (McGowan, 2014: 202), Bakhtin (1984) examines how it is the carnivalesque which displays comedy's utopian potential, offering the possibility for social hierarchies, and those in positions of authority, to be questioned and their stations subverted. Here, the carnival could 'unsettle power structures, ... making them visible in the first place and opening them up for further negotiation' (Kamm and Neumann, 2016: 6–7). However, the suspension of this social hierarchy and the inversion of social roles were only temporarily performed (McGowan, 2014), with the carnival failing to offer any sustained internal challenge to this authority (Heller, 2005). As a result, the open acknowledgment of authority's self-ridicule relied upon a cynical distance that separated those in power from their own self-ridiculousness.

Therefore, an underlying concern in Critchley's (2002a) (and Bakhtin's) approach is the extent to which his view of comedy echoes this cynical detachment/distance, which fails to elicit an internal challenge to those in authority. Today, this can be identified in the array of late-night television hosts, such as John Oliver, who, in their frequent mocking of the US President Donald Trump, merely invoke a cynical distance that ensures that such authority remains unchallenged ('dusting the balls of power, rather than castrating them' (Žižek, 2018)). Of greater concern is that these comedians encourage a sense of liberal arrogance, with many of their associated Trump jokes inadvertently mocking the working-class communities who voted for him.

Furthermore, central to Critchley's (2002a) approach is the slight revision that he confers on Freud's notion of the 'superego'. Indeed, if, under Freud, the superego refers to the moral codes and ethical impulses that manage the ego, then:

> in humour, we see the profile of 'super-ego II', a super-ego which does not lacerate the ego, but speaks to it words of consolation. This is a positive super-ego that liberates and elevates by allowing the ego to find itself ridiculous. If 'super-ego I' is the prohibiting parent, scolding the child, then 'super-ego II' is the child that has become the parent: wiser and wittier, if slightly wizened.
>
> *(Critchley, 2002a: 103)*

This is continued when, in accordance with his work on ethics and the subject, Critchley (2012) elaborates an understanding of the superego ('super-ego II') as a benevolent force which helps to inversely constitute the subject in its accepted failure. In other words, for Critchley, 'the notion of the subject as constituted by its recognition in an unconditional ethical Call engendered by the experience of injustice and wrongs' (Žižek, 2017: 340) is, in part, achieved through comedy's ability to modestly ground the subject with the realisation of their own imperfections. Consequently, 'Instead of installing anguish and despair, this superego enables us to laugh at our limitations, failures, and false pretensions' (Žižek, 2017: 341).

Yet, such benevolent power which Critchley bestows upon the superego ('super-ego II'), fails to account for those examples where humour can be both 'brutal' and 'sadistic' (Žižek, 2017). Žižek (2017) highlights how the superego is not a benevolent, ethical force, but one that often encourages a sense of irrational guilt amongst 'survivors', such as Jewish survivors of the holocaust. Here, the superego maintains a malignant form that negatively torments the subject. Accordingly:

> When Critchley emphasizes how the subject always fails with regard to the Call of the ethical Thing, he seems to fully endorse this dimension, this failure as constitutive of subjectivity. There is, however, a crucial accent to be added here: it is totally wrong to directly identify this failure of interpellation – the fact that the subject never rises to the level of its responsibility towards the Call of the Good – with the subject.
>
> *(Žižek, 2017: 344)*

In other words, Critchley's account works to locate the subject as that which emerges from 'its' inability to meet the superego's ethical demands (Žižek, 2017). Instead, it is the subject's *inability* to settle with the *excess* of being which points towards a far more positive appraisal of the subject, as Wood asserts: '[Žižek's] key insight … is that because the subject … is split, it always *remains inherently opposed* to the process of ideological subjectivization' (2012: 26 [italics in original]). As a consequence, it is this 'split' which continually gnaws away at the interpellation of the subject: 'the infinite force of negativity called by Freud the "death drive"' (Žižek, 2017: 344). The significance of this Žižekian subject will be returned to below; for now, however, we will continue this discussion of the subject in the work of Heller.

Agnes Heller

In Heller's (2005) work on comedy, incongruity becomes apparent when we consider that the effects of comedy occur 'when the times are out of joint' (Murphy, 2006: 68), and when something that was once considered natural now seems unnatural. There is, in this instance, an overlap with Critchley's perspective on how the self proves contradictory to the injunctions of the superego. Heller elaborates upon this contradiction in relation to Kant's understanding of the joke:

> Human existence itself is the essential incongruence. That is, incongruence is the essence of human existence. We are born in order to die. Everything we live for or against, … our cognitions and emotions, the very fact that we are always involved in something, is incongruent with nothing. And death (not dying, which is something) is nothing. Kant described the joke as a play of thoughts that suddenly ends in nothingness. Human life is like a joke. It is like

> a novel or a drama which ends in nothingness; it is a comic novel or drama: the human comedy.
>
> *(2005: 213)*

It is clear from Heller's (2005) account that comedy and incongruity prove an integral feature of the human condition and, more importantly, as a way of engaging with the extent to which all humans are 'thrown' into being. To help clarify this, Heller draws the following distinction: 'Philosophically speaking, there are two initial a priories in human life: the social a priori (the world into which each is thrown) and the genetic a priori (the inherited endowments of the thrown being herself)' (2005: 201). These two a priories prove integral to the 'essential incongruence' which underscores Heller's understanding of the subject (2005: 213). That is, while every individual is endowed with a *genetic a priori*, which is brought to bear through their own unique genetic code, it is this code which allows the human to be a social being. It is in this sense that 'all people are "thrown" into a concrete social universe' – the *social a priori* (Heller, 2005: 201). The social a priori is what comes to mediate between the singular and the universal and can be considered as the cultural values, norms and beliefs that constitute one's culture (Heller, 2005). Indeed, this relation between the social and genetic a priori is clearly visible in everyday examples, such as:

> Whenever we are sitting in a train or subway and we smile at an unknown infant, the child either smiles back or does not, yet the reaction of this 3–5-month-old will be the same whether white or brown or black, Chinese or Indian, American or German, and at the same time, it will be a very individual reaction. No sign of culture can yet be detected in the behaviour of so young a child; this appears only later. In a one-year-old child, one can easily detect the signs of a particular culture.
>
> *(Heller, 2005: 21)*

Whereas the social a priori is neither fixed nor static, it is contingent on the genetic a priori that one is endowed with and, as result, it is in the imperfect relation – or tension – between the two a priories that the subject's experience of historical contingency is founded.

Heller elaborates upon this imperfect tension when she refers to the 'abyss' that exists between the genetic and social a priories. This abyss lasts throughout our life and is where laughter emerges. Indeed, the gap between the genetic and social a priori finds no symmetry, but instead the two remain asymmetrically aligned, as Heller explains:

> The dovetailing between the social/cultural and the genetic a priori is never entirely completed. To some degree, dovetailing is usually a success. After all, the newborn is also coded for social life without qualification, since whenever dovetailing ends in a total failure, the newborn cannot grow up and cannot

> survive on its own in the social world into which he or she was thrown. On the contrary, if dovetailing ends in total success and no gap remains, then nothing short of a natural catastrophe could make the world (any world) change; there would be no ethics, history, or culture in its broader sense.
>
> *(2005: 22)*

This failure to achieve any complete dovetailing underscores human existence and our sense of being in the world. It is the incongruity between the two a priories, indeed, the impossibility of bridging our social and genetic a priories, that results in either laughter or crying (Heller, 2005).[3] Thus, for Heller, there is an abyss which stands between the two a priories and it is this incongruity between the two which explains both the omnipresence of laughter as well as the historical contingency of humour. Certainly, Heller is not suggesting that laughter exists solely in our 'genetic' make-up; rather, 'the dovetailing of the two a priories is an exquisitely human task' (2005: 23) and it is a task that antagonistically occurs throughout our lives.

To summarise, we can, drawing upon the work of Heller, begin to see how our genetic and social a priories present 'an unbridgeable abyss' from which comedy emerges as part of our own existential predicament (2005: 201). Echoing Critchley (2002a), this provides another variation on what can be conceived as the inherent distance which is prescribed by the 'abyss' that exists between the social and genetic a priori. Even if one was embedded entirely within the social a priori (an example of over-confidence, self-righteousness or fanatical obedience), the effect of laughter is what occurs in the distance *between* this individual and the laughing observer. What remains pertinent to such distance, however, is the difficulty in determining whether laughter emerges solely from this tension or from an individual who occupies a *specific* genetic or social position. This is a point of contention that remains in Heller's assertion that, 'We laugh and cry from the position of the social a priori *and/or* the genetic a priori' (2005: 213 [italics added]). In fact, in other instances, Heller notes:

> Laughter is always about leaping over the abyss. The joke is the only genre which is 'specialized' to elicit and solicit laughter; it allows us to leap over the abyss. The abyss, of course, remains there, for we must also stop laughing, and what remains in the aftermath of laughter is an awareness of the sense of senselessness, the very presence of the abyss, and the recognition that it remains there, whatever we do.
>
> *(2005: 155–156)*

Accordingly, do we conceive of laughter and comedy as residing *within* the tension between the genetic and social a priori or in *transiting* the abyss which exists between them?

Therefore, what remains prominent across both Critchley (2002a) and Heller's (2005) accounts is the sense of *distance* which is prescribed *between* the subject and the social setting, and, more importantly, *between* the subject and their symbolic identity. In both cases, it is the externalisation of the subject which causes comedy; an argument which ignores comedy's ability to endear a reflexivity that works on *both* the subject and social setting. Instead, the following will argue that comedy is truly subversive when it encounters a shift in perspective that allows the subject to realise the incongruity which is shared *within* the subject and society. It is comedy's ability to perform this inherent incongruity which avails it a significant subversive potential.

Comedy: A materialist critique

Despite the previous criticisms of Heller's (2005) approach, her attention to the 'abyss' bears a certain affinity with Lacan's notion of the Real. Indeed, in the same way that the Real is enveloped with our symbolic-imaginary constructions, continuously dislodging and disrupting any sense of unity (Žižek, 2006d), for Heller, it is an underlying sense of 'Incongruity [which] points at the abyss' within the human condition (2005: 156). It is in this way that *we* are enveloped with a sense of comic tension, reflected in comedy's ability to 'promis[e] something that is senseless, something that makes sense in its senselessness' (Heller, 2005: 156). In doing so, comedy:

> assures us … [that] [w]e overcame, for a moment, a human condition that cannot be overcome. The 'relief,' even in sexual jokes, does not come from our crossing the proper boundaries of sexual behavior, but from crossing thereby and simultaneously the boundaries which divide our desire (the genetic a priori) and the rules presented by our world (the social a priori), in general.
>
> *(Heller, 2005: 156)*

Key here is the 'crossing of boundaries' which reveal but also 'speak' to 'the limits of our finitude'. It is not necessarily the case that the notion of the 'abyss' stands between 'our desire' (genetic a priori) and 'our world' (social a priori), but that such tension, which underscores our existential condition, is inherent to reality *and* the subject.

This tension is what provides comedy its incongruity, and can also reveal a decidedly subversive edge. Indeed, in the same way that comedy presents a certain sense in senselessness, we can begin to see how, in the case of authority, 'for all authority figures [… who] stand for a kind of rationality', it is 'Jokes [which] challenge those rationalities while making fun of them, in the name of reason' (Heller, 2005: 156). This subversion of authority, and the rational ridiculing of rationality itself, posits a strange logic to Heller's thesis, one that can be envisioned as akin to a Mobius strip. Accordingly, rather than separating rationality and irrationality, comedy's subversion allows it to reflexively render what is rational through what may at first seem to be a path of irrationality. We can observe this as integral to the comic genre. Indeed:

> Comic genres make us laugh; this is their intention. But this is not their sole intention. They do not intend to make us laugh for laughter's sake alone (only stupid sitcoms do this, and only then to make a buck), but in order to invite us to take their position of assessment, their position of judgment, their evaluation of character, situation, and action. The comic genres invite us to change our regard. They ask us to notice from a distance something in which we may have been too immersed to see, our own follies included.
>
> *(Heller, 2005: 210)*

In addition, Heller notes:

> We look at something or someone from a distance, as irrational or ridiculous, yet also with involvement, as someone worth loving, hating, pitying, despising, or empathizing with. Still, something important happens through the alienating regard: with it, we see things we had not seen before, take note of circumstances that have otherwise escaped our notice.
>
> *(2005: 211)*

While remaining critical of the 'distance' which underscores Heller's approach, what these two examples reveal is the ontological shift that comedy can provide – that moment where we observe something which before was not observed. For Heller, comedy is therefore integral to philosophical inquiry, exposing that which 'can make us laugh at the human condition itself' and which 'can tell us in words what laughter cannot express in words, namely the unspeakable' (2005: 29). It is in exposing these expressions that comedy's subversive potential can be performed.

To continue this line of inquiry is to remain within the confines of comedy's incongruity, an incongruity, which, for the remainder of this study, will be driven by a materialist critique. Here, comedy's incongruity does not occur when two differences are joined together, but rather from comedy's ability to draw attention to that minimal difference which paradoxically constitutes the irrational in the rational and the sense in senselessness. In following this path, this analysis will turn to the work of Alenka Zupančič and her adoption of Hegel's concrete universal (Zupančič, 2008). As Pound asserts, Zupančič's materialism is not one which seeks to critique idealism, but which, via 'the comic mode', reveals 'the very point at which the ideal appears directly as the material' (2010: 9). Indeed, 'it is this paradox – *this incongruity* – which generates the truly subversive comic mode of comedy' (Pound, 2010: 9 [italics added]). Importantly, however, such incongruity is not predicated on the distance between the self and superego, as per Critchley (2002a), or the genetic and the social a priori, as per Heller (2005), nor is it grounded in the difference between reality and non-reality, but rather such incongruity can be considered as 'a "pure" or "minimal" difference incarnated in reality itself' (Karlsen and Villadsen, 2015: 531). Therefore, in what follows, attention will be given to Žižek's (2006a) parallax view and how, when considered alongside

Zupančič's (2008) adoption of the concrete universal, comedy's subversive significance can be performed.

Comedy, Hegel and the concrete universal

Whereas scholarly work on the significance of Hegel's approach to comedy remains limited, it is Hegel's *Phenomenology of the Spirit* (1998)[4] that, for Zupančič (2008), offers particular significance for examining comedy's form. Indeed, while Hegel's (2010) *Science of Logic* has led scholars to consider the extent to which Hegel succeeds in outlining a system of dialectics, from which abstract universals are transposed into concrete universals (Baumann, 2011; Kisner, 2008; Stern, 1997), it is this system of dialectics which Zupančič (2008) draws upon in order to examine comedy's subversive significance. Here, 'comedy enables us to confront the division within authority and gain purchase on it' (McGowan, 2014: 213).[5] However, by way of confronting this division in Hegel's interpretation of the universal, we can also turn to how it has been politically conceived in the work of Žižek (2006a, 2010). [6]

A universal notion can refer to any law, norm or moral injunction (such as 'thou shalt not kill' or 'be polite') or to a neutral term that seeks to contain a collection of shared particulars (such as 'the people'). Universals can appear self-evident, performing a determinative role in orientating a range of different particulars, each of which are contained or classified under the universal (McGowan, 2018). Key here is that the universal stands opposed to the particular: 'universals denominate or identify particulars, but they do not fully express what they are – and are thus also different from or abstract against them' (Baumann, 2011: 74). As a result, universals are frequently viewed as 'abstract' containers, with various particulars falling within a certain abstract notion (Baumann, 2011).

Whereas Hegel's work is often viewed through his account of dialectical *synthesis*, in the case of the universal, we can begin to see how any universal injunction ('thou shalt not kill', 'be polite', 'don't steal') is inherently contradictory and decidedly dialectical. Benhabib notes how:

> For Hegel, there is more to a form of life than what the participants can grasp in thought. Immanent critique unfolds through the contradictions they face as they aim to understand a world they can only imperfectly grasp; this dialectic of thought can only be stilled when, as Hegel supposed would happen in a fully rational form of life, thought and actuality are reconciled.
>
> *(2018)*

It is against such reconciliatory synthesis, however, that Žižek (2006a, 2015) focuses attention on the dialectical contradictions and tensions that are brought to bear in Hegel's philosophy. In fact, following Chapter One, we can begin to see how Žižek's political writings have frequently shown how 'liberalism relies on an imaginary notion of universality as a disengaged, shared and neutral "open space" for compromise' (Wood, 2012: 18). Opposing such a notion, Žižek outlines how no universal can remain 'neutrally' separated from the concrete immediacy of day-to-day life as well as to the antagonisms and tensions that frame particular political divisions (Wood, 2012). In sum, there cannot be a general universal which in some way brings together a number of different particulars; on the contrary, any universal is limited in its application, thus bringing to contention its own universality. It is this limit, conceived through contradiction and antagonism, which is dialectically emphasised in the site of a problem-deadlock that constitutes any particular rendering of the universal (Kapoor, 2018). As a result, Žižek's universalism 'neither pretends to transcend the particular nor imposes a positive universalized norm' (Kapoor, 2018: 5). Instead, Žižek notes that 'not only does the universal Idea always appear in a distorted or displaced way; this Idea is *nothing but* the distortion or displacement, the self-inadequacy, of the particular with regard to itself' (2012: 535).

It is in this regard that any universal notion is, fundamentally, 'divisive … [and] always fail[ing] with respect to its concretization …, because no response, no individual can be universal absolutely' (Zimeri, 2010: 35). In this case, Žižek's (2006b) universal is one that is aware of, yet grounded in and enacted through, its own exceptions. We can see this reflected in recent LGBTQIA+ debates which have centred on the use of public bathrooms by non-cis individuals (Thorn, 2016). Though many of these criticisms fail to acknowledge Žižek's (2018) Lacanian inspired Hegelianism – an approach which he applies directly to the 'bathroom debates' – his calls for there to be a 'general gender' bathroom aptly highlight his considered approach to the inherent deadlock which underscores debates on 'gender' and the various (particular) failures to answer this deadlock (Žižek, 2015). Here, Kapoor explains how Žižek's appeal for:

> A 'general gender' or 'gender as such' toilet would thus not stand beyond difference but enact sexual difference as such (before its specific determinations); it would embody the universal antagonistic dimension (Real) of sexuation, underlining the impossibility and failure of categorization.
>
> *(Kapoor, 2018: 15)*

Notably, this example details how it is the antagonism itself which cuts across gender differences, with the 'general' toilet symbolically encapsulating the inherent tensions and contradictions that constitute sexuation.

What remains important in Žižek's contention is the extent to which any 'universal' is just another assertion grounded in a particular position/perspective. When a Christian or Jew debate religion or when a deconstructionist or analytic philosopher disagree, it becomes clear that they don't just share certain differences and that each particular position harbours its own universal perspective; rather, it is that each position views these *differences* differently (Terada, 2014; Žižek, 2017). Cinematically, we can see how such an understanding of difference is portrayed in Spike Lee's effective use of the montage in *Do the Right Thing*

(1989). By bringing together various sequences, each depicting their own racial epithets, Lee is able to portray the *shared* racial antagonisms that underscore urban environments. However, what is significant in Lee's use of the montage is that each sequence is able to show these 'racial' differences from the *different* perspectives of each 'racial' group. Brought together, it becomes clear that the 'universal' is that which becomes visible in the inherent antagonisms that exist *within* and *across* each group.

Consequently, in the case of identity politics, we can refrain from 'focus[ing] on how each (ethnic, religious, sexual) group should be able fully to assert its particular identity', under some shared sense of 'neutral' universality, and instead propose 'the much more difficult and radical task … to enable each group to access full universality' (Žižek, 2018: 91) – a universality locked in the *shared* antagonism of each group. It is along these lines that we can begin to assert that:

> it is the abstract universal itself that is, by definition, imperfect and limited, because it lacks the moment of self-consciousness, of the self, of the concrete; it is universal and pure only at the price of being ultimately empty. The turn or shift at stake here is thus not a shift from the universal to something else, but a shift within the universal itself. … It is only as a concrete self that the universal comes to its own truth via the gap of self-consciousness.
>
> *(Zupančič, 2006: 188)*

In the concrete universal, it is the *differences* across various particulars that are transposed to the universal, so that, rather than the universal uniting the particular differences, it is the particularity of the concrete form which constitutes this *difference* (Stern, 1997). To help explain this process, we can turn to McGowan's example of 'marriage equality':

> Universality does not consist in the achievement of access to marriage for all. We don't achieve universality at the mythical point when all are included. … Universality becomes evident rather in the claim made by proponents of marriage equality that the ban on gay marriage violates universal equality. By pointing out what is missing for the symbolic field – gay marriage – they articulate universal equality. By saying 'gay marriage is marriage,' they say what is missing within the particularity of heterosexual marriage.
>
> *(2018: 206–207)*

From the particular position of gay marriage, it becomes clear that there is something wrong, something inconsistent or inherently missing from the universal injunction that marriage is for all. The significance of this approach is that the 'gap' between the universal and the particular is encompassed in the particular, so that it is the claims made by gay marriage proponents which perform the 'gap' (that which is missing) in the universality of marriage equality. If the 'gap' was located in the universal (in this case a form of marriage that doesn't include gay marriage), then the distinction between the universal and particular would obtain a hegemonic function akin to Laclau's (2000) notion of an 'empty' hegemonic universal, which simply draws upon a particular content to stand in for the universal (Žižek, 2000a). In this instance, the universal remains an empty container forged upon a certain particular that has, through some form of political mobilisation, won the right to claim the place of universality over all others (McGowan, 2018).[7]

On the contrary, in the case of the concrete universal, it is each particular exception that announces its own position of enunciation and which subsequently presents the 'work of the negative' inherent to the universal and to *that* point of exclusion within each particular (Žižek, 2018: 189). This:

> suggests that the important element of universality *is not* the abstract point of identification but, rather, what must be excluded to create this point. Because it is this point of exclusion that establishes the field of universality, it is also this point that holds the greatest threat to that order: its intrusion into the symbolic order threatens the coherence of that order.
>
> *(McMillan, 2013: 46 [italics added])*

It is this 'threatening' constitutive exception which exposes the 'differences' at the heart of the universal, so that 'the only "reconciliation" between the universal and the particular is that of the *universalised exception*' (Žižek, 2010: 23). Here, the 'gap' between the universal and particular becomes located in the particular and, thus, in doing so, embodies its own universal exception, a 'minimal difference' – or, as we will discuss later, a 'parallax gap'. This short circuit prescribes a form of reflexivity, whereby the universal is enacted through its own 'exception'. Accordingly, it is 'When subjects fail to register within the field of symbolic recognition, [that] their absence aligns them with universality' (McGowan, 2018: 208).

As the following discussion will seek to elaborate, it is through this universal exception that comedy can obtain a subversive significance. Here, Zupančič's (2008) analysis of comedy, and her attention to the inherent 'gaps', antagonisms and differences that are performed in the concrete universal, can help to expound upon comedy's subversive significance. However, in order to better understand this significance, let us consider in closer detail Zupančič's false and true comedy distinctions.

True and false comedy

In her approach to comedy, Zupančič (2008) distinguishes between two forms: false comedy and true comedy. With regard to the first, Zupančič notes how in various cases comedy is often perceived as:

> a genre that strongly emphasizes our essential humanity, its joys and limitations. It invites – or even forces – us to recognize and accept the fact that we are finite beings. It teaches us that we are only human, with all our faults,

> imperfections, and weaknesses, and it helps us to deal affirmatively and joyfully with the burden of human finitude.
>
> (2008: 47)

Such appraisals may seem largely positive, especially when one considers how former analyses of comedy draw attention to its ability to render our humanness palpable and to remind us that we are 'only human' (Critchley, 2002a). However, Zupančič (2008) is critical of such approaches, primarily for the fact they propose an underlying conservativism that fails to challenge abstract, universal notions of socio-symbolic status.[8] In such instances, examples of false comedy rely on the distance *between* the universal and concrete:

> False, conservative comedies are those where the abstract-universal and the concrete do not change places and do not produce a short circuit between them; instead, the concrete (where 'human weaknesses' are situated) remains external to the universal, and at the same time invites us to recognize and accept it as the indispensable companion of the universal, its necessary physical support. The paradigm of these comedies is simply the following: the aristocrat (or king, or judge, or priest, or any other character of symbolic stature) is also a man (who snores, farts, slips, and is subject to the same physical laws as other mortals). The emphasis is, of course, precisely on 'also': the concrete and the universal coexist, the concrete being the indispensable grounding of the universal.
>
> (*Zupančič*, 2008: 30)

This is apparent in the extent to which, while submitting figures of authority to ridicule, ultimately, such practices maintain their power. As a result, in false comedy 'it is the logic of domination that is allowed to operate freely, not in spite but because of efforts to undermine it' (Bonic, 2011: 97).

To this extent, false comedy maintains the status quo: it is conservative, not subversive (Zupančič, 2008). Often, such support stems from humanist accounts, whereby 'comedy gets turned into a drab lesson meant to show us our mere humanity – to teach us that we are not perfect, that after all we are only human, that we should simply accept our weaknesses, limitations and imperfections' (Kottman, 2008: 4). This, according to Zupančič (2008), misses the subversive potential of comedy. Instead, Zupančič's (2006, 2008) approach requires that we examine not just the content of comedy but, more importantly, its form.

To illustrate this formal significance, Zupančič draws upon former US President George W. Bush, who would deliberately 'mock his own presidential self', so that while such mocking, in most instances, comedically 'portraying the inflexible war President as "the guy next door"' fully 'aware of his faults and imperfections' (2008: 33), these gestures would ultimately serve to *distance* Bush from his own (real) concreteness. That is, the distance *between* Bush – the self-depreciating man (concrete) – and Bush – the President of the United States, head of state, head of government and commander-in-chief of the US Armed Forces (universal) – was constituted in a media strategy that benefitted Bush through his comic 'human' failings. Here:

> The direct parody of oneself and one's beliefs can flourish very well within the conservative paradigm of *combining* the concrete and the universal. It can successfully promote the very ideology whose human side and weaknesses are being exposed. There are plenty of examples in several veins of Hollywood comedy, in which derision of our own beliefs and of the 'American way of life' produces the very distance necessary to sustain these very same beliefs and this very same way of life.
>
> *(Zupančič, 2008: 33 [italics added])*

As a form of false comedy, this conservative tendency 'relies on the peaceful co-existence of the abstract and the concrete in its attempt to remind us that even the elites are only human' (Ladegaard, 2014: 117). Accordingly, in the case of Bush, while his comic displays sought to engender sympathy, in doing so, his symbolic identity, and the power structures that maintained his symbolic authority, remained preserved and unchallenged (Ladegaard, 2014).

In contrast, true comedy occurs when the universal, in both its abstract and actual dimensions, is brought together in a particular concrete example that provides a short circuit (a change of places) between the universal and concrete. It is by displaying the *universal in its concrete form* that the gaps and inconsistencies in the abstract universal are transposed to particular instances that render visible its own inherent inconsistency. With regard to Zupančič's example of the baron who slips on a banana peel, the comedy of this scene is not drawn from the fact that anyone – even a baron – can slip on a banana peel, but, instead, it is when the baron stands up and presumptuously continues to appear *to himself* as a 'baron' that true comedy is performed.[9] In the latter, it is the symbolic title, 'baron', which proves comic. As a result, comedy becomes truly subversive when it highlights how the universal's essential ideas, values and forms are incongruously rendered in concrete instances. Therefore, according to Zupančič, 'The real comedy of George W. Bush can be seen at times when he makes no effort to be funny, but solemnly appears as an American President *who believes that he really is an American President*' (2008: 34 [italics added]).

This latter contention underscores Zupančič's (2008) argument that it is the particular/concrete which affects a non-coincidence in the universal, dissociating it of any metaphysical significance (Pound, 2010). That is, while telling a joke can be used to relieve tension, build coherence and maintain the stability of a particular situation, in contrast, Zupančič's (2008) Hegelianism points to those jokes which confer a different perspective on a particular situation or, as noted earlier, present the particular's universal exception (Žižek, 2000a). For Pound:

> This argument is developed with a materialist thrust: if jokes have traditionally been on the side of materialism …, usurping the universal in favour of the

> particular (i.e. jokes target the false elevation of subjectivity as in the example of the man slipping on the banana skin), [... Zupančič's] point is that these jokes don't go far enough. A joke may bring us back to earth with a thud, but it still leaves the possibilities of the heavens intact.
>
> *(2015: 180–181)*

As mentioned, such failure fuels the impotency of false comedy, which simply presents an ironic or cynical stance. Instead, for Zupančič, 'true comedy' is 'not so much involved in unveiling and disclosing the nudity or emptiness behind appearances as [it is] involved in constructing emptiness (or nudity)' (2003: 166–167). In doing so, '"true" comedy, ... exposes the fundamental incongruity between men and their fantasies in all its concrete materiality' (Ladegaard, 2017: 183).

Indeed, it is in performing this incongruity that comedy can render the concrete universal. In view of Žižek's (2012) understanding of the universal – as constituting those deadlocks that fail to accurately perform the universal in its particularity – we can begin to examine how our universal notions are frequently undermined through moments of comedy. Central to this claim is the concern that it is *through the universal itself* that we can identify the subversive potential of comedy. For example, consider the universal notion that we should, as best as possible, 'be polite' to others (evident when any parent encourages their child to say 'please' and 'thank you') and then imagine this universal notion in its concrete form: two people stand on a train platform, the train arrives, the doors open and, at the same time, both politely gesture to the other, 'after you', with each sharing the reply, 'no, after you'. Very quickly we see how this imaginary situation poses a comic sequence as the two individuals politely prevent each other from getting on the train, culminating in the inherent inconsistency of the universal (politeness) being enacted through the failure of its concrete performance.

In such instances, comic pleasure emanates from the realisation that the universal fails; that the universal, much like the symbolic/big Other, is inconsistent and that such failure is 'funny'. Indeed, it is this incongruity in the concrete universal which highlights comedy's subversive potential, not by ridiculing the universal, but by *performing* the universal's ridiculousness through the incongruity of the particular concrete example. For the baron who slips on the banana peel, 'Rather than the slip itself, the funny thing is that the baron continues his walk as if nothing had happened' (Ladegaard, 2017: 182), all the time remaining confident in his own universal importance.

As an adjunct to Zupančič's (2008) baron example, we can consider how the 'slip on a banana peel' does not necessarily have to evolve around a figure of obvious authority but can posit a formal significance that underscores the comic performance. The well-known 'Del falls through a bar' scene from the British comedy *Only Fools and Horses* (1981–2003) provides a notable example. Indeed, it is through 'the ebullient, ever cheeky Derek "Del Boy" Trotter', a comic character 'always with a new joke on the tongue and a new girl on his arm' (McKenna, 2015: 200), that we observe the same presumptuous authority as the baron who believes he is a baron. In fact, much like the baron, there is not much to confirm Del's (David Jason) image, apart from his excessive attempts to belong to a symbolic order which confers such authority. This is emphasised when we consider that the series was set during 1980s Thatcherism. While the social context was very rarely acknowledged in the series, 'the rise of the yuppie and the struggle of working class communities to scrimp and scrape in face of the neoliberal onslaught' (McKenna, 2015: 200) was a narrative that proved salient in the show's storylines and its lead characters: Del Boy and Rodney Trotter (Nicholas Lyndhurst). It is against this context that, rather than be excluded from this world, Del seeks to be a part of it, and it is in this way that Del's comic performances work to highlight the inherent inconsistences and modes of excess of the period. In fact, McKenna notes that Del is often seen in 'red braces, gaudy gold chains and yuppie Filofax' (2015: 200), an amalgamation of the 1980s 'loadsamoney/yuppie' aesthetic. Moreover, Del is a character who, despite his London-working class background, desperately seeks to be viewed as an intelligent entrepreneur, adept at the art of business, widely admired by women and respected by men. Throughout the show's series he dreams up and concocts various schemes to 'make money', with the added surety of his own entrepreneurial abilities. Indeed, Del's unbridled confidence is often contrasted against his less-sure younger brother, Rodney. Notably, however, it is in the famous bar scene that we witness Del's presumptuous attitude concretely performed.

In the scene, Del stands at the end of a bar with his friend Trigger (Roger Lloyd Pack), with Del explaining to Trigger the type of 'man' that women 'go for'. In an attempt to prove his mature sophistication, and 'natural' ability to charm the opposite sex, Del seeks to attract the attention of one of the many women who are in the bar. With one arm on the bar, Del looks out across the room and catches the eye of an attractive woman, who gives him a certain look. Taking a breath, Del lifts his arm from the bar, stands straight and says to Trigger: 'We're on a winner here, Trig. Alright, play it nice and cool son, nice and cool, you know what I mean…' Unawares to Del and Trigger, a waiter has just left the bar via the flip-up counter-top which Del had previously had his arm resting on. As he finishes speaking to Trigger, he leans back against the counter-top which is now raised. With drink in hand, Del falls through the gap in the bar. In a continuation of the scene's comic performance, Trigger, who is much taller than Del, fails to notice the fall and does a full-circle to see where Del has gone (he fails to look 'down' where he would clearly see Del on the floor of the bar). While Trigger spins around, shocked at Del's sudden disappearance, Del jumps up off the floor, disheveled and wet from his spilt drink. With a 'cool' nonchalant shrug of the shoulders, Del re-establishes his composure and states to Trigger:

DEL BOY: Drink-up, Trig. Drink-up, we're leaving.
TRIGGER: Ain't you gonna try for those birds?
DEL BOY: (*masking an injury from the fall*) Nah mate. You're cramping my style… cramping my style.

Here, Del's symbolic identity – a confident, charming, suave 'ladies' man' – is concretely performed in his sudden comic fall. Again, much like Zupančič's (2008) baron, this example is not significant for the fact that anybody could, while attempting to impress, fall through a bar, slip down a manhole, or slide on a banana skin – examples that would all give the impression that Del is just like anybody else – but rather it is the manner in which Del quickly asserts his assumed symbolic status that proves truly comical. Despite his fall, which is then followed by the retort: 'you're cramping my style', Del defers his embarrassment onto Trigger and continues to go on his way (and out the bar), all the while holding onto the belief that he is still a charming, sophisticated 'ladies' man'. In this particular scene, it is Del's universal impotence which proves comical.

Furthermore, we could posit a feminist reading of the performance. That is, through the comic display we see the assumption that a woman would be attracted to a man such as Del. In the scene, the subtle, ambiguous look from the woman who attracts Del's attention could quite as easily have been thinking… 'what an idiot!' Instead, Del's presumptuous confidence and his self-assured certainty is concretely performed and, ultimately, comically subverted.

In what follows, attention will be given to extending Zupančič's (2008) analysis of the concrete universal with two additional perspectives: Todd McGowan's analysis of comedy as dialectically predicated on lack and excess and Žižek's notion of parallax (McGowan, 2017; Žižek, 2006a). While Žižek's (2006a) parallax view has not been applied specifically to analyses of comedy, in the following discussion it will be used to highlight the 'shift in perspective' that occurs when the universal is concretised. Before this, however, we will turn to McGowan's lack and excess.

Comedy's lack and excess

According to McGowan:

> Comedy occurs when we are surprised by a conjunction of lack and excess. An excessive response to lack or the emergence of lack occasioned by excess reveals how every lack is excessive and every excess is lacking. When the coincidence of lack and excess surprises us, this is the comic event.
>
> *(2017: 13)*

Importantly, both lack and excess should not be seen as disparate terms, but rather viewed as providing an 'intimate relation' that, when exposed, can reveal a comic effect (McGowan, 2017). Indeed, the notion of 'lack' will be returned to in our discussions on the subject and the other (see Chapter Three); for present purposes, however, it is important to outline how McGowan's (2017) approach bears a resemblance to the subject's 'excessive' capacity to rebuke its interpellation – as noted in Žižek's (2017) critique of Critchley (2009) – as well as the inherent inconsistencies that underscore the various ways in which the universal is concretely performed (Dean, 2006).

In either case, it is a perception of wholeness which underscores both the subject and the universal. That is, while it is a sense of imaginary wholeness which structures the subject's sense of self, it is this same sense of wholeness that is enacted by the universal in its various attempts to obscure those inherent exceptions that undermine its universality. For the latter, however, 'Wholeness is not inimical to exclusion but depends on it because the exclusion provides the external point of reference that enables the structure to define itself as a [universal] whole' (McGowan, 2014: 206). As a result, such exclusion is often enacted through an 'Excess … of the distortion that lack produces' (McGowan, 2017: 16). It is from this 'lack' that both the subject and the universal can be considered.

It is in this vein that McGowan (2017) highlights how our everyday routines are framed through the regulated separation of lack and excess: we lack excitement during the working week, only to then partake in excessive forms of enjoyment at the weekend (drinking, eating with friends, going on a night out, taking drugs). For McGowan, 'comedy arises from a direct statement that identifies a lack with an excess that disrupts our everyday existence' (2017: 37). This relation between lack and excess can be examined in McGowan's (2017) analysis of *Monty Python and the Holy Grail* (1975) and *The Silence of the Lambs* (1991), both of which provide a comic rendition on the topic of 'death'.

For example, when McGowan notes that 'There can … be funny scenes of death, as long as someone responds to this literal lack with excess' (2017: 13); in the case of *Monty Python* and *Silence of the Lambs*, it is the dismemberment of The Black Night (John Cleese) and the remarks from Dr Hannibal Lecter (Anthony Hopkins) that help to illustrate this distinction. With regards to *Monty Python*:

> As he [The Black Knight] loses each of his arms and legs, he continues to insist on his own inevitable victory in the struggle. After the loss of the first arm, he proclaims, 'T'is but a scratch.' When he loses the other arm, he insists that it is only a 'flesh wound.' … Even in the midst of a horrific dismemberment, the Black Knight never deviates from his belief in his own superiority or his devotion to continuing the fight. The more of his body the Black Knight loses, the surer he is of his eventual victory and the more he taunts his opponent with his own superiority. He thus embodies lack and excess simultaneously. It is this disparate connection that provides the key to grasping the comic.
>
> *(McGowan, 2017: 13)*

Much like Zupančič's (2008) presumptuous baron, it is The Black Knight's own presumptuous desire to carry on fighting that is comically performed. Certainly, in comparison with the character of Hannibal Lecter, The Black Knight's loss of limbs stands in clear opposition to the various instances where Hannibal sadistically divulges how he eats his unfortunate victims. Yet, note how, in the following scene, 'While talking on the telephone to FBI agent Clarice Starling (Jodie Foster), he tells her, "I'm having an old friend for dinner"'; McGowan adds:

> the film cuts to a shot of his former jailor and tormentor, Dr. Chilton (Anthony Heald), arriving by plane at what seems like a tropical island where Lecter is hiding out. Lecter's final joke implies that he intends to eat Chilton. Spectators can find the comedy in this statement because they have seen Chilton's arrogance, sexual aggression toward Starling, and cruelty toward Lecter. In other words, the film presents Chilton as a figure of excess, and this enables us to chuckle (even if uncomfortably) at Lecter's pun about eating him. Chilton's demise contrasts with that of the other characters in the film only insofar as he is excessive. In this sense, he is the cousin of the Black Knight.
>
> *(2017: 14)*

Accordingly, whereas McGowan (2017) draws attention to the change in victim, it is the formal relation between lack and excess which is important. Indeed, it is here that we can draw connections with the inconsistencies that Zupančič (2008) highlights in her account of the concrete universal.

In accordance with the previous discussion of the universal, we can begin to trace how the universal and its exceptions can be perceived through the irrational excess which works to obscure and distort the inherent lack of the universal form (Dean, 2006). In fact, Murphy draws attention to how 'The most instantly recognizable kind of social distortion is excess', adding that:

> There are various kinds of excess. Firstly, there are the excesses of the intellect. Pomposity, conceit and vanity are the typical comic faults of the professor. Then there are material excesses. Avarice is the typical comic failing of the wealthy. There are also the excesses of identity. The envious person wants to be someone else. The jealous person wants to control someone else. Each comic excess brings forth a deficit. Conceit encourages pedantry, avarice produces meanness, and jealousy produces blindness. All these faults seem to inspire around them a lack of courage and a lack of sense. Is there anything more comically disreputable than cowardice or stupidity?
>
> *(2006: 70)*

These excessive elements are often ideologically framed through examples of fantasy, which condense such excess in a particular feature or individual. Most notably, this is reflected in the role of the Jew in anti-Semitism, whereby 'the "Jew" condenses in a unique figure the excessive nature of capitalism – its wild profiteering, etc. – as well as its proletarian subversion – the "Jewish-Communist plot"' (Žižek, 2008a: 152 [parenthesis removed]).

In addition, further connections can be drawn between McGowan's (2014) comic excess and Zupančič's (2008) account of false comedy in order to highlight how 'the task of conservative comedy is one of constituting the wholeness by way of the exclusion' (McGowan, 2014: 206). Such a fantasy of wholeness – a fantasy that deliberately seeks to obscure the inherent lack – is conducive to forms of authority which draw upon examples of false comedy in order to maintain their status. Often, their use of comic excess seeks to uphold the distinction between the universal and the concrete (as noted in the Bush examples). Accordingly, with regards to the representation of black Americans in US comedy, McGowan notes how, 'A large portion of American entertainment is rife with images of black comic excess created for the purpose of creating the image of American society from which this black is excluded' (2014: 206).

Indeed, this management of excess echoes Bakhtin's notion of the carnival, via the temporary suspension of everyday routines and hierarchy, which radically uses comedy to mock and/or subvert those in authority (McGowan, 2014). Equally, such assertions echo Critchley's (2002a) own contentions that humour, comedy and jokes can offer a suspension of reality, from which the subject's being is brought to light. However, for both Bakhtin (1984) and Critchley (2002a), the temporality of such humour is evident in the return to normalcy which proceeds the carnival/joke. Instead, what is required is a form of humour that, as Zupančič's (2008) true comedy suggests, produces comedy through the *performance* of this authority itself. This can be seen in Žižek's reference to the significance of The Marx Brothers' *Duck Soup* (1933), which does not 'reside in its mockery of the totalitarian state's machinery and paraphernalia, but in openly displaying the madness, the "fun," the cruel irony, which are *already present* in the totalitarian state' (Žižek, 2017: 342). It is here that 'The Marx brothers' "carnival" is the carnival of totalitarianism itself' (Žižek, 2017: 342). In other words, it is the excessive 'carnival' of totalitarianism which is brought to light through its concrete materialisation.

Moreover, if we consider that the best way to use comedy's subversive potential is through deliberately performing the excesses of the universal, then we can follow McGowan's (2016) lack-excess distinction by examining two comic examples which he uses to highlight how such excess is intricately tied to examples of social inclusion and exclusion. Here, McGowan (2016) draws upon the comic performances of Charlie Chaplin and his famous comic character the 'Little Tramp', as well as the films of Buster Keaton. With regards to Chaplin, McGowan notes how the Little Tramp is 'an excessive disturbance of the social order that exiles him' (2016: 604). That is, the Tramp is what is excluded from the social system through the excesses of capitalism; his comedy is what excessively draws attention to the exclusions of this system. This is made apparent in the opening scene of *City Lights* (1931) which:

> involves the unveiling of a monument dedicated to 'Peace and Prosperity.' As the civic leaders lift the cover from the new monument, the Little Tramp appears asleep on the monument. The initial minutes of the film depict the authorities trying to remove the Little Tramp from the monument and he trying to extricate himself. His presence on the monument reveals that despite the presence of the new monument the city has not

> actually attained peace and prosperity for all. The Little Tramp is the stain in the unveiling of the monument, a stain that gives the lie to what the monument proclaims.
>
> *(McGowan, 2016: 604)*

The unveiling of the statue and the comic surprise which follows from witnessing the Little Tramp fast asleep at the foot of the monument provides a concrete universalisation of what capitalism seeks to exclude. Furthermore, the Tramp's excessive appearance – 'Chaplin brings together the lower class absence of wealth with the upper class attire' (McGowan, 2016: 604) – disturbs the social order. In so doing:

> The Little Tramp shows us the social leftover, what society cannot use and what has no place in society – and yet what stands out excessively. He is the ultimate figure of lack: he typically does not have a home or a job, and he often does not have enough to eat.
>
> *(McGowan, 2016: 604)*

We also witness this 'excluded' excess in Ricky Gervais's *Derek*, a British comedy-drama, which aired between 2012 and 2014. In this series, Gervais played a care worker, Derek, who works at a care home for elderly residents. Derek is socially awkward and presents a childlike naivety and, despite his role as a care worker, shares many of the social exclusions that his elderly friends are subject to. In view of McGowan's analysis of the included/excluded excess of comedy, we can consider McKenna's assessment that:

> by focusing on a group of elderly people living in a retirement home, *Derek* is drawing attention to those who fall outside the remit of the cycle of capital expansion and are therefore outsiders by the very fact of their social being. Even the helpers in the care home – such as Derek himself – are people, for the most part, who would struggle to secure conventional employment; together, their care home community comes to form an 'excluded other', a group which is located outside the organised social field of capital reproduction.
>
> *(2015: 201)*

McKenna's reference to both Derek and the elderly as an 'excluded other' ('those who fall outside the remit of the cycle of capital expansion'), highlights how, much like Chaplin's Little Tramp, there remain those who are excluded from the workings of capitalism. In the same way that the Little Tramp is both homeless and jobless, the inherent inconsistencies of the capitalist social order are excessively framed throughout the series, with both the residents and its staff living and working under the constant fear of neoliberal 'cut-backs'. For McKenna, Derek and the elderly are subject to:

> a sleek, refined, steely sharp model that in the pursuit of capital expansion, more and more eliminates from its remit any extraneous, 'unproductive' baggage. In such a climate, the elderly are most at risk because they are figures who have ceased to sell their labour power – that is, they have ceased to be the 'productive' creators of new value in the precise Marxist sense. In one way, they are even more vulnerable than the children in society, for the children have the capacity to evolve into future wage labourers, and they are from this purview more valuable.
>
> *(2015: 201)*

It is in such instances that the comedy of the series is often performed through the relations between Derek and the elderly, both of whom reflect an excluded excess (McKenna, 2015).

However, while Chaplin, and the residents of Derek's care home, constitute the excess that emerges in their exclusion from the social order, it is important that such comic portrayals do not present a picture of wholeness by simply including the excluded within the society that rejects them. Indeed, such assertions would merely serve to uphold the universal, by including its own exclusion: the very exclusion which is required in order to maintain the universal. Although McGowan (2016) steers us away from such assumptions, he comparatively draws upon the example of Buster Keaton in order to highlight how Keaton's *inclusion* reflects a different form of excess.

In comparison to Chaplin's Little Tramp, which depicts the *excessive exclusion* of the social order, Keaton's various characters reflect the *excessive inclusion* of the social order through performances that, in comparison with Chaplin, comparatively reveal the inherent instability of the social order. That is, 'Whereas Chaplin finds excess outside the social structure, Keaton finds it within, and it acts as an obstacle for him' (McGowan, 2016: 611). As a result:

> Keaton is the contingent excess that internally troubles every social order. His comedy reveals that social success depends on contingency, and in this way he destroys all myths of proper social hierarchy, whether earned through birth, through merit, or through hard work.
>
> *(McGowan, 2016: 616)*

It is here that we can extend Zupančič's notion of the concrete universal by seeking to identify those moments of universal excess which prove comically disruptive for the social order. In fact, while reflecting upon the political significance of both Chaplin and Keaton, McGowan asserts that 'Despite Chaplin's more radical politics, Keaton creates a more radical comedy because it illustrates how the social order subverts itself rather than trying to subvert it from the outside' (McGowan, 2016: 612). In much the same way that Zupančič (2006, 2008) draws attention to those particular instances, when the universal is shown to be inconsistent via its concrete manifestation, 'the failure of the social order derives from its own contradictions, and Keaton's films direct our attention toward these contradictions' (McGowan, 2016: 612). However, in order to elaborate upon this process, the following section will seek to draw attention to the dialectical tensions which underscore the concrete universal and how this can transpose the inherent gaps within the universal. To do so, we will turn to Žižek's notion of parallax and to the effects of comic repetition.

Comic repetition and the division of the 'One'

If we consider Zupančič's (2008) reference to comic repetition and the 'joint articulation' of the One with *itself*, then it is apparent that comic sequences follow a formal structure whereby a sense of continuity is achieved through discontinuity. That is, when we expect something different but get a version of the same repeated to us. This version of the same represents an 'inner connection' between discontinuous parts, which can present 'a moment of "radical negativity"' from which 'the gap that momentarily suspends the Order of Being' is affirmed (Moolenaar, 2004: 273). While Moolenaar applies such affirmation to Lacan's distinction between the 'discourse of the Master' and the 'discourse of the Analyst', for present purposes, it can be used to reveal that such 'radical negativity' can 'be regarded as something "positive" or productive' (Moolenaar, 2004: 273). It is in this light that Zupančič's material conception of comedy can be conceived:

> not [... because] it reminds us of, and insists upon, the mud, the dirt, dense and coarse reality as our ultimate horizon (which we need to accept), and as a condition of our life [... but] because it gives voice and body to the impasses and contradictions of this materiality itself.
>
> *(2008: 47)*

These impasses and contradictions become apparent when we consider how comedy and jokes perform the division of the One. Importantly, this is not a One split into two, but a One that, through a comic shift, reveals its own internal division and its own inherent lack, thus resulting in the *appearance* of two. This appearance is drawn from the failure of the One to fully coincide with itself and, as a consequence, bears a formal significance akin to comedy's incongruity.[10]

This approach stands opposed to those that conceive of comedy as being grounded in multiplicity. Murphy details how 'Comedy is not monist. It always summons up more than one reason and more than one kind of rationality' (2006: 66). This 'rationality' is underscored by Murphy's concern that comedy performs 'a delicious, frenetic, spirited combat, in which neither side triumphs' (2006: 66). Instead, 'Via the dazzling swing shift, the warring sides are yoked in matrimony. They are joined in a third-party comic entity. Humour united them in a paradoxical antithetical union' (Murphy, 2006: 66). Murphy's (2006) latter comments draw attention to comedy's ability to 'marry' together two opposing and contradictory distinctions, with the disjuncture it provides echoing Critchley's (2002a) views on comedy's disruptive potential. Yet, if we consider these remarks through a dialectical lens, then we can begin to envisage how such a marrying together of two disparate elements can be reinterpreted as a division of the One. Here, the 'third-party comic entity' emerges as that fantasmatic-comic element which obfuscates such antagonisms, and which proves to be the excessive surplus of such division (the *objet a*) (McGowan, 2017; Murphy, 2006). In fact, to refer to Murphy's examples of the relationship between comedy and identity:

> the swing shift from one rationale to another [... is] [d]ramatically ... symbolized by a change of identity. Trading places, confusion of identities (*Rosencrantz and Guildenstern*), cross-dressing (*Some Like It Hot, Tootsi*), authors denying their authorship (*Don Quixote*), and shipwrecked locales (*Gilligan's Island*) where identities are subverted in the very act of trying to maintain them – all are comic devices for exploring how the human self becomes a stranger to itself.
>
> *(2006: 72)*

As can be seen, Murphy's remarks deny a simple marrying together of two disparate elements by acknowledging the self-estrangement which underscores 'how the human self becomes a stranger to *itself*'. This same division of the One is echoed in McGowan's lack and excess, which, as he notes, 'are nothing but different forms of expression for the same structure' (2017: 20). Equally, within the comic word play of The Marx Brothers we frequently see how forms of speech paradoxically emerge from the unexpected contortion of language *itself*.

Certainly, the division in these examples is not simply One divided into two, in the sense that the 'two' correspond to a yin-yang style relation (Dolar, 2012). In this way, the two would equal One. Rather, what is suggested in the division of the One is that there is a One *and the Other*, and the two hold no symmetrical relation. Instead, the Other is that which allows the One to be counted as One. Accordingly, the One divided *from itself* does not create symmetry but, instead, asymmetry.

Furthermore, the division of the One is not an attempt to apply a simple monism. Indeed, 'The reply of a materialist theory is to show that this very One already relies on certain exclusions: the common field in which plural identities disport is from the start sustained by an invisible antagonistic split' (Žižek, 2006c: 35). It is in this sense that Žižek (2006b, 2006c) argues that it is the multiple that obfuscates the initial division of the One from itself, with such multiplicity disguising the inherent limits and forms of excess which underscore this multiplicity. For example, 'In Lacan's terminology, the establishment of the symbolic law, the (systemic) totalization of a signifying structure, cannot take place without producing a remainder, an excess, a dimension of the real that marks the limit of formalization' (Shepherdson, 1995: para. 47). This limit is what posits any totality as non-All and, thus, from a dialectical/materialist perspective, it is this limit which lays bare the contradictions that underscore any totality; these contradictions, in short, are what remain inherent to the division of the One.

Moreover, these contradictions point to a certain lack/excess within the totality, presenting an engagement with the Real (Kunkle, 2012). This is echoed in the work of Daly (2010) who has argued for a return to the notion of 'totality' in order to better equip our understandings of subversion. Though Daly cautions that 'a totality is at its strongest when it is able to circumscribe the very terms of its own subversion' (2010: 10) – that is, hegemonic control is maintained by managing the contradictions inherent to any totality – it is, nevertheless, through identifying this 'split-ness' (this division of the One) that comedy's subversive significance can be identified. To help elucidate on this process, we can turn to Žižek's (2006a) notion of parallax.

Comedy and parallax

Žižek's (2006a) parallax view is an elaboration on his dialectical materialism and Hegelian influences. As previously noted, Žižek's (2012) use of dialectics stands opposed to traditional interpretations of Hegel, which perceive his dialectical process as grounded upon an evolutionary logic. According to Žižek, 'For a proper dialectician, there is no moment of maturity when a system functions in a non-antagonistic way' (2015: 377). Instead, antagonism is central to the existence of any system and dialectics is how we acknowledge contradiction as an internal logic in both the subject and object (Chow, 2014). It is in this way that Žižek 'replace[s] … the polarity of opposites with the concept of the inherent "tension," gap, non-coincidence, of the One itself' (2006a: 7). It is this 'gap' which is reflected in the term 'parallax'. Importantly, this gap is not subsumed or integrated, but reveals an underlying 'One', which is itself comprised of two opposing perspectives. Acknowledging these perspectives is what underscores parallax: the ability to observe two incompatible perspectives of the same object – a parallax view.

This is echoed in optical illusions such as the well-known silhouette which depicts both an old *and* young woman. What is important, however, is that such images are not 'illusions', but a single image that can be seen from two perspectives and from which each perspective changes the image itself. To this extent, Žižek's notion of parallax 'changes the perspective of an object supposedly known previously … and shows a perspective that, albeit already there, was necessary to be shown again' (Garcia and Sanchez, 2008). It is in this way that, when 'Arguing from a parallax position', Žižek believes we 'should be in a position to ask the right questions; questions which are posed from the perspective of two incommensurable points of view' (Mangold, 2014: 8). Central to such contentions is the ability to live with certain paradoxes and, more importantly, apply these paradoxes as part of a short circuit. Indeed, 'in short circuiting two incongruent dimensions' we can 'reframe our perspective and thus our very reality' (Kunkle, 2012). In so doing, 'reality' itself appears as dialectical via the inability to ever truly 'separate our understanding *of* reality from reality' (Wood, 2012: 12).

Furthermore, it is in approaching this reality that Žižek's (2006a) parallaxical account can be married with Zupančič's (2006, 2008) material approach to comedy and, specifically, to the division of the One. As Wood explains, 'The parallax gap is not only a shift between (or juxtaposition of) two perspectives; more fundamentally, it is the pure, minimal difference or incommensurability that even divides one perspective or one object *from itself*' (2012: 241). That is, it is the minimal difference inherent to the One, which intrinsically divides itself from itself. Importantly, it is in accordance with this understanding that Žižek's notion of parallax echoes the previous discussion on the inherent inconsistencies of the universal and the various (comic) excesses which seek to obfuscate reality's own inherent lack. Here, 'Symbolic identity and symbolic reality – any "One" – is ruptured by the odd juxtaposition of the parallax gap' (Wood, 2012: 17).

In fact, 'It is this logic of the "minimal difference," of the constitutive non-coincidence of a thing with itself, which provides the key to the central Hegelian category of "concrete universality"' (Žižek, 2006a: 30). As noted above, this concrete universality is comically performed when individuals, such as Bush, or, to adopt a more recent example, US President Donald Trump, unquestionably 'perform' themselves. In other words, it is only when these personalities adhere to their symbolic identities, that they in fact reveal or, more appropriately, perform, their own 'minimal difference', their own inherent inconsistency. It is in this sense that they *really* are funny. This minimal difference can also be identified in Zupančič's reference to the line from Plautus's play, *Amphitryon*: '*I swear to you, I was there before I had arrived*'. Indeed, such a 'line is funny or comical precisely because the play makes it possible, since it is not simply meaningless, or an abyssal logical paradox, but the most accurate description of the facts' (Zupančič, 2008: 78).

To return briefly to a television example, we can observe how the notion of parallax is performed in the 'satirical' comedy of Charlie Brooker and his widely acclaimed *Newswipe* (2009–2010). In contrast to the previously mentioned examples of satire in British comedy (most notably, *Brass Eye*, a satirical mockumentary, and *The Thick of It*, a satirical comic-drama), Brooker's comedy is notable for the particular approach it takes to deconstructing popular media narratives. Here, Brassett and Sutton detail how:

> Interestingly, much of Brooker's output is addressed to the audience of media: the individual subject, who watches the news and seeks to comprehend global events. So, in addition to the presenter and the first person narrator, Brooker also appears as a television viewer, who is sat in his living room on a comfortable sofa. This attempt to define and personalise the audience suggests a degree of identification – breaking down the illusory barrier between performer and audience – and a provocation, asking us: do you see it this way? Do you challenge or question what you are told? Such a reflexive conception of the audience subject suggests an unstable performance: there is a possibility for disagreement, ignorance, denial or even involvement.
>
> *(2017: 256)*

What remains crucial to Brassett and Sutton's (2017) analysis is the sense in which Brooker's comedy performance – depicted through his first-person narrations – dissolves any distinction *between* the audience and the media and, more importantly, between Brooker (including his critical approach) and 'us' the audience. Notably, Brooker's media derisions are not just critical assessments of the media but also include moments where he takes the media's message literally, often for comic effect. To this end, Brooker's comedy is not centred on a critical distance – a satirical performance of media narratives, rendered in a fictional setting (such as the fictional studio used in Morris's *Brass Eye*) that requires no participation from the audience – but instead provides a parallaxical approach whereby the audience are *included* in the deconstruction itself. That is, through a form of 'minimal difference', Brooker's sofa-critiques present the audience as 'split' in their role as agents of viewership (they maintain the choice to watch Brooker or change the channel) *and* in their observance of this viewership being performed to them. Here, Brooker's comedy takes on a far more subversive significance in that his performance *of the audience to the audience* encourages a level of reflexivity from which the audiences' own position is inconsistently performed (are we watching Brooker? Is Brooker watching/performing us?)

Inducing such a para-logical vision is central to Žižek's use of jokes and comedy by way of highlighting important cultural, political and economic antagonisms. In fact, it is through the use of jokes that Kunkle believes Žižek's work allows us 'to change our orientation to the reality we think surrounds us and … open up a space for a critique of universals that emerge out of the particular cases themselves' (Kunkle, 2012). For our present purposes, it is here that we can draw a more fundamental connection between Žižek's (2006a) parallax view and Zupančič's (2008) concrete universal.

Comedy and the Real

As previously noted, it is Zupančič's (2008) contention that true comedy functions by performing the concrete universal. It is in this sense that the universal and concrete shift places, so that in performances of true comedy, we witness a comic performance that lays bare the inconsistencies of the universal or, as discussed above, the division of the One. To this end, it has been argued that it is through adopting a parallax view that comedy induces such a 'shift' via forms of comic surprise that deliberately *involves* 'us' the audience. Importantly, such comic surprise occurs when we expect something different but get the same repeated to us. As evidenced in Žižek's (2006a) parallax view, such minimal difference is brought to bear in those moments where instead of One becoming Two, we get One + One. Here, Dolar explains:

> In every repetition there is already, in a minimal way, the emergence of that which escapes symbolization, the haphazard contingent object appears which spoils the mere repeating of the same, so the same which returns is never the

> same although we couldn't tell it apart from its previous occurrence by any of the positive features or distinguishing marks.
>
> *(Dolar, 2005: 200)*

This contingency in repetition is used by comedy in order to 'perceive a certain duality where we have so far perceived only a (more or less) harmonious One' (Zupančič, 2008: 121). It is such duality that reflects a 'minimal difference', indeed, 'a split at the very core of the same' (Zupančič, 2003: 168). It is this 'split' – conceived as a 'parallax gap' – which is subsequently revealed in the minimal difference that joins together two heterogeneous orders, two incompatible perspectives that can be observed through a comic repetition (Žižek, 2006a).

It is also these moments which bear a relation to the Real. Indeed, whereas 'tragedy confronts us with the Real', in the case of comedy, 'Comedy, ... does not confront us with the Real, it repeats it' (Zupančič, 2008: 179). This repetition is reflected in those excessive elements and fantasy formations that, in trying to mask and obfuscate an inherent lack, repeatedly encounter the same underlying Real in often surprising ways (McGowan, 2017). If we consider the formal logic of this suggestion – bearing in mind that the One is non-identical with itself (with the *One* and *itself* transiting a minimal difference), and that any symbolic order is grounded in difference – then, rather than 'Repetition [... being] the recontextualization of any positive content', of something that is novel and therefore 'surprising', comic repetition can be used to reveal that it 'is the repetition of a Real antagonism or negativity that is left out of (repressed from) the symbolic order' (Wood, 2012: 50). Indeed, 'Because that which is repressed always returns', then to 'repeat' is to draw attention to the underlying antagonisms which perform 'the same unrepresentable X' (Wood, 2012: 50) – something always-already there. It is in this sense that comic surprise offers something different to novelty, by highlighting how 'We can be surprised at something that we know very well, even expect[,] yet when it happens [again], it surprises us' (Zupančič, 2008: 181 [parenthesis removed]). It is this functioning which allows us to laugh at comedy's ability to surprise us with what we already expect, but in an unexpected way.

We can see this 'surprise' in comic sequences, such as mistaken identities where the notion of repetition plays an important role in that, very rarely, is repetition simply an identical reoccurrence. Instead, it is us – the audience – who are often aware of the 'mistake' and subsequently it is the repeated performance of this mistake which makes a particular sequence comical (Zupančič, 2008). Such repetition is also visible in examples of hyperbole, slapstick and double entendre. Certainly, this is not to deny a level of conservatism in the comic performance. As Zupančič highlights, comedy which centres on 'mistaken identities' is frequently denounced as being conservative due to the fact that by the end of the sequence, the mistaken identities are rectified and everything returns to normal: 'it turns the world order upside-down only in order ultimately to reestablish it in its full force, with no cracks to speak of' (2008: 90). Instead, if we consider that, for Zupančič (and Lacan), the Real is impossible (the unpresentable X), then, in her words, 'The

Real as impossible means that there is no right time or place for it' (2003: 177). Here, any antagonism is an excess of the Real, as it is translated and repeated in the symbolic. As a traumatic encounter, it is an impossibility that happens, and this is what makes it traumatic. The significance of comedy is that it is this impossibility which is laid bare.

Consequently, what this discussion has led to is an underlying connection between the Real and comedy's ability to approach this Real via a parallaxical short circuit based upon the minimal difference which underscores comic repetition. As Žižek explains:

> the comic effect proper occurs when, after the act of unveiling, we confront the ridicule and the nullity of the unveiled content: in contrast to the pathetic scene of encountering, behind the veil, the terrifying Thing, too traumatic for our gaze, the ultimate comical effect occurs when, after removing the mask, we confront exactly the same face as the one on the mask. This is why the Marx Brothers' 'This man looks like an idiot and acts like an idiot; but this should not deceive you – he is an idiot!' is properly comical: when, instead of a hidden terrifying secret, we encounter the same thing behind the veil as in front of it, this very lack of difference between the two elements confronts us with the 'pure' difference that separates an element from itself.
>
> *(2006a: 109)*

More importantly, this minimal 'pure' difference, observed through a shift in standpoint, is the Real or, at least, in the case of comedy, our way of engaging with the Real through comedy – a way of 'looking awry' (Žižek, 1991).

It is in this manner that the effects of true comedy occur through a repetition which provides a short circuit (a parallax shift) that is grounded in the surprise we receive when we expect something different, but get the same (Analisi, 2016). Here, 'Comedy does not consist simply in the imaginary One falling apart, splitting into multiplicity or into two' – this describes false comedy, where the concrete and universal remain divided (One into two) – 'but begins only at the moment when we see how these two can precisely not separate or part completely, and become simply "two ones"' (Zupančič, 2008: 78). As a result, 'There is something like an invisible thread that keeps linking them, and it is this very thread that constitutes the true comic object' (Zupančič, 2008: 78).

This 'thread' is comically performed in the ontological inconsistency that underscores our social identities and universal notions. Notably, we see this inconsistency performed when a character contingently embodies a symbolically constructed and universally defined notion (a 'King', 'priest', 'judge', 'President'), without any acknowledgment of the incongruity between their symbolic investment and their actual, concrete, material embodiment. Accordingly, we do not laugh at the baron because he is human, we laugh at the human because he is a baron. Again, to revamp Zupančič's (2008) Bush example: it is when Donald Trump believes he is a US President that he becomes truly comical.

What this discussion has drawn attention to is the importance of examining the formal structure of comedy and, specifically, its material basis. Through the splitting of the One, it is argued that comedy can shed light on the inconsistencies of this materiality, as evident in comedy's repetition of the Real. In the final part of this chapter, attention will turn to exploring this inconsistency in action. First, by examining the difference between the joke and the comic sequence; and second, by exploring the performance of comedy via the comedy character.

The joke and comedy sequence

In her analysis of comedy, Zupančič makes a point of distinguishing between the formal structure of jokes and a performed comedy sequence, with specific attention being afforded to how the two forms of humour maintain a temporal and structural difference. According to Zupančič:

> a joke is always situated (exclusively) in the *instantaneity* of the moment at which its point passes. The pleasure in jokes is instantaneous and very much confined as to its time, which does not mean, however, that it cannot be repeated. If we pass the joke on, it will again produce satisfaction. … We can find pleasure in the same joke only if we change partners. Comic pleasure is different in its temporality: it is not instantaneous, but stretches over a certain lapse of time.
>
> *(2008: 136)*

To help expound upon this distinction, Zupančič draws upon Lacan's Master-Signifier in order to highlight that, when a joke is told, it is the 'punchline' which retroactively determines the joke's narrative. In other words, it is the final statement which emerges from an unexpected place and which subsequently redefines the joke's narrative, causing laughter. For Zupančič, it is this aspect of the joke that gives it a sense of surprise and it is this sense of surprise that 'shed[s] some light on the specific temporal modality of jokes: … In this way, we get a completely different story out of the same elements' (2008: 133). It is these 'same elements' which allow us to consider how the formal structure of the joke echoes the divided One: a One which is retroactively perceived as two. For example, if we consider that, for Critchley (2002a), the joke reveals an incongruity *between* the joke and the social context, imbuing humour with a 'distancing' significance, then it is the release of tension forged in the 'distancing' between the joke and social context which provides 'comic relief'. Alternatively, if we view the significance of the joke as revealing the One divided, then rather than 'distancing' the listener from their social surroundings, what the joke retroactively performs is the division *within* the joke's formal narrative – a 'different story out of the same elements' (Zupančič, 2008: 133). It is this difference which exposes the gap made visible via the joke's parallax effect.

Therefore, while on the one hand, jokes can be distinguished for using Master-Signifiers to help retroactively create a sense of surprise – producing the laughter that occurs when we hear a good joke – on the other hand, the comedy sequence presents a different temporal form. Here, Zupančič elaborates:

> It is very important for the construction of a comic sequence that the signifying objects produced in it, including the comic pleasure that sticks to them, are used as the material and the means of its further construction, not simply released as such. Some could be released as jokes or gags that remain just that, but most have to be kept within the comic field and used as possible passages to further events with which to construct the comic sequence. This is why a series of consecutive jokes and gags, with no inner connection, is not enough to qualify as comedy – it does not fulfill one of the crucial conditions of comedy, … continuity that constructs with discontinuity.
>
> *(2008: 147)*

To this extent, a comic sequence is that which 'holds on' to some 'inner connection' across a particular sequence of events. If we recall that comedy does not confront the Real, but repeats it, then we can begin to see how such repetition forms part of the continuity of the comic sequence, yet one which is forged through its discontinuity. As noted in the previous reference to the comic sequences which involve mistaken identities, such sequences achieve their 'comedy' via a 'surplus *jouissance*' that is produced by the original 'mistake' and which is then discontinuously performed and re-performed (repeated) in various ways over the course of the comic sequence. In contrast to jokes, therefore:

> Master-Signifiers enter the scene of comedy not in order to have the last word, but in order to be repeated there (as well as subjected to other comic techniques). Their repetition is not simply their affirmation. An identical reaction (of a character) repeated ten times necessarily has its repercussions on the stability of the Master-Signifier involved. And the repercussions of this kind of comic repetition usually point not in the direction of stabilizing the repeated position but, rather, in the direction of shaking it.
>
> *(Zupančič, 2008: 177)*

If we consider the sense of 'surprise' that is afforded when one tells a joke – a process that retroactively determines the joke's preceding signifiers, organising them in a different and surprising way – and if we take note of how the comic sequence reveals a continuity through discontinuity – that is, the comic object (in this case, the joke itself) is discontinuously repeated – it is possible to provide a parallaxical account of these two key distinctions: continuity through discontinuity, in the case of jokes, and 'repetition', in the case of the comedy sequence. In fact, whereas for Chow, 'both Freud and Zupančič make the mistake of putting too much emphasis on the punch-line or the new Master-Signifier resolving the void in meaning, rather than retroactively causing us to see the very break in meaning it produces' (2014: 227), it is through a parallaxical perspective that such (dis)continuity can be achieved via the joke's repeated performance in a comic sequence. What the comedy sequence subversively draws attention to is the very void in meaning which is exposed as a discontinuous 'break' in meaning itself. Furthermore, if we consider that such a 'break', 'void' or 'gap' in meaning is brought to light retroactively, then it is also important that we recognise the significance of the Master-Signifier as that 'which designates one's place in the social hierarchy' (Žižek, 2005a: 136). Indeed, it is through such designation that we can draw attention to the subversion of this social hierarchy *in* the comedy character.

The comedy character

> A patient in a large hospital room with many beds complains to the doctor about the constant noise and cries other patients are making, which are driving him crazy. After the doctor replies that nothing can be done if the patients are like that, that one cannot forbid them from expressing their despair since they all know they are dying, the patient goes on: 'Why don't you then put them in a separate room for dying?' The doctor replies calmly and glibly: 'But this is a room for those who are dying...'
>
> *(Žižek, 2005b)*

The above example neatly highlights the self-negativity that underscores the subject's relation to itself. As evident from the story, it is only in 'the final twist [... that] the patient's subjective position is undermined: he finds himself included into the series from which he wanted to maintain distance' (Žižek, 2005b). This same 'realisation' can be found at the end of M. Night Shyamalan's *The Sixth Sense* (1999), where the character Malcolm Crowe (Bruce Willis) suffers a similar realisation.

Notably, this negative self-relation stands opposed to Critchley's (2012) 'positive' (yet, arguably, negative) view of the subject, a subject that emerges from its failed moral sublimation. In much the same way that Zupančič's (2008) Master-Signifier retroactively frames the joke's formal structure, in the above story, the final revelation poses a similar function for the terminal patient, in that their self-negativity or self-estrangement is constitutive of the effects of the Master-Signifier in designating the subject's position in the symbolic order. Accordingly, Žižek details how such designation reveals the 'gap' which is inherent to the subject, the:

> same gap [which] is also exemplified by the two names of the same person. The pope is at the same time Karol Wojtyla and John Paul II: the first name stands for the 'real' person, while the second name designates this same person as the 'infallible' embodiment of the Institution of Church – while the poor Karol can get drunk and babble stupidities, when John Paul speaks, it is the divine spirit itself which speaks through him.
>
> *(2004: 392)*[11]

In this example, we see how any identity and, in the case of the Pope, any position of authority, is 'displaced from itself' (Wood, 2012: 147). Such displacement is what ties the subject to the Real; as that which provides 'a reflexive asymmetry in the world picture' (Wood, 2012: 26). In fact, it is this asymmetry which, following the previous critique of Critchley's (2002a) self/ego stands to present the subject as that which 'always *remains inherently opposed* to the process of ideological subjectivization' (Wood, 2012: 26). This self-relating negativity is not simply an 'imaginary distance towards symbolic identification' (Žižek, 2000b: 259), as the positing of such a distance is the very form in which interpellation can occur (it succeeds by allowing the subject to believe that they are more than *that*) (Žižek, 2000b). Rather, the subject ('barred subject') is 'a dimension of self-relating negativity which a priori eludes the domain of *vécu*, of lived experience' (Žižek, 2000b: 259). This negativity is constitutive of the gap from which 'the self' emerges; a misunderstanding akin to the patient in the hospital (Žižek, 2000b, 2005b).

Key here is the dialectical relation between alienation and separation. That is, while the subject is alienated from their 'being', by way of being barred by language, they are, at the same time, provided a window of opportunity from which their own negation of this process provides a form of separation from the signifier – a separation which locates the subject in the gap itself.[12] It is this alienation-separation which underscores the subject's inherent 'split' or, in accordance with the above discussion on comedy and the One, exposes the subject's 'empty' location within the self-divided social order.[13] Indeed, to help clarify this, we can draw from a literary example, namely Dolar's (1991) consideration of the 'Monster' from Mary Shelley's *Frankenstein*. In the novel:

> the creature created by Frankenstein is a monster without a name, and his basic problem in the novel is precisely that he cannot find his double. It is a creature without filiation or a genealogy, without anybody who would recognize or accept him (not even his creator). His narcissism is thus thwarted from the outset, and the main part of the plot actually springs from his demand for a partner, somebody like him, a wife, so that he could start a line, a new filiation.
>
> *(Dolar, 1991: 16)*

It is the Monster whom bears no inherent split: 'He is One and Unique, and as such he cannot even have a name – *he cannot be represented by a signifier* (which absence is often "spontaneously" filled in by his "father's" name), he cannot be a part of the symbolic' (Dolar, 1991: 16). More to the point, the Monster achieves no *self*-separation to the Other/symbolic order, the Monster is unable 'to present itself as the object of the desire of the Other, an object to fill its lack' (Dolar, 1998: 24), and, as a result, suffers its own form of subjective destitution (the Monster can never ask: 'what am I for the other?'). The Monster is prevented from being provided that which, through a certain symbolic gesture (the act of naming), would retroactively locate the Monster (the subject) in the symbolic order. In doing so,

Dolar (1991) effectively captures the importance of the divided One (the divided subject) and of a whole that is 'not-All' (without exception). In fact, it is the Monster's 'wholeness' which leads to his own played-out frustrations. As a result:

> Whereas the imaginary *ego* functions as a fantasy of unity, the subject as Real is the *gap* of being. The subject in this sense … is the empty place in the symbolic structure; this is why the subject as parallax gap is distinct from the process of symbolic subjectivization and ideological indoctrination.
>
> *(Wood, 2012: 237)*

This 'gap of being' can help elucidate the relationship between the subject and comedy. That is, it is in the comedy character that the inherent contradictions, antagonisms and impasses of the social order are concretely performed. In other words, the comic character is not just a representation of a particular 'fictional' persona, but a performance of the divided subject – of the subject as Real.

For example, if we consider the case of tragedy, then it is apparent that our ability to believe the performance of the actor – their *representation* of a particular persona – is one in which the quality of the actor-subject's performance is tied to the character they play (think of well-known and widely lauded performances such as Robert De Niro *as* Travis Bickle in *Taxi Driver* (1976), or Marlon Brando *as* Colonel Kurtz in *Apocalypse Now* (1979)). In dramatic forms such as tragedy, what we see is:

> an organic fusion or synthesis of the actor-subject and the character precisely because the subject *represents* the character (and the better the representation, the more powerful will be the feeling of a fusion of these two, of the individual and the universal).
>
> *(Zupančič, 2008: 35 [italics added])*

What is key in Zupančič's account is that such performances are 'a fusion of … two' (2008: 35), with the credited actor performing the universal (the 'tragic' character). The actor (concrete) *and* the universal are brought together through a fused coincidence, with the actor's performance measured by their ability to *represent* ('perform') the universal. It is this formal structure which is reflected in instances of false comedy and in those politicians who 'imitate' or represent their own comic selves (Žižek, 2018; Zupančič, 2006, 2008). In the UK, one is reminded of politicians such as Boris Johnson, whose comic persona and various gaffes have proven a formative feature of his *political persona*.

In the case of false comedy, it is the 'lack' which is both acknowledged and performed as part of the performance. As a result, figures of authority can subject themselves to witty, self-depreciations in order to highlight, as McGowan does in relation to a king, 'that he has the ability to appear as a lacking subject in order to prove that he isn't' (2014: 208). In doing so, 'the wittiness functions precisely as a way of distancing oneself from one's own concreteness' (Zupančič, 2008: 33).

These false comedy gestures serve to maintain one's symbolic authority, as evident in 'the White House Correspondents' Dinner, a banquet where authority openly mocks itself' (McGowan, 2014: 208). The dinner is notable for offering the US President a light-hearted opportunity to mock both himself, his office and the Presidential cabinet. The effect of this open mockery, however, is that it never confronts the President's universal symbolic authority, but in satirising the role, serves to maintain its position of authority through a satirical self-distancing. Accordingly, while 'the individual actor *represents* the universal character he plays' (Žižek, 2005b [italics added]), in the same way, the 'comic' US President *represents* a humble, self-mocking, 'everyday' individual (who nonetheless remains a US President). Ultimately, the subject-actor representing the tragic persona and the US President representing a 'normal' person rely upon a synthetic fusion of both the 'real' (human individual) and the symbolic (tragic persona/President).

In contrast, for a true comic character, it is 'in a comedy [that] *he immediately is this character*' (Žižek, 2005b [italics added]). This reveals how 'The comic work takes the hero's position seriously, accepts it, and follows it to the point where it reveals its own absurdity and so destroys itself' (Roche, 2002: 415). Here, the inconsistencies of the universal are repeatedly performed *in* the comic persona (Donougho, 2016), so that in the case of true comedy, 'some universality ("tramp," "worker," "misanthrope"...) has to let a subject in all his concreteness shine through it' (Zupančič, 2008: 37). It is the concrete subject which immediately *is* the universal.

Therefore, it is in the case of the true comedy character that we can trace the subversive significance of the comic character. For example, if 'Authority grants the figure of authority status within the symbolic structure and confers wholeness on this authority', then 'By abandoning the authoritative position of enunciation, one also abandons this recognition and joins the mass of the excluded' (McGowan, 2014: 212–213). It is in such instances that 'one incurs ostracism, vilification, and even condemnation', so that '*One is divided against oneself*' (McGowan, 2014: 213 [italics added]). Moreover, it is this sense of self-division, or self-estrangement, which is enacted in the comedy character, highlighting 'why so few in authority are able to take this step in the direction of a genuinely critical comedy. Critical comedy, authored by an authority figure, costs this figure its authority' (McGowan, 2014: 213).

We can observe examples of this in Ricky Gervais and Stephen Merchant's *Extras* (2005–2007). Through the show's portrayal of 'real' celebrities, as 'surreal, bizarre, and sometimes even tyrannical' (McKenna, 2015: 205), Gervais and Merchant were able to position a number of well-known actors, musicians and television personalities in situations that allowed them to perform exaggerated versions of their celebrity image. In one notable scene from series two, episode four, we watch the show's lead character, Andy Millman (Ricky Gervais), filming a charity appeal advert. After filming his short segment, Chris Martin, lead singer of the band Coldplay, enters the room to film a similar segment. Upon speaking to one of the directors it becomes clear that Martin is only interested in promoting Coldplay's new album, a greatest hits compilation. Accordingly, he asks if the backdrop could contain an image of the new album; he suggests that perhaps Coldplay's music could accompany the advert; and, when told that neither of these suggestions would be possible, he turns to the camera and unbuttons his coat in order to reveal a picture of Coldplay's (fictional) greatest hits album printed on his t-shirt – the words 'out now' clearly visible. The scene is certainly funny, with the segment playing off the fact that, rather than genuinely wishing to help the charity's benefactors, Martin is instead using the opportunity to promote his own music.

Notably, the scene echoes a later Gervais sketch – involving the 'real' Gervais – which was used for the UK's 2007 'Comic Relief' appeal. In the sketch the audience are led to believe that Gervais is filming a short segment in a Kenyan shanty town in order to visit its impoverished inhabitants, who will, pending our donations, benefit from the relief's fundraising (the film's style mimics the format of 'real' charity segment, involving celebrities who visit the world's impoverished areas). It is here that we meet 'Daniel' a resident of the shanty town. However, once the director shouts 'cut' it becomes clear that Gervais is in a film studio, with a green-screen, and hasn't actually visited Kenya. Again, much like the Chris Martin scene, it becomes evident that Gervais is using the opportunity to promote his own celebrity image. In what follows, Brassett notes how:

> Ricky ironically suggests that he is one of the world's greatest living comedians. He claims *The Office* 'changed the genre' and compares himself favourably to John Cleese. He finishes with the suggestion of what people at home will think of him: 'hold on though, we love everything he's done, but has he got a heart of gold? *He's in Africa, the answer is yes!…* If he's doing that then we'll continue to buy his DVDs'. Convinced of the argument, Steven Merchant decides to take part in the video. Then Jamie Olivier – who 'hasn't been seen on TV caring about anything for at least 3 days' – also joins in. The progress is completed when Ricky sees a 'homeless' 'smack-head' that turns out to be Sir Bob Geldof. While Geldof initially describes it as a 'fucking disgrace', he is eventually persuaded to take part because he has a single coming out. When filming is finished, Daniel takes off his mask to reveal that he is in fact Bono, dressed up as an African, attempting to promote the U2 singles album which is coming out.
>
> *(2009: 238)*

For Brassett, 'the interventions of Ricky Gervais in campaigns like Comic Relief and Make Poverty History' present a form of 'irony [which] serves as a vital and creative resource for thinking through the "limits" of global ethics, on a mass public stage' (Brassett, 2009: 237).

While such scenes clearly highlight the 'limits' of global ethics, it is, unfortunately, through such 'ironic' gestures that the subversive significance of these scenes is undermined. Indeed, what becomes evident, in both the Gervais and Martin scenes, is the ways in which a number of famous celebrities are *performing* a comic version of themselves, in much the same way that certain politicians (Bush, Johnson) perform their 'comic' selves. In the case of Martin, we have Chris Martin, the real musician, *and* Chris Martin, the exaggerated comic persona. The scene's comedy relies upon him representing a comic persona that maintains a clear separation between the 'real' Chris Martin and the 'fake' Chris Martin. In fact, once completed, the real Chris Martin can walk off set, safe in the knowledge that his 'satirical' performance leaves the 'real' subject intact (even Chris Martin can have a laugh at himself).

If we compare this to those comic performances which rely upon certain 'generic' character types, such as Chaplin's Tramp, then it is apparent that although the 'character is perfectly stereotypical and has been seen hundreds of times … at the same time it would be hard to find something more concrete, subjective, and universal in the same gesture as precisely the Tramp' (Zupančič, 2008: 37). It is here that Zupančič (2008) draws attention to the character of 'Borat', played by the British comedian, Sacha Baron Cohen. Zupančič highlights how:

> Borat is … a good example of the fact that comic characters are not simply represented by (different) actors, and that their link goes 'beyond representation' in the usual sense of the term: it reminds us that it is by no means uncommon for comic characters (actors) to carry on with their 'act' beyond the fictional framework (stage, movie) to which they belong. The promotion tour of Borat was done by Borat himself. This made it much more effective (and appropriate) than a promotion in which Sacha Baron Cohen talked about (t)his character, about how and why he created it, and thus posited himself as the subject behind Borat. On the other hand, it is rather difficult to imagine, say, a promotion of a new production of Hamlet being done by Hamlet himself, that is to say, by the actor carrying on as Hamlet in the 'outside' world.
>
> *(2008: 38, f/n 3)*

Indeed, what we observe in Borat is a sublimation between the actor and their comic persona, whereby the 'gap' is transposed into the comic character. It is in such instances that 'we cannot say that the subject-actor *represents* a (comic) character for the spectator' – this would reflect the actor's performance of a character in tragedy – 'but that the subject-actor *appears* as that gap through which the character relates to itself, "representing itself"' (Zupančič, 2008: 35 [italics added]).

Such a 'relating to itself' can be seen in various instances where comic characters 'break the fourth wall'. In fact, 'breaking the fourth wall' is not unique to TV sitcoms, with the tactic being seen in the comedy series *Fleabag* (2016–2019), where the lead character, 'Fleabag' (note, we are never given a 'real' human name), frequently glances at, speaks to and acknowledges the camera ('us', the audience). Over the course of the series we learn that this camera-acknowledgment forms part of the character's own psychic estrangement as she comes to terms with the death of her best friend and the guilt that she suffers by playing a part in her death. What is significant, however, is that it is *in* the performance of the comic character 'Fleabag' that we observe the subject's self-estrangement, as demonstrated in the following example from Žižek:

> Recall the immortal Lucy from *I Love Lucy* whose trademark gesture when something surprised her was to bend her neck slightly and cast a direct fixed gaze of surprise into the camera – this was not Lucille Ball, the actress, mockingly addressing the public, but an attitude of self-estrangement that was part of 'Lucy' (as a screen persona) herself.
>
> *(2006a: 106 [parenthesis removed])*

Notably, *in* the comic performance of Lucy, we do not get Lucille Ball *and* Lucy, but 'Lucy' as a 'pure difference', as that which separates herself *from* herself. Therefore, if we follow the Lacanian contention that the subject is marked by an inherent lack, which, for Žižek (1998), is what constitutes the subject as Real, then, in the case of comedy, it is this lack/'gap' which appears through the character's concrete materiality and which reflects the subject's self-estrangement within a symbolic order that, nevertheless, serves to designate the subject's position (Zupančič, 2008). This endows comedy a level of efficacy which 'exposes the incompleteness of the social order and of the subject who exists within this order' (McGowan, 2014: 205). This incompleteness, or lack, is excessively performed *in* the comedy character (McGowan, 2017).

To return to Zupančič's (2008) use of the concrete universal, it is here that we can begin to outline how, through a parallax shift, comedy allows us to view the inherent inconsistencies, antagonisms and impasses which structure the subject and symbolic order. In the case of true comedy, it is not 'the ridiculous contingencies of our earthly existence' which are performed, but rather 'the full assertion of universality, the immediate coincidence of universality with the character's/actor's singularity' (Žižek, 2006a: 107). This 'immediate coincidence' is reflected in the division of the One, so 'that what the universal and the individual share is the very split or ontological difference that runs through both of them' (Wood, 2012: 38). Rather than 'exist[ing] in a separate transcendent realm', true comedy reveals that 'It is only when universality becomes embodied or enacted within a physical being that it actually becomes universality' (McGowan, 2017: 61). It is here that our 'humanness' stems from our ability to concretely perform abstract universals, comically. That is, it is not the 'human' – the baron, the miser, the local wide-boy entrepreneur, or the US President – which is brought back 'down to earth' by the concrete puddle, banana skin, countertop or witty remark, but the symbolic identities and universal notions that humans perform in all their ridiculousness. It is the 'true' comedy character who embodies the abstract universal in their own concrete actions.

In the following chapter, it will be considered how the Real and the concrete universal can be brought to bear in examples of comedy which seek to build a shared sense of obscene solidarity with the other. What should be drawn from this chapter, however, is the extent to which comedy can subversively present the universal at work (Zupančič, 2008). In the case of racist jokes and their associated racist meanings, this can offer a unique way of exploring comedy's subversive potential.

Notes

1 For such a discussion, I recommend Berger (2014).
2 See also Karlsen and Villadsen (2015).
3 This is brought to bear when we consider those 'who identify themselves entirely with some social a priori (without having leapt over the abyss) [and who] are incapable of laughing and crying' (Heller, 2005: 201).
4 Hegel (1998) situates his discussion of comedy in his section on art, religion and other dramatic forms, including 'epic' and 'tragedy'. Hegel (2004) also considers comedy in relation to the development of art in his Aesthetic lectures (see Roche, 1998). Yet, it is in the *Phenomenology* that Hegel provides a dialectical reading of comedy. This approach, as will be shown, bears particular significance to the work of both Zupančič and Žižek.
5 See also Pound (2010, 2015) and Zupančič (2008).
6 See also Dean (2006), McMillan (2013) and Sharpe and Boucher (2010).
7 Later, this discussion will be supplemented with McGowan's (2018) assertion that such a universal echoes Lacan's notion of the Master-Signifier. Importantly, for Laclau (2000), the empty signifier is the universal, it stands for the universal: 'the metonymic act that substitutes a particularity for universality is also how a group becomes representative of broader society, and therefore achieves hegemonic status' (Salter, 2016: 121).
8 See also Freud (2003).
9 This particular scene goes as follows: 'a toffee-nosed baron slips on a banana peel (thus demonstrating that even he is subject to the laws of gravity), yet the next instant he is up again and walking around arrogantly, no less sure of the highness of His High-ness, until the next accident that will again try to "ground" him, and so on and so on' (Zupančič, 2008: 29).
10 This non-coincidence of the One works in contrast to those considerations which view the ontological foundations of reality as grounded in multiplicity (Deleuze and Guattari, 2004).
11 Wojtyla was Pope John Paul II from 1978 to 2005.
12 Verhaeghe elaborates on this process, noting that 'The important thing about the subject is that it has no essence, no ontological substance. Its production is by the signifiers, coming from the field of the Other, but it would be a mistake to assume that a subject is identical to the produced signifier(s). A fixed identification with several signifiers presents us with the ego. In this sense, the Lacanian subject is exactly the opposite of the Cartesian one. In the formula "I think, therefore I am" Descartes concludes from his thinking that he has a being, whereas for Lacan, each time (conscious) thinking arises, its being disappears under the signifier' (Verhaeghe, 2018: 375).
13 This self-division is reflected in the subject, which is itself divided (Žižek, 2008b).

References

Analisi, S. 2016. Comedy, repetition and racial stereotypes on television. *Cinergie*, 9, 103–116.

Apocalypse Now. 1979. Film. United Artists.

Bakhtin, M. 1984. *Rabelais and His World*. Bloomington, NI: Indiana University Press.

Baumann, C. 2011. Adorno, Hegel and the concrete universal. *Philosophy & Social Criticism*, 37 (1), 73–94.

Benhabib, S. 2018. Below the asphalt lies the beach [online]. *Entkunstung*. Available from: https://entkunstung.com/below-the-asphalt-lies-the-beach [Accessed 5 January 2019].

Berger, P. L. 2014. *Redeeming Laughter: The Comic Dimension of Human Experience*, 2nd edn. Berlin, Germany: De Gruyter.

Bergson, H. L. 2008. *Laughter: An Essay on the Meaning of the Comic*. Rockville, MD: Wildside Press.

Bonic, N. 2011. Psychoanalysis and comedy: The (im)possibility of changing the socio-symbolic order. *S: Journal of the Jan Van Eyck Circle for Lacanian Ideology Critique*, 4, 91–108.

Brassett, J. 2009. British irony, global justice: A pragmatic reading of Chris Brown, Banksy and Ricky Gervais. *Review of International Studies*, 35, 219–245.

Brassett, J. and Sutton, A. 2017. British satire, everyday politics: Chris Morris, Armando Iannucci and Charlie Brooker. *British Journal of Politics and International Relations*, 19 (2), 245–262.

Chow, B. 2014. The tickling object: On Žižek and comedy. In: B. Chow and A. Mangold, eds. *Žižek and Performance*. Basingstoke: Palgrave Macmillan, 224–252.

City Lights. 1931. Film. United Artists.

Critchley, S. 2002a. *On Humour*. London: Routledge.

Critchley, S. 2002b. Did you hear the one about the philosopher writing a book on humour? *Think*, 1 (2), 103–112.

Critchley, S. 2009. *Ethics-Politics-Subjectivity: Essays on Derrida, Levinas and Contemporary French Thought*. London: Verso.

Critchley, S. 2012. *Infinitely Demanding: Ethics of Commitment, Politics of Resistance*. London: Verso.

Daly, G. 2010. Causes for concern: Žižek's politics of loving terror. *The International Journal of Žižek Studies*, 4 (2), 1–23.

Dean, J. 2006. *Žižek's Politics*. New York, NY: Routledge.

Deleuze, G. and Guattari, F. 2004. *Anti-Oedipus: Capitalism and Schizophrenia*. London: Continuum.

Derek. 2012–2014. TV Series. Channel 4.

Do the Right Thing. 1989. Film. Universal Pictures.

Dolar, M. 1991. 'I shall be with you on your wedding-night': Lacan and the uncanny. *October*, 58, 5–23.

Dolar, M. 1998. Cogito as the subject of the unconscious. In: S. Žižek, ed. *Cogito and the Unconscious: Sic 2*. Durham, NC: Duke University Press, 11–40.

Dolar, M. 2005. Comedy and its double. In R. Pfaller, ed. *Schluss mit der Komödie!/Stop That Comedy!*Vienna: Sonderzahl, 181–210.

Dolar, M. 2012. One divided into two. *e-flux*, 33, 1–12.

Donougho, M. 2016. Hegelian comedy. *Philosophy and Rhetoric*, 49 (2), 196–220.

Duck Soup. 1933. Film. Paramount Pictures.

Extras. 2005–2007. TV Series. BBC Two; BBC One; HBO.

Fleabag. 2016–2019. TV Series. BBC Three; BBC Two; BBC One.

Freud, S. 2003. *The Joke and its Relation to the Unconscious*, trans. Joyce Crick. London: Penguin.

Garcia, G. I. and Sanchez, C. G. A. 2008. Psychoanalysis and politics: The theory of ideology in Slavoj Žižek. *The International Journal of Žižek Studies*, 2 (3). Available from: https://zizekstudies.org/index.php/IJZS/issue/view/9 [Accessed 30 November 2020].

Giappone, K. B. R. 2018. *The Punk Turn in Comedy: Masks of Anarchy*. Gewerbestrasse, Switzerland: Palgrave Macmillan.

Hegel, G. W. F. 1998. *Phenomenology of the Spirit*, trans. A. V. Miller. Delhi, India: Motilal Banarsidass Publishers.

Hegel, G. W. F. 2004. *Introductory Lectures on Aesthetics*. London: Penguin.

Hegel, G. W. F. 2010. *The Science of Logic*. Cambridge: Cambridge University Press.

Heller, A. 2005. *Immortal Comedy: The Comic Phenomenon in Art, Literature, and Life*. Lanham, MD: Lexington Books.

Kamm, J. and Neumann, B. 2016. Introduction: The aesthetics and politics of British TV comedy. In: J. Kamm and B. Neumann, eds. *British TV Comedies: Cultural Concepts, Contexts and Controversies*. Basingstoke: Palgrave Macmillan, 1–22.

Kant, I. 2007. *Critique of Judgement*. New York, NY: Cosimo.

Kapoor, I. 2018. Žižek, antagonism and politics now: Three recent controversies. *The International Journal of Žižek Studies*, 12 (1), 1–31.

Karlsen, M. P. and Villadsen, K. 2015. Laughing for real? Humour, management power and subversion. *Ephemera: Theory & Politics in Organization*, 15 (3), 513–535.

Kisner, W. 2008. The concrete and universal in Hegel and Žižek. *The International Journal of Žižek Studies*, 2 (2), 1–35.

Kottman, P. A. 2008. Slipping on banana peels, tumbling into wells: Philosophy and comedy. *Diacritics*, 38 (4), 3–14.

Kunkle, S. 2012. Embracing the paradox: Žižek's illogical logic. *International Journal of Žižek Studies*, 2 (4). Available from: http://zizekstudies.org/index.php/IJZS/issue/view/10 [Accessed 30 November 2020].

Laclau, E. 2000. Identity and hegemony: The role of universality in the constitution of political logics. In: J. Butler, E. Laclau and S. Žižek, eds. *Contingency, Hegemony, Universality: Contemporary Dialogues on the Left*. London: Verso, 44–89.

Ladegaard, J. 2014. Laughing matters: Four Marxist takes on film comedy. In: E. Mazierska and L. Kristensen, eds. *Marx at the Movies: Revisiting History, Theory and Practice*. Basingstoke: Palgrave Macmillan, 102–122.

Ladegaard, J. 2017. The comedy of terrors: Ideology and comedy in Marlowe's *Doctor Faustus*. *Textual Practice*, 31 (1), 179–195.

Little Britain. 2003–2006. TV Series. BBC Three; BBC One.

Mangold, A. 2014. Introduction: Performing Žižek: Hegel, Lacan, Marx, and the parallax view. In: B. Chow and A. Mangold, eds. *Žižek and Performance*. Basingstoke: Palgrave Macmillan, 1–12.

McGowan, T. 2014. The barriers to a critical comedy. *Crisis and Critique*, 1 (3), 201–221.

McGowan, T. 2016. The location of silent comedy: Charlie Chaplin's outsider and Buster Keaton's insider. *Quarterly Review of Film and Video*, 33 (7), 602–619.

McGowan, T. 2017. *Only a Joke Can Save Us: A Theory of Comedy*. Evanston, IL: Northwestern University Press.

McGowan, T. 2018. The absent universal: From the Master Signifier to the missing signifier. *Problemi International*, 2 (2), 195–214.

McKenna, T. 2015. *Art, Literature and Culture from a Marxist Perspective*. Basingstoke: Palgrave Macmillan.

McMillan, C. 2013. *Žižek and Communist Strategy: On the Disavowed Foundations of Global Capitalism*. Edinburgh: Edinburgh University Press.

Modern Times. 1936. Film. United Artists.

Monty Python and the Holy Grail. 1975. Film. EMI Films; Cinema 5.

Moolenaar, R. 2004. Slavoj Žižek and the real subject of politics. *Studies in Eastern European Thought*, 56, 259–297.

Morreall, J. 1982. A new theory of laughter. *Philosophical Studies*, 42 (2), 243–254.

Murphy, P. 2006. The comic agon-comedy and philosophy. *Budhi: A Journal of Ideas and Culture*, 10 (3), 61–77.

Newswipe with Charlie Brooker. 2009–2010. TV Series. BBC Four.

Nikulin, D. 2014. *Comedy, Seriously: A Philosophical Study*. New York, NY: Palgrave Macmillan.

Only Fools and Horses. 1981–2003. TV Series. BBC One.

Pound, M. 2010. Comic subjectivity: Žižek and Zupančič's spiritual work of art. *The International Journal of Žižek Studies*, 4 (4). Available from: http://zizekstudies.org/index.php/IJZS/issue/view/20 [Accessed 30 November 2020].

Pound, M. 2015. Political theology and comedy: Žižek through rose tinted glasses. *Crisis and Critique*, 2 (1), 171–191.

Roche, M. W. 1998. *Tragedy and Comedy: A Systematic Study and a Critique of Hegel*. New York, NY: State University of New York Press.

Roche, M. W. 2002. Hegel's theory of comedy in the context of Hegelian and modern reflections on comedy. *Revue Internationale De Philosophie*, 3 (221), 411–430.

Salter, L. 2016. Populism as a fantasmatic rupture in the post-political order: Integrating Laclau with Glynos and Stavrakakis, Kōtuitui. *New Zealand Journal of Social Sciences Online*, 11 (2), 116–132.

Sharpe, M. and Boucher, G. 2010. *Žižek and Politics: A Critical Introduction*. Edinburgh: Edinburgh University Press.

Shepherdson, C. 1995. History and the Real: Foucault with Lacan. *Postmodern Culture*, 5 (2). doi: doi:10.1353/pmc.1995.0015.

Stern, R. 1997. Hegel, British idealism, and the curious case of the concrete universal. *British Journal for the History of Philosophy*, 15 (1), 115–153.

Swabey, M. C. 1961. *Comic Laughter: A Philosophical Essay*. New Haven, CT: Yale University Press.

Taxi Driver. 1976. Film. Columbia Pictures.

Terada, R. 2014. Universal/particular. In: R. Butler, ed. *The Žižek Dictionary*. London: Routledge.

The Silence of the Lambs. 1991. Film. Orion Pictures.

The Sixth Sense. 1999. Film. Buena Vista Pictures Distribution.

Thorn, R. 2016. Why toilets are a battleground for transgender rights [online]. *BBC*. Available from: www.bbc.co.uk/news/uk-england-36395646 [Accessed 7 March 2019].

Verhaeghe, P. 2018. Lacan's answer to alienation: Separation. *Crisis and Critique*, 6 (1), 365–388.

Westwood, R. 2004. Comic relief: Subversion and catharsis in organizational comedic theatre. *Organization Studies*, 25 (5), 775–795.

Wood, K. 2012. *Žižek: A Reader's Guide*. Chichester: Wiley-Blackwell.

Zimeri, S. 2010. Slavoj Žižek on the dialectic of the universal and the particular [online]. Available from: https://filosofisksupplement.no/wp-content/uploads/2010-slavoj-Žižek-dialectic-universal-particular.pdf [Accessed 4 March 2019].

Žižek, S. 1991. *Looking Awry: An Introduction to Jacques Lacan through Popular Culture*. Cambridge, MA: MIT Press.

Žižek, S. 1998. *Tarrying with the Negative: Kant, Hegel, and the Critique of Ideology*. Durham, NC: Duke University Press.

Žižek, S. 2000a. Class struggle or postmodernism? Yes, please! In: J. Butler, E. Laclau and S. Žižek, eds. *Contingency, Hegemony, Universality: Contemporary Dialogues on the Left*. London: Verso, 90–135.

Žižek, S. 2000b. *The Ticklish Subject: The Absent Centre of Political Ontology*. London: Verso.

Žižek, S. 2004. The structure of domination today: A Lacanian view. *Studies in Eastern European Thought*, 56, 383–403.

Žižek, S. 2005a. *Iraq: The Borrowed Kettle*. London: Verso.

Žižek, S. 2005b. The Christian-Hegelian comedy. *Cabinet Magazine*. Available from: www.cabinetmagazine.org/issues/17/Žižek.php [Accessed 10 March 2019].

Žižek, S. 2006a. *The Parallax View*. Cambridge, MA: The MIT Press.

Žižek, S. 2006b. Preface to the paperback edition: The big other between violence and civility. In: R. Butler and S. Stephens, eds. *Slavoj Žižek: The Universal Exception*. London: Continuum, vii–xxxii.

Žižek, S. 2006c. Why we all love to hate Haider. In: R. Butler and S. Stephens, eds. *Slavoj Žižek: The Universal Exception*. London: Continuum, 33–41.

Žižek, S. 2006d. *How to Read Lacan*. London: Granta Books.

Žižek, S. 2008a. *The Sublime Object of Ideology*. London: Verso.

Žižek, S. 2008b. *The Plague of Fantasies*. London: Verso.

Žižek, S. 2010. *Living in the End Times*. London: Verso.

Žižek, S. 2012. *Less Than Nothing: Hegel and the Shadow of Dialectical Materialism*. London: Verso.

Žižek, S. 2015. *Absolute Recoil: Towards a New Foundation of Dialectical Materialism*. London: Verso.

Žižek, S. 2017. *In Defense of Lost Causes*. London: Verso.

Žižek, S. 2018. *Like a Thief in Broad Daylight: Power in the Era of Post-Humanity*. London: Allen Lane.

Zupančič, A. 2003. *The Shortest Shadow: Nietzsche's Philosophy of the Two*. Cambridge, MA: MIT Press.

Zupančič, A. 2006. The 'concrete universal', and what comedy can tell us about it. In: S. Žižek, ed. *Lacan: The Silent Partners*. London: Verso, 171–197.

Zupančič, A. 2008. *The Odd One In: On Comedy*. Cambridge, MA: MIT Press.

3

COMEDY, RACE AND RACISM

Television, comedy and race

Since the end of the Second World War, British television schedules have played host to a wide variety of comedies that have sought to draw upon social anxieties regarding 'race', ethnicity and cultural difference. Beginning in the late 1960s and continuing throughout the 1970s, sitcoms such as *Curry and Chips* (1969), *Love Thy Neighbour* (1972–1976) and the previously mentioned *Till Death* served to portray the UK's changing social dynamics through a genre that proved adept at representing the everyday realities of immigration and cultural diversity within the UK. Though these characters and storylines would help provide ethnic minority groups some form of representation on television, many would remain indebted to stereotypical depictions and cultural clichés. Indeed, these tensions have continued throughout contemporary discussions on race, racism and the use of cultural stereotypes in British comedy.

Certainly, while many comedians would confidently deride the use of open racism (Quirk, 2018), a number of well-known British comedians have frequently criticised the extent to which Acts of Parliament, such as the Racial and Religious Hatred Act (2006), seek to infringe upon the civil liberties of the public (Kamm and Neumann, 2016). Notably, when these criticisms are not directed at specific Acts of Parliament, they inevitably resort to derisions of political correctness (Buchanan, 2014). As a result, attempts to regulate or censure celebrated TV comedies often become enveloped within debates on political correctness and the impact of its commanding dictates. Kamm and Neumann assert:

> There is arguably a grave danger involved in policing TV comedies in whatever fashion because they are artistic in the sense that they lend expression and

> give a voice to dispositions and anxieties at the time of production, which although 'edgy and quite hard-hitting' expose such tensions to laughter.
>
> *(2016: 16)*

Nevertheless, it is clear that such limits and their transgression are historically relative, with certain comedies being retroactively censored. In 2013, an episode of *Fawlty Towers* had a line depicting the difference between 'Niggers' and 'Wogs' removed (Kamm and Neumann, 2016).

Accordingly, while the case of *Fawlty Towers* serves to expose how examples of racism have been used in a number of well-known comedy storylines, in other instances, the representation of ethnic minorities posits a far more ambiguous framing. Here, the ambiguity of certain racial stereotypes can both assert as well as undermine racial prejudices (Norris, 2014). In this respect, the representation of race in comedy tends to revolve around the use of racist stereotypes to either support racist views, via generalisations that seek to characterise a particular ethnicity, or through examples that seek to undermine these stereotypes by drawing attention to the inherent contradictions that inevitably limit such generalisations. In fact, for British comedian Stewart Lee, 'the exploration of boundaries, of social limits and their transgression in comedies is and has always been at the core of the genre' (Kamm and Neumann, 2016: 15).

These boundaries would prove integral to the popularity of *Till Death* with its depictions of cultural/racial differences being used to comment upon the UK's post-war racial diversity. Here, Bebber (2014) details how particular scenes would often involve the black or Pakistani character making a reverse comment directed towards Alf which was subsequently used to emphasise his racial prejudice (of greater concern here was the fact that the Pakistani character was played by a white actor). Accordingly, by turning Alf's racism against him, these scenes 'had the overall effect of hardening the notion of racial difference … and more fundamentally, of naturalizing the use of racial epithets among all Britons' (Bebber, 2014: 265). Reflecting a form of reverse racism (Weaver, 2010), such remarks could encourage 'mutual mistrust' between ethnic groups, eliciting encounters grounded in an aggressive animosity and potential violence.

To this extent, the use of offensive language 'to supposedly highlight ignorance can too often be used as way to reassert old traditions under an often opaque, protective shell' (Norris, 2014: 97).[1] Drawing upon the work of Medhurst and Tuck (1996), Norris details how:

> In … sitcom this practice simultaneously can offer both regressive and progressive areas of discourse, which admittedly may reinforce dominant ideologies and stage minorities for their comic value alone, but can also work as a valuable processing space for communities and creates a necessary visibility for marginal presences
>
> *(2014: 88)*

In such instances, the use of stereotypes can support forms of ironic commentary, which, 'as a well-intentioned response to political correctness' can 'backfire through an unnuanced reading or simply be over-ridden by the offence caused when weighed against the cultural history of a particularly tired construct' (Norris, 2014: 107).

Yet, to simply censure certain jokes and comic performances on the grounds of political correctness can result in reactionary forms that deliberately seek to undermine such regulations in favour of a return to ignorance. With regards to the British comedian Roy Chubby Brown, Quirk notes how:

> [Brown's] freedom to joke is given priority over more politically correct sensibilities that might try to rectify wider societal power imbalances. Brown's comments are typical of the mind-set that his 'old school' tribe brought to the justification of their work: a joke is a joke, not a political act, and the ability to say what you like in the context of joking is held sacred.
>
> *(2018: 29)*

In her analysis, Quirk (2018) highlights how Chubby Brown's disdain for the institutionalisation of political correctness was justified by his incitement of 'working-class' frustrations steered towards those political elites, whose desire to promote political correctness was reinforced by their position as benefactors of neoliberal globalisation and their cosmopolitan outlook. What remains significant, however, is that these same frustrations could also be found in the comic sketches of the Oxbridge-educated Harry Thompson and Shaun Pye (writers of the animated comedy *Monkey Dust*). In their series, Thompson and Pye took aim at the political establishment as well as 'taboo' topics, such as pedophilia, bestiality and suicide, as well as satirically commenting upon contemporary issues including immigration, terrorism, and a popular culture driven by celebrity and hyper-commercialisation.

To this end, whether one attempts to intentionally de-politicise politically incorrect humour by telling a racist joke in an ironic fashion, or if one refrains from the racist joke altogether, in both cases one is left with a form of ignorance that either overlooks the joke's racist significance, or alternatively seeks to bury it. In either case, we lose the subversive potential of comedy. Whereas the intention in this study is not to assume nor promote the victimisation of those groups who are believed to be ridiculed by certain stereotypes (to a certain extent, the comedy in *Till Death* is unique in its ability to subvert the minority-as-victim trope), what can be considered is the inherent ambivalences and underlying ambiguities which underscore comedy's formal structure. Indeed, while it has been argued that certain stereotypes are grounded in a level of 'truth' (Brown, 1995), it is not necessarily the case that these stereotypes should be proven as either 'true' or 'false', but rather that specific attention should be given to the *ways* in which these 'truths' are stereotypically employed and to the cultural and/or personal idiosyncrasies which they reveal. In this sense, the performance of certain stereotypes can be subversively used to highlight the inner ridiculousness of any stereotype which is subsequently attributed to a specific group, but also, at the same time, proves idiosyncratically reflective of that group's sense of difference. It is in this way that analyses of comedy can follow a process of identifying those inherent inconsistencies and forms of failure which underscore relations with the other.

Accordingly, in contrast to Lockyer and Pickering's contention that 'when a joke is critically evaluated as sexist or racist, by definition, the joke fails and becomes severely devalued as comic discourse' (2008: 811), this chapter will provide specific attention to identifying those 'racist' elements that underscore certain comic performances, and which, while deliberately drawing upon racial stereotypes, serve to 'devalue' these stereotypes as part of the comic performance. To do so, a brief consideration of the comedy of Sacha Baron Cohen and his Ali G and Borat personas will help provide some 'comic context' to the present chapter.

Ali G: A comedy parallax

Sacha Baron Cohen, and his comic portrayal of the fictional characters Ali G and Borat, offers a clear example of the concrete universal in action. With regard to the character Borat, Zupančič (2008) details how, in one episode, Borat enters a gun store in the US and asks the store owner whether the gun he is presented with is good at killing Jews (Borat is a fictional Kazakhstan Muslim). In such instances, Borat does not challenge us to 'laugh' at the act of killing Jews or even of US gun laws, but rather his comedy comes from his complete acting out of US gun law – the immediate concrete performance of an abstract universal that invariably constitutes US society ('the right to bear arms' remains the Second Amendment to the United States Constitution). Borat does not encourage 'us to laugh at the seriousness with which we take our own codes, precepts, values and beliefs' (Littlewood and Pickering, 1998: 291), but instead seriously *performs* these 'codes, precepts, values and beliefs' in all their concrete and comic ridiculousness.

Indeed, Cohen's comedy has sought to blur and even 'mongrelize' racial classifications, most notably in the character Ali G (Gilroy, 2004). Cohen's performances can be, and have been, considered 'racist', as evident in his performance of certain racial stereotypes (Brockes, 2016; Gibson, 2000). Accordingly, though 'Baron Cohen has altered the terrain on which British comedy interacts with racial representation', Weaver asks whether:

> On the one hand, Baron Cohen has reintroduced race into the mainstream, in a not unproblematic way. On the other hand, through the complexity, irony and multiplicity of the material, perhaps he has advanced cultural criticism, which will make older forms of race representation in comedy far less likely to appear.
>
> *(2011: 262)*

To this end, there was in the Ali G performance a 'complex layering [... to] his persona' (Lockyer and Pickering, 2008: 815). This complexity:

> revolved around the question of who was impersonating whom in the Ali G persona and whether this subverted or perpetuated the possibilities of black stereotyping. Was Ali G a white, Jewish, or Asian wannabe? Alternatively, was he a white man pretending to be an Asian pretending to be black, or a Jewish man pretending to be an Asian pretending to be a white man pretending to be black?
>
> *(Lockyer and Pickering, 2008: 815)*

Notice how a parallaxical understanding of the contravening interpretations that are appropriated to the character Ali G are brought to bear in the contradiction between Cohen's problematic reintroducing of race *and* his ability to advance cultural criticism. While for Lockyer and Pickering (2008), the Ali G character was clearly ambiguous in his ethnic impersonations, their proposed questions emphasise how the character served to embody these differences as part of his comic display. Ali G was neither one thing nor another, but rather served as a conduit – a divided One – through which the UK's multicultural differences and inconsistencies could be performed.

What emerges from discussions on Cohen's comedy is the way in which he 'surprisingly' acknowledges racial distinctions, both performing them and, in many ways, distorting them (Alonso, 2016; Gilroy, 2004; Weaver, 2011). One could even venture the assertion that the man from Staines (UK), who loves his 'Julie' and smoking his 'herb', was, in the accompanying film, *Ali G Indahouse* (2002), a better proponent of the UK's cultural diversity, especially when compared to the pompous politicians that he encountered during his time in Westminster politics. Gilroy highlights:

> Ali G was not homophobic, macho, aggressive, or antisocial. He obeyed the speed limit, believed in the healing power of God's green herb, and had identified the terminal duplicity of all forms of politricks. He was loyal, decent, and honest. When punched by Charles Dance's repellent deputy prime minister, his response is to cry. These admirable qualities were entirely lost on the positive-image school of cultural critique.
>
> *(2004: 146)*

Notably, there was nothing 'new' in Cohen's performances, not in the sense that what he performed was 'novel', but rather was simply a 'repeated' version of the UK's already existing multiculture. As a result, he performed (or, spectacularised), quite literately, the spectre of race in its most unshielded and Real form. Again, in comments echoing the self-estrangement of the comedy character (discussed in Chapter Two), Gilroy notes:

> I have no doubt that many people would also have been laughing at what Ali G showed us about British culture. They laughed louder and longer because he revealed it to be alien, eccentric, and absurd in its snobbery, stupidity, and perverse attachment to numerous forms of destructive hierarchy – class, race, religion. Those dismal qualities were not being exposed from the outside by a stranger but explored from the inside in a daring act of patriotic love. By imagining himself as a stranger in his own country, Ali G refined a systematic estrangement from local habits and turned it into an art.
>
> *(2004: 149)*

However, rather than acknowledging Ali G's exposition of Britain's post-imperial culture, criticisms of Cohen vehemently admonished his performances, with many denunciations suggesting that his displays offered a covert portrayal of political incorrectness (BBC, 2002; Campbell, 2017; Elsworth, 2006; Saunders, 2007; Waxman, 2007; Weaver, 2011). In light of these criticisms, we can ask: did Cohen get too close to those 'ethnic' attributes that the multicultural subject seeks to keep hidden? Rather than simply *respecting*, did Cohen cross a line when he performed these differences? And, if so, what were the cultural differences that he was performing?

In view of such questions, what Cohen's performances emphasise – in fact, what was built into them – was the fundamental negativity at the heart of identity and of the antagonistic split at the heart of the One. In doing so, Ali G rendered precisely the fundamental antagonism which both structures and underscores our understandings of difference. This was achieved by deliberately performing and undermining those cultural distinctions that symbolically framed the very notion of cultural difference (Kapoor, 2018). With regard to these differences, the following chapter will pay specific consideration to examining how this inherent negativity forms a constitutive feature of social interaction and, in light of wider analyses on race, racism and political correctness, can allow us to re-approach the study of race as it pertains to comedy.

Seeing 'race'

As touched upon in the above introduction, Žižek's ideological critique lays claim to the notion that 'there exists a "spectral" underside of ideology …, which more forcefully attaches the subject to the symbolic surface of ideological propositions' (Flisfeder and Willis, 2014: 10). While this line of inquiry is extended in Žižek's (2008a) application of Lacan's *objet a*, as well as his work on fantasy (Žižek, 2008b), for present purposes, it is suggested that this '"spectral" underside of ideology' can be effectively rendered in critical interpretations of political correctness, race and racism (Flisfeder and Willis, 2014: 10). In particular, it can allow us to examine how the persistence of race and racism remains situated 'in the unavoidable human practice of classifying and discriminating kinds of things' (Mitchell, 2012: 38).

Certainly, this does not suggest that we simply accept race as an uncontested 'pseudoscientific illusion' (Mitchell, 2012: 38). Instead, as Mitchell notes:

> Flesh and bone – skin color and physiognomy – have consistently played a primary role in the visual perception of racial identity. They provide a set of visual schematisms that allow one to differentiate types of people, sometimes with prejudice, sometimes without. When we 'see race', we are actually seeing through a screen composed of stereotypical search templates and labels. We are not, in other words, seeing 'flesh and bone', but a matching of certain sensory data with pre-conceived linear profiling and color codes.
>
> *(2011: 408)*

Rather than ignoring 'race', Mitchell's approach emphasises the 'paradoxes and enigmas' which underscore our 'racial identities' (Lane, 1997). If we consider Mitchell's contention that 'the major problem to be explained in the so-called post-racial era, ... is the persistence of race as a political and economic issue, as well as a term linked to the all-too-durable phenomenon of racism' (2012: 22), then approaching race in all its symbolic, illusory and fictional mediations can help to realign our engagement with racism (Hook, 2008). In fact, in an example that draws connections between the work of Jacques Lacan, Paul Sartre and Frantz Fanon, Mitchell highlights that, 'Lacan's remark on the inexistence of woman has always, ... resonated with echoes of Sartre's claim that "the Jew does not exist", and Fanon's remark that "the black man does not exist"' (2011: 407). In effect, while 'saturated with irony [... and] not to be taken literally' these statements reflect how our symbolic identities present 'a declaration of non-existence in the face of undeniable existence' (Mitchell, 2011: 407–408). In other words:

> race is an illusion, a fantasy, a myth, and yet it is also a palpable, functional reality, one that cannot be abolished or negated by any declaration or scare quotes. It is like ideology itself, a camera obscura in which the world appears upside down.
>
> *(Mitchell, 2011: 408)*

Certainly, Lacan's 'There is no sexual relationship' and 'Woman does not exist', as well as Fanon (1952) and Mitchell's (2011) appropriation of this logic, should not be conceived as asserting that race (or gender) doesn't exist, or that race should be considered as in some way abject. Rather, Lacan's phrase highlights how the symbolic categories that we use to conceive 'woman'/'black' are detrimental to understanding the significance of these classifications. Something always persists which distorts, negates or dislodges any classification and it is our recourse to using 'racial' classifications which subsequently frames our social antagonisms. In this sense, there is 'no relation' between the body and the symbolic classification used to 'classify' it; instead, it is our symbolic framing of race that fundamentally distorts its appearance, and which dictates the conditions on which 'race relations' are contoured and shaped. Flisfeder and Burnham provide further clarification, with specific reference given to interracial/multicultural relationships:

> Consider what happens when one is in an interracial or multicultural relationship: when one is black and has a white girlfriend, is Hispanic and has an Asian boyfriend, is Jewish and has a Catholic girlfriend, and so on through other various permutations of so-called mixed relationships (including cross-class relationships). When (if) the relationship ends, does one not soon hear from one's family or friends that it was doomed because of that racial or ethnic difference? ... The point, of course, is that such (racist) fetishes of ethnic difference as a cause of relationship failure, ... are a way of disavowing the fundamental incommensurability that Lacan theorized as 'there is no sexual relationship' (and its corollary, 'there is a non-relationship').
>
> *(2017: 35)*

Ultimately, this suggests that 'race relations' (and 'sexual relations') are framed by an absence that fundamentally determines these relations. This is not to imply that 'race relations' are inherently bounded to perpetual violence, ignorance and resultant racism, but that 'race' is itself marked by an impossibility – the Real – that is often obscured through fantasy projections of a perfect harmonious (racial) totality. It is here that, rather than viewing racial alterity as innate (Lane, 1997), we can instead conceive 'Difference [... as] real-impossible – something that eludes and resists the symbolic grasp' (Žižek, 2016). We can see this interpretation of 'difference' (as constituted antagonism) reflected in Žižek's account of class antagonisms and the excessive elements which unsettle any 'harmonious' relationship:

> If the division of the social body into two classes were complete, without the excessive element (Jew, rabble ...), there would have been no class struggle, just two clearly divided classes. This third element is not the mark of an empirical remainder that escapes class classification (the pure division of society into two classes), but the materialization of their antagonistic difference itself, insofar as this difference precedes the differentiated terms. In the space of anti-Semitism, the 'Jew' stands for social antagonism as such: without the Jewish intruder, the two classes would live in harmony... Thus, we can observe how the third intruding element is evental: it is not just another positive entity, but it stands for what is forever unsettling the harmony of the two, opening it up to an incessant process of re-accommodation.
>
> *(2013: 6)*

In applying this understanding, it becomes apparent that race is often 'the most readily available "solution" to approaching the Real' (Hook, 2008: 150). However, as will be argued below, comedy can provide a unique role in eliciting and approaching this Real and for providing a certain dexterity in traversing the symbolic and fantasmatic 'solutions' that constitute race. For now, however, the following sections will draw together key strands from the above discussion. Primarily, this will engage with psychoanalytic/Lacanian approaches to race and racism (Frosh, 2013; Hook, 2004, 2008; Mitchell, 2012; Žižek, 1998a), Žižek's (1997, 2006a, 2006b, 2010) account of the other and Hsiao's (2010) race as spectacle and spectre.

Race, racism and the Real

By way of navigating the trap of political correctness, we can re-approach race's socio-symbolic significance as central to an understanding of racism as Real (Mitchell, 2012). In fact, with regards 'to the tenets of liberalism', Gilroy argues that:

> Because 'race' ought … to be nothing, it is prematurely pronounced to be of no consequence whatsoever. Racism either disappears at this point or lingers on as a marginal issue, an essentially prepolitical event that should not be addressed by any government worthy of the name.
>
> *(2004: 159)*

In view of this disappearance, we can turn to Mitchell's application of the Real as a way of distinguishing between race and racism. For Mitchell, 'The Real, … is the location not of race but of racism. Racism is what hurts. … Race is the set of symptoms or signs – the diagnostic tool – that provides access to the disease known as racism' (2012: 17). As a result, instead of viewing 'the root term as primary and the "-ism" as the derivative phenomenon', Mitchell reverses this signification, stating that, 'Racism is the brute fact, the bodily reality, and race is the derivative term, devised either as an imaginary cause for the effects of racism or as an attempt to provide a rational explanation' (2012: 19). It is clear, from Mitchell's account, that racism is afforded a disruptive potential, much like that of the Real. It is in this way that Mitchell considers race to be 'the Symbolic-Imaginary construction of a fragile "reality" used to explain, contain, and manage the Real known as racism, and sometimes to unleash it in unimaginable acts of violent hatred' (2012: 19). Certainly, this approach does not ignore the significance of racism, by deferring it to the Real, but rather draws attention to how examples of racism are reflected in racial signs which are brought to bear through a 'racialised' body.

If we associate, as Mitchell (2012) does, the Real with racism, then it becomes possible to consider how the effects of racism continue to have 'violent effects' on both the body and the symbolic order (the process of symbolisation) (McMillan, 2013). Here, 'the Real … is nothing but a reaction to the body entering symbolization' (McMillan, 2013: 124) and, as a consequence, while the body is both socially and discursively constructed, it is the body's location within this process of symbolisation that serves to highlight how forms of racial oppression maintain an affective and embodied significance. As a result, racism is not located solely in the discursive realm but, in a very Real sense, ex-sists in a 'pre-discursive' bodily form

(Hook, 2004, 2008). Hook offers further clarification when he argues that while 'the "real" of the body … should not be taken as a license to an easy universalism', and although 'This "real" is not completely independent of the flux of historical and discursive construction', it is evident that 'The "real" is that which represents a recurring deadlock of comprehension in different historical eras' (2008: 143). Such 'deadlock' reveals how the body prescribes a certain intensity that fails to provide any complete symbolic representation; revealing itself to be formed by a 'constitutive irresolvability' (Hook, 2008: 150).[2] It is this 'irresolvability' which perpetrates the 'more than' quality of the subject,[3] and it is through the imposition of a symbolic order on 'the body' that we can begin to consider how race refers to those symbolic differences that 'colonize' the body. Indeed, while such inquiries follow 'the great Lacanian motif of symbolization as a process which mortifies, drains off, empties, [and] carves the fullness of the Real of the living body', Žižek supplements this symbolisation with the concern that 'the Real is at the same time … the excess which escapes symbolization and is as such produced by the symbolization itself' (2008a: 191).

By locating racism beyond the discursive, we can also identify how the body is not necessarily torn between the symbolic and the Real but intertwined within a discursive/symbolic register that is disrupted and fragmented by the Real. That is, while the body remains tied to its signification within the symbolic order – a signification with its own historical connotations – it is also distorted, divided and undermined by its own impossibility; indeed, by the fantasies that continually frame yet fail to effectively 'racialise' the body in its entirety. Here, the Real can be attributed to those remaining effects which escape the body's irresolvable symbolisation and which elicit forms of racist fantasy. It is along these lines that Hook proposes that we should direct attention to 'what is produced in the impossible attempt to mediate this "real"', by examining the fantasies and symbolic differences 'that are called upon to reconcile this constitutive irresolvability' (2008: 150).

When conceived as a mode of the Real, it is racism which serves as the effect-cause of racial difference, with racialised discourses and fantasies occurring as a response to this irresolvable difference. In contrast to the racist fantasy, there is not 'one' single 'race' above all others, but rather it is the nonexistence of a unified and non-divided 'One' which is depicted in examples of racism. It is in this way that racial differences can be absolved from their associated (and, clearly false) anatomical/biological differences, towards a critical understanding of the effects of these 'differences' in distinguishing between different 'racialised' bodies.

To this extent, while for Mitchell (2012), racism is located in the Real, it is 'race' which is located in the symbolic-imaginary and which is both constructed and encoded in distinguishing between 'black' or 'white'. Importantly, this is not an attempt to reduce all racial experiences to a white-black binary. In her (de)construction of race in American literature, Keating notes how:

> theorists who attempt to deconstruct 'race' often inadvertently reconstruct it by reinforcing the belief in permanent, separate racial categories. Although

> they emphasize the artificial, politically and economically motivated nature of all racial classifications, their continual analysis of racialized identities undercuts their belief that 'race' is a constantly changing sociohistorical concept, not a biological fact.
>
> *(1995: 902)*

Clearly, while Keating's (1995) remarks refer to discussions of race in America, they nevertheless serve as a clear reminder of the biological-sociological distinctions which underscore accounts of race and which inevitably lead to simple white-black binaries. Accordingly, though many remain open to 'the realization that "race" is a biological fiction' (Lane, 1997: 7), Keating's (1995) critique remains indebted to the significance of 'race' and to the 'demand that it have political and symbolic importance' (Lane, 1997: 7).

Consequently, whereas forms of simple 'deconstruction' are clearly opposed by Keating (1995), it is also apparent that attempts at 'deconstructing' racial binaries should not lapse into simple conclusions, which merely assert that everything is constructed, non-fixed and socially and historically relative. While agreeing with the fact that race bears a socio-historical significance, it is important to remember that attempts to 'multiply' our understandings of race can just as easily be used to erect and, in some instances, solidify racial categories. What is ignored in these attempts is the significance of the Real.

In order to highlight this significance, we can briefly turn to The Frankfurt School and their objections to the social and historical revisionism of Freud's 'unconscious', which bears a similar critique. In short, Žižek notes how – most notably in the work of Fromm – 'Freud is reproached for projecting into the "eternal human condition" features which are strictly dependent on specific historical circumstances' (2005a: 10). Arguing against this historical revisionism of Freud, 'members of the Frankfurt School, particularly Theodor Adorno and Herbert Marcuse, fought this "revisionist" tendency from the very beginning in the name of a strict historical-materialist approach' (Žižek, 2005a: 10). Here, Žižek considers:

> What, then, were the Frankfurt School's objections to this revisionist attempt to 'socialize' Freud[?] … While 'revisionism' replaces 'nature' ('archaic', 'pre-individual' drives) with 'culture' (the creative potential of the individual, his alienation in contemporary 'mass society'), for Adorno and Marcuse, the true problem resides *in this 'nature' itself.* In what appears as 'nature', as biological or, at least, phylogenetic heritage, critical analysis must unearth the traces of historical mediation.
>
> *(2005a: 10)*

In directing the question towards 'this nature itself', a clear Hegelian gesture is enacted, from which critical attention is afforded to the historical emergence of the 'concept', *nature* (Žižek, 2005a). In part, this explains how 'cultural' arguments can take on a 'quasi-natural' significance, whereby our 'inherently' stable natures are hampered by a repressive society that serves, paradoxically, to promote a deconstructionist/contextual analysis that simply 'historicizes' our sense of alienation (Žižek, 2005a). In other words, in order to propose a 'cultural', deconstructionist understanding, one has to accept a relatively fixed, or at least stable, understanding of 'nature', from which such cultural assessments can be made. Instead of resorting to either 'nature' or 'culture', which, as the above suggests, simply replaces one for the other, what is required is a critical perspective which considers *how* this understanding *is* 'the adequate manifestation of a historical reality which is itself "false"' (Žižek, 2005a: 11 [italics removed]).

Importantly, this 'nature-culture' debate within The Frankfurt School can be given further emphasis when we consider the work of Judith Butler and how, in her renowned *Gender Trouble* (1999), Butler theorises the extent to which sex (biology) and gender (culture) differences are 'always-already "posited"' and that 'the line separating "culture" from "nature" is always determined by a specific cultural context' (Žižek, 1998a: 128). Indeed, it is this 'cultural context' that endows us to locate the subject as the site for a variety of discursive practices, through which the 'subject' is performed. Yet, what is ignored in 'This cultural overdetermination ... is precisely the deadlock of the Real' (Žižek, 1998a: 128–129). In fact, 'because the opposition between nature and culture is always-already culturally overdetermined, i.e., that no particular element can be isolated as "pure nature," does not mean that "everything is culture"' (Žižek, 1998a: 129); instead, for Žižek, '"Nature" *qua* Real remains the unfathomable X which resists cultural "gentrification"' (Žižek, 1998a: 129).

Accordingly, what we see through converging the Frankfurt School with Butler (1999) is how our nature-culture binaries can be easily tied to examples of cultural overdetermination. This becomes evident when we consider the various ways in which nature is stabilised and fixed through idealised forms of cultural representation that mask or obscure nature's inconsistency. It is here that the various subjectivities that can be radically performed, as noted by Butler (1999), are merely multiple forms of being that ultimately rely upon a 'stable' nature from which these identities can be enacted.

If we consider this alongside issues of race, we can see that, while remaining critical of reducing race (and gender) to biology, it is just as unhelpful to reduce these terms to forms of cultural relativism and discursive (re)production. It is following this path that, as evidenced in the previous criticisms of political correctness and its ability to draw from a position of liberal universality *and* 'colour-blindness', examples of 'whiteness' can very easily be presented 'as a pseudo-universal category that hides its specific values, epistemology, and other attributes under the guise of a nonracialized, supposedly colorless, "human nature"' (Keating, 1995: 904). Such a 'nonracialized' position simply avoids the impasses of racial difference; ignoring that 'unfathomable X' which belies any simple determination – i.e. the Real (or, in Butler's case, the 'trouble' at the centre of her gender analysis (Žižek, 1998a)).

Consequently, when discussions on race, racial classifications and racial stereotypes can, via a process of deconstruction, simply reify racialised meanings, at the same time – and here we can return to Keating – what begins as an interrogation of 'whiteness' or 'blackness' *should* very easily 'tur[n] into an interrogation of "race"' (1995: 916). What these conclusions draw attention to is the significance of these binaries in the first instance, and to the various ways, and the various failures, that occur when trying to symbolise 'race' through a crude biological reductionism, which fundamentally ignores the symbolic order, as well as an equally crude cultural determinism which overlooks how our pre-symbolic biological codes are subject to forms of symbolic and imaginary construction that permit a continual self-questioning. It is in this vein that our interrogations of race can 'touch' the Real, as Keating alludes to:

> The point is not to encourage feelings of personal responsibility for the slavery, decimation of indigenous peoples, land theft, and so on that occurred in the past. It is, rather, to … more fully … comprehend how these oppressive systems that began in the historical past continue misshaping contemporary conditions.
>
> *(1995: 915)*

Significant here is the comprehension of past 'oppressive systems' that *continue* to misshape contemporary society. It is this ongoing misshaping which avers the Real.

Accordingly, what this approach seeks to draw attention to is the significance of such a simple white-black binary in constructing and imagining race and, more importantly, how this binary confers a symbolic and imaginary significance *which aims to symbolise race*. It is this 'symbolic-imaginary' significance which is produced in Boakye's reflections on being black/not-black. Indeed, while asserting, 'I'm not black. … I'm probably something closer to raw cocoa, or coffee, or flat Coca-Cola', Boakye adds that, 'The … problem with being black is that *it is absolutely, at least symbolically, true*. Because, if nothing else, one thing I can confirm is that I am not-white' (Boakye, 2019). To this extent, we can conceive of 'race … as a medium that weaves together the symbolic and imaginary to form a "reality" (or a fantasy) known as race' (Mitchell, 2011: 406) – what Boakye (2019) refers to as that 'invisible lens'. Moreover, this reality is never whole nor consistent, but contradictory: 'a complex knot of pride and insecurity' (Boakye, 2019). As previously noted, the symbolic is characterised by its inconsistencies and as a result constitutes a 'fragile reality' that is amiable to the disturbing effects of the Real – that which 'denigrates just as much as it defines' (Boakye, 2019). Indeed, as 'the site of trauma, and the unpresentable', it is the Real which 'becomes the site of racism' (Mitchell, 2011: 406), so that while it is through the mediation of race (conceived as symbolic-imaginary) that we are continually required to manage the violent acts of hatred which result in racist trauma (conceived as the Real), it is nonetheless these effects, and all their troubling significance, which is obfuscated and masked through examples of cultural tolerance, reconceived as 'identity politics'.

Importantly, it is the Real which continually dislodges any objective classification or perspective. This Real tension is reflected in Keating's comparative appraisal of Toni Morrison's *Playing in the Dark* (1992) and Aldon L. Nielsen's *Reading Race* (1988), both of which Keating examines with regards to how a 'simplistic binary between fixed definitions of "blackness" and "whiteness" occurs in literary interrogations of "whiteness"' (1995: 914). According to Keating, while 'Morrison ... begins blurring the artificial boundaries between "blackness" and "whiteness" by exploring what "white" representations of "blackness" tell us about literary "whiteness" ... Nielsen focuses almost entirely on "white" poets' racist stereotypes of "blacks"' (1995: 914). Consequently, 'Although [Nielsen] acknowledges the fictional, contradictory nature of these "white" representations of "blackness"', his 'constant focus on the stereotypes themselves inadvertently reifies the racist imagery he tries to undercut' (Keating, 1995: 914). What is significant in Keating's (1995) analysis is that no blurring of the boundaries is exempt from a 'white' or 'black' perspective, regardless of the position one takes in achieving this perspective. In any interrogation of either 'white' or 'black' one is left with blurring the distinction *or* reproducing the distinction in the pursuit of interrogation itself. In either instance, we get the return of the Real, so that both Morrison's (1992) and Nielsen's (1988) analyses reflect two approaches – two symbolic and interpretative perspectives – whose difference is marked by the Real.

It is in this sense that we can begin to account for 'racism's notorious recalcitrance in the face of historical, discursive, institutional and ideological change' (Hook, 2004: 677).[4] By ensuring that we approach and 'grapple with racism['s] uncanny logic of return' (Hook, 2004: 673), we can consider how it is this 'uncanny logic' which stands opposed to discursive/constructionist approaches that, although valuable in highlighting 'how racism is linked to processes of social, political and economic domination and marginalisation', and while 'shed[ding] light on how such phenomena come to be naturalised within society at trans-individual and extrapersonal levels' (Hook, 2004: 673, 677),[5] nonetheless fail to effectively consider how examples of racism have proved historically and culturally *pervasive*. Hook considers:

> why is it that one could (theoretically) change the concerned social constructions of race and racism, transform the terms of public discourse, change even the material and structural conditions of society such that there is no longer any palpable reward for being racist and ... racism would conceivably nevertheless persist?
>
> *(2004: 678)*

We can relate such criticism to the efforts of political correctness itself. That is, while arguing against racism and attempting to reframe and regulate our approach to race, examples of political correctness have nevertheless failed in preventing the persistence of racism, with the possibility that it may have even encouraged discursive forms of racism. To this end, and while drawing upon Žižek's (1998b) account of otherness, Hook highlights that it:

> is … when socioeconomic analysis fails to account for some key feature of racism, [that] critics evoke a need to supplement it with an analysis of the cultural context, and vice versa. They cannot, as such, provide a complete account of the analysed phenomenon. What is required is the more careful designation of the link between social structures and psychical consequences
>
> *(2004: 677)*

Instead, it is racism which is often conceived as the 'ground' from which particular political circumstances arise (Žižek, 1998a, 1998b). The effect here is that political circumstances are seen as bringing to the fore latent forms of racism, with racism perceived as the underlying cause in examples of political antagonism. While Žižek (1998a) originally based this understanding on his critique of Western-European interpretations of the Balkan War – from which Serbian aggression was misconceived as the ethnic-cause, rather than the struggle for power in a post-Communist Yugoslavia – this same dynamic can also be seen in Žižek's assertion that:

> The ongoing civil war in the Central African Republic between the Christian south and the Muslim north is not just an explosion of ethnic hatred. Rather, this explosion was triggered by the discovery of oil in the north of the country: France (linked to Muslims) and China (linked to Christians) are fighting for the control of oil resources through their proxies.
>
> *(2017a: 43)*

What these examples highlight is the need to reverse the 'racism as cause argument' in order to consider racism as the *effect-cause* of political circumstances which provides the ground from which racist attitudes are performed. This is not a subtle reversion to the previously critiqued discursive/constructionist approach, which privileges cultural/contextual reductionism, but rather, as can be seen in Hook's (2004) application of the work of Young (1990a, 1990b), sets out to provide a more focused 'concern … with forms of racism that manifest in what we might term a symptomatic manner, in patterns of habitualised dislike, avoidance, discomfort, or aversion' (Hook, 2004: 681). What is more, we should not merely reverse the cause of racism so that these 'symptoms' are simply attributed as the effects of political circumstances and/or social structures, but, in a double reversal, seek to examine how, today, certain 'racist effects' can work to incorporate their own causal justification.

In fact, this can be identified in one notable example, drawn from an interview with the actor Liam Neeson, who, while responding to a question regarding his ability to play violent roles, began to describe the story of a friend who was raped (*The Independent*, 2019). Upon being told of the attack, Neeson admitted to asking his friend 'what colour' the rapist was, from which she replied he was black. In an example of reality mimicking fiction, with Neeson clearly channeling his later performances in the *Taken* (2008–2014) films, he went on to detail how he subsequently patrolled the streets at night in order to provoke a random 'black bastard' whom he could 'kill' in retaliation for his friend's rape (*The Independent*, 2019). In the process of the interview, Neeson recited the incident as an example of how he sought to draw upon an experience of 'primal' anger, which, rather helpfully, allowed him to get 'into' character for his (then) forthcoming film (Michallon, 2019).

As noted by the historian David Olusoga, it is important that Neeson's actions are not viewed as some innate form of 'primal' racism; indeed, 'The characterisation of racism as "primal" goes to the heart of what racism is and what it is not' (Olusoga, 2019). Notably, Olusoga's 'is' and 'is not' bear a Lacanian significance in that, while not asserting the 'primal' or 'instinctive' nature of racism, such remarks shed light on the ways in which symbolic constructions of race and racialisation point to a symbolic dis-order (a Real-impossible) that bears a semblance with Boakye's (2019) black/not-black 'tension'. However, although Olusoga (2019) contends that racism is socially learned, directing attention towards Neeson's socially learned disposition can just as easily be used to excuse his desire to seek revenge as a reflection of his social background and/or 'generation' (Žižek, 2005b). Instead, we can conceive of Neeson's response as bearing a Real significance, especially when we consider how it is encountered through a symbolic-imaginary form – a fantasy frame which seeks to bring a level of fantasmatic 'wholeness' to a particular situation (in this case, racial revenge).

To this end, if we remember that 'Within any symbolic system, the real is what cannot be signified' (McGowan, 2007: 64), then, in the case of both Neeson's remarks and Olusoga's analysis, it is apparent that, rather than offering any complete form of symbolisation, we see the relative struggle of trying to provide Neeson's racism a form of signification that would confer some form of meaning. In the days following the interview, such confusion was matched by the strange sense of 'reflexivity' that Neeson's account presented. In commenting upon this reflexive mode, Žižek notes that:

> modernism still clings to the illusion that reflection somehow radically affects its object. That is, … after one explains to a racist the true causes of his hatred for foreigners, this hatred should disappear… [… Alternatively] a post-modernist takes into account that, even if my racism is 'reflexive', it still remains racism pure and simple, and, even worse, that a first-level racism can only become operative when accompanied by a second-level reflection that contains and disavows its true scope.
>
> *(1996: 511–512)*

In view of Neeson's open acknowledgment of the incident we can see how it is through 'reflexively' acknowledging one's racism that one can both 'contain' and 'disavow' one's racist intent.

Unsurprisingly, the interview garnered a large degree of public shock, with Olusoga highlighting that:

> What shocked many black people [and white people] was having someone step through the line of thinking that can and does lead to racial violence and racialist murder. … Neeson's second question to the victim was to ask her the race of her attacker. Why go from the individual to the entire race, from the singular to the group, from the guilty to the innocent? We know why. That is how racism works. That is racism in action. What appalled many was that, when recounting that critical leap of illogic, Neeson did so, seemingly, without analysis or acknowledgement.
>
> *(2019)*

Contra Olusoga (2019), it is suggested here that Neeson was fully aware of the racism that underscored his revelation, if only by the fact that he knew what he was saying was 'racist'. By sharing the incident, Neeson's account served as a source of disavowal that, in some way, mitigated against its racist significance. Predictably, in the days following the interview, the inevitable 'I'm not a racist' narrative was proclaimed by Neeson (BBC, 2019), with additional help from actress Whoopi Goldberg, who defended Neeson's candid admission (Horton, 2019). Yet, what Neeson's admission reveals is exactly how (postmodern) forms of racism can work to disavow their racism through openly and *reflexively* acknowledging their racist intent. That is, by fully acknowledging an incident of former racism, and then retracting its intent (therefore, appearing non-racist), Neeson's comments could effectively *be* racist.

This is in no way intended to let Neeson 'off the hook' nor limit racism's significance by removing it from the process of signification; instead, it is to draw attention to the Real and to its vivid elicitation when foreclosed from the symbolic. Accordingly, rather than proving 'illogical', as per Olusoga (2019), paradoxically, Neeson's shocking 'racist' revelation bared its own logic in that it allowed him to support and maintain his 'not-racist' image (a 'non-sense' that, for Neeson, existed within a symbolic structure of 'sense'). Here, Neeson's racism 'elude[d] explanation by sole reference to either conscious precepts or social history' (Lane, 1997: 4), and, while not resorting to easy explanations – which relegate Neeson's racism to an attribute of his personality (a maladapted form of deviancy inherent to his psychology) or to his social background (Hook, 2004) – ultimately, Neeson's response revealed how the disavowal of racism in the symbolic returns in the Real of a fantasmatic justification grounded in racist vengeance. This points to the Real antagonism of racial difference as it is located in various assumptions which continually defy 'objective' classification. In order to better understand this Real, we can turn to Hsiao's (2010) spectacle and spectre distinctions.

The spectacle and spectre of race

In his analysis of black-minstrelsy, Hsiao (2010) highlights how, historically, the performance and visibility of race has often occurred during periods where political discussions on race were noticeably absent. That is, Hsiao asks:

> As visible as racial differences – or physical characteristics of a certain race in the eye of another – were, why did they appear invisible in the dawning moments of modern (western) democracy, *invisible* in the sense that the enslaved race was not even considered part of the socio-political order premised on equalitarianism?
>
> *(2010: 161)*

Drawing specifically upon the blackface performances of the Caribbean performer Bert Williams, Hsiao (2010) relates this paradox to the fact that despite William's being black, the Real effects of his 'blackness' were ignored and obscured through the spectacle of his racialised blackface performance. Indeed, whereas 'the notion of something being hidden by virtue of its very visibility is well recognized within literature' (Taylor, 2010: 113), for Hsiao (2010), it is the presentation of a black man performing blackface minstrelsy, behind a black mask, which helps to reveal how the spectacle of race is closely intertwined with its spectral supplement. In other words, while we often 'see race' (Mitchell, 2012), it is also haunted by forms of in-visibility. As a result, 'the specter of race lurks in the backdrop of the spectacle, as an indissoluble remainder in the wake of a certain political mobilization' (Hsiao, 2010: 173).

We can continue this line of inquiry in view of Žižek's (2008a, 2008b) writings on anti-Semitism and how the displacement of the 'Jew' 'generate[s] the false impression that society is (or can be) free of antagonisms, insofar as its possible corruption is located in its outside' (Vogt, 2007: 62). As Vogt notes it 'is precisely through this dissimulation that the spectral presence of the "Jew" becomes decipherable as a symptom, that is, a repressed Real of (anti-Semitic) society' (2007: 62). What is notable is that while the fantasy-image of the 'Jew' seeks to locate society's antagonism as *outside* society itself, it is the spectral presence of the 'Jew' that avers the Real *within* society (an obscured class antagonism). We see this same formal structure in Hsiao's (2010) spectacle and spectre distinctions. Here, the spectacle of race creates a form of displacement that works to obfuscate race's political significance. What is notable is that such displacement occurs as part of the spectacle, as evident in forms of racial ignorance and racial in-visibility. As a result, and in a similar fashion to Neeson's racist admission, it is through race's spectacle that its *spectral* presence can become, to a certain extent, hidden in plain sight. It is not that the displacement of race can simply be 'removed', as in the violent repression and murder of Jews in the case of Nazi Germany, but that race's symbolic manifestation is just as easily displaced through its spectacle. It is in this way that one can begin to think of those numerous 'cultural' celebrations that, while applauding racial diversity, nonetheless fail to 'remove' or curtail pervasive forms of systemic racism.

Viewing race as spectacle and spectre does not merely provide a more elaborate attempt to focus on 'black' racial identity as opposed to 'white'. Indeed, the spectre of race can cut across both distinctions by drawing attention to the non-acknowledgment of race through forms of open obfuscation (i.e. race's spectacle). In so doing, the implementation of racial boundaries exists within race's absent-presence, as Keating highlights in the case of 'racialized' literary genres, such as the Harlem Renaissance:

> Although scholars generally conceptualize the Harlem Renaissance as a 'black' literary movement (I suppose because those identified as 'Harlem Renaissance writers' were people of African descent), they do not conceptualize Transcendentalism as a 'white' movement, even though – to the best of my knowledge – the Transcendentalists were all people of European descent. In our 'multicultural' era, we have studies of 'Chicano' narrative, 'Asian American' novels, 'Native American' poetry, and so on. But imagine a course or a book devoted exclusively to white-skinned writers (as so many courses and books still are) that acknowledged this fact in its title: Say, 'Classics of the White Western World,' 'The White American Experience,' or 'White Regional Writers.'
>
> *(1995: 905)*

Notice how the open demarcation of 'black' literature acknowledges 'race' in such a way that it apoliticises its significance; a process echoed by the fact that the apoliticisation of 'whiteness', that is, its non-acknowledgment, works from the assertion that such a distinction need not be made.

The specific form of this approach stands in contrast to any biological interpretation of race, which views race as in some way innate or genetically defined, as well as discursive/constructionist approaches, which seek to locate understandings of 'race' in different socio-historical contexts. Instead, by considering the spectre of race one can begin to outline how the mediation of 'race' by the symbolic is continually rendered incomplete or unbalanced. It is this 'unbalancing' which racist ideologies seek to rectify, and which are subsequently grounded in 'racist' fantasies that prescribe simple 'us' and 'them' narratives. In doing so, the Real of racism is encountered in the effects of its own symbolic failure. It is the failure of this symbolisation, and its supplementing fantasies, which subsequently obfuscate the spectre of race, but which nonetheless implies its spectral significance.

It is here that we can draw a connection between Mitchell's (2012) racism as Real and Hsiao's (2010) spectacle and spectre distinctions. That is, if we consider that 'The Symbolic can never saturate the Real and so, consequently, there is always some part of the Real which remains unSymbolized' (Myers, 2003: 74), then what cannot be accommodated reveals a positing of the Real which disrupts and distorts any imaginary or symbolic construction, as evidenced in its non-accommodation. Notably, it is this 'unSymbolized' element which presents a certain co-dependence between the Real and the spectre of race, reflected in the various ways in which our accounts of 'race' – even when ignored – remain tied to racial descriptions which lay bare its presence. It is this spectral presence which provides race and racism a material and immaterial significance, so that any racial depiction – any 'spectacle' – is shadowed and haunted by its spectre. This spectre is exemplified in racial or cultural faux pas, but also in more obvious forms of racist aggression. Consequently, for Hsiao, it is the spectre's:

> resistance to becoming-conscious despite the efforts of 'raising consciousness' by the official ideology and despite also the staging of racial difference as spectacle, … [that] [t]he traumatic effects of such a specter can be instantiated by its persistent and recurrent haunting, even in the displaced and disguised form of spectacle.
>
> *(2010: 161–162)*[6]

Such 'recurrent haunting' points to the centrality of race as a 'medium' or 'spectacle' through which the symbolisation of racial differences is never complete nor fully symbolised and, as a result, is always maintained by some form of 'symbolic debt' (Žižek, 2012b). This debt is reflected in Lane's contention that 'Every citizen of Europe and North America is haunted by the specter of racism' and that 'Despite our concern to restrict this specter to traumatic chapters of history', examples of racism continue to 'revisi[t] contemporary society in shocking and surprising forms' (1997: 3). As can be seen, it is racism's 'haunting' effects which constitute that 'part of the Real that returns to haunt reality in the guise of the spectral supplement' (Myers, 2003: 74–75). This haunting is supported by the fact that while 'The Real needs mediating … it continues to bubble under the surface of the Symbolic and Imaginary constructions we use for that mediation' (Taylor, 2010: 70).

Accordingly, if we remember that, for Mitchell (2012), racism is Real, then the spectre of race is what 'emerge[s] in this very gap that forever separates reality from the real' (Žižek, 2012b: 21). It is in this way that the traumatic effects of racism continue to underscore the spectacle of race, so that rather than hiding or ignoring racial differences, they instead provide safeguarded displays that occlude and conceal that which exceeds race's symbolic representation (i.e. the Real). In such displays, racism is a mode of the Real which returns via the spectre of race and is brought to bear through its traumatic effects (Hsiao, 2010; Mitchell, 2012; Myers, 2003). It is, in short, the spectral significance of race – its immateriality, in-visibility – which constitutes that 'part of reality that remains non-symbolized' (Žižek, 2012b: 21 [parenthesis removed]), but which, more importantly, remains at the limit of reality itself.

Following this line of inquiry, we can begin to consider how it is through race's spectacle (its mediation in the symbolic) that the inherent limits of race's symbolisation (its spectral supplement) produce its own fundamental antagonism:

the Real of racism (Mitchell, 2012). This relation between the spectre of race and the Real of racism can be related to Gilroy's contention that 'the very attempt to hold "racism" together as an object to be analyzed' is central to 'disput[ing] racial common sense' (2004: 10). In view of the preceding argument, what becomes clear from Gilroy's concern is that such an analysis requires recognising, in our 'racial common sense', the spectral supplement that sustains the fantasmatic formations which structure and underscore 'racial *common sense*'. This recognition can be achieved when we consider how this spectral counterpart works off a certain redoubling that is brought to light in the inherent fictionality of racial fantasies (Žižek, 2012a). Indeed, we can observe how a process of redoubling – a 'duality of symbolic fiction and spectral apparition' – is reflected in examples where the smooth, non-antagonistic functioning of society is based upon fantasy's fictional/spectral co-dependence (Žižek, 2012a: 685).

Here, any fantasy is dialectically 'split' or redoubled in the co-dependence which is achieved *within* fantasy's fictional vision (fantasy_1) *and* that corresponding spectral element (fantasy_2) that serves to prevent or inhibit this vision, so that 'Those who are alleged to realize fully fantasy_1 (the symbolic fiction)' require 'recourse to fantasy_2 (spectral apparitions) in order to explain their failure' (Žižek, 2012a: 685). In the case of Nazi anti-Semitism, we see this co-dependence in the fantasy of a Germany free of social antagonisms (fantasy_1) and the subsequent prevention of this fantasy in the Jewish plot (fantasy_2) (Žižek, 2012a). The point is that it is *within* the symbolic fiction and its spectral supplement that we get the redoubling of fantasy: we get *both* its beautifying and horrifying aspects (Salter, 2016).

This redoubling draws attention to how the Real of racism, while not being approached directly, can be averred through traumatic experiences that posit the spectre of race. Bearing in mind that traumatic experiences can never be approached directly, but require, on behalf of the subject, a certain 'traversal' which re-renders the effects of trauma (Edkins, 2003), then, paradoxically, rather than openly deriding or ignoring examples of racism – a process that, in the case of post-race debates, simply maintains an underlying (non-)racist fantasy – we can instead acknowledge the inherent failure (the 'gap') and inconsistency of race's symbolisation(s) through the 'redoubling' that fantasy's fictional vision and spectral element present (Mitchell, 2012; Žižek, 2012a). To explore this, we can return to our previous criticisms of political correctness.

Political correctness and race as spectacle

What is often seen in debates and discussions on multiculturalism and cultural difference is how the spectacle of race remains 'predicated on the invisibility of race even in those instances when it manifests itself through the staging of racial elements and/or the figurations of race' (Hsiao, 2010: 161). It is in 'the spectacle of race, … [that] the spectral existence of racial trauma is occluded or concealed precisely by means of exposing racial difference in full view' (Hsiao, 2010: 182). In similar fashion, examples of political correctness work by turning race into a spectacle through which forms of tolerance, although acknowledging racial discrimination, pervasively maintain the spectre of race as unacknowledged and 'silently ignored' (Lentin and Titley, 2011; Žižek, 2006c). This is evidenced in Žižek's (2006c) example of the *burakumin*. In Japan:

> the caste of the untouchables is called the burakumin: those who have contact with dead flesh (butchers, leatherworkers, gravediggers), who are sometimes even referred to as eta, 'much filth'. Even today, in our supposedly enlightened times, when they are no longer openly despised, they are still silently ignored. Not only do companies still avoid hiring them and parents refuse to allow their children to marry them, but, under the 'politically correct' pretence of not offending them, ignoring the issue altogether is the preferred course of action.
>
> *(Žižek, 2006c: 185)*

What is suggested here is that, in accordance with Hsiao's (2010) spectacle and spectre distinctions, forms of political correctness, tied to proponents of liberal multiculturalism, openly ignore the spectre of race in all its 'traumatic', 'shocking' and 'surprising' forms. In other words, it is in making race visibly-invisible (in-visible) that its significance is ultimately masked resulting in examples of racism going unperturbed and unacknowledged. Here we can begin to see how the frenetic activity to turn political struggles into racial struggles serves to obfuscate the effects of racism by ensuring that both individuals and groups remain open to cries of 'racism', enacted through public scandals, or, alternatively, ignored and/or dismissed under instances of 'not-racist' (Lentin, 2018). It is through the pronouncement of political correctness that the Real of racism becomes marginalised, ignored and hidden. It is here that the spectre of race – that which truly acknowledges and approaches the other's difference, with all the incongruity that Real human interaction requires – is ignored and made absent.

Accordingly, by way of ensuring that our behaviours and forms of interaction are regulated and managed and that our knowledge of a diverse range of cultures (their tastes, values and customs) are recognised, we can begin to consider how examples of political correctness remain embedded in an underlying desire to 'prevent some traumatic thing, the real thing, from happening' (Žižek in Taylor, 2009: 177). As a result, rather than preventing forms of harassment, political correctness spectacularises the differences which underscore such forms of harassment. This can result in a rather complicated and paradoxical situation, whereby one is required to be aware of racial/ethnic differences, while also being fully composite with the 'correct' ways of thinking, talking and referring to these differences. Here, Swaim neatly captures the frustrations this can cause:

> You must consider every facet of life in light of racial sensitivities, sexual politics or some kind of cultural imperialism; but you'd better not talk

> openly about any of these things unless you're prepared to negotiate their exquisite complexities and unless you're up to date on all the latest banned phrases.
>
> *(2016)*

To this end, Mitchell asserts that:

> What we cannot do is to make race disappear by putting it in scare quotes or declaring ourselves to be in a post-racial era. *We need to regenerate the concept of race in new terms as part of an anti-racist strategy.*
>
> *(2011: 407 [italics added])*

Through outlining this 'anti-racist strategy', Mitchell argues for 'a way of seeing through race to its racist origins, taking account not only of its sources in inequality, bondage, and xenophobia but also of its creative, productive capacity to generate new communities of resistance and structures of feeling' (2012: 37). Notably, rather than ignoring race, Mitchell (2012) imbues race with a critical and subversive significance. Here, Mitchell's contentions chime with wider criticisms of 'post-racial' societies, noting that 'The whole unfolding of the conception of race as a scientific and political-cultural concept must be remembered and reframed, especially at a time of racialization run wild' (2012: 32). It is in such instances that 'the subtle and intricate dynamics of racism' can be observed and subverted (Mitchell, 2012: 32). Indeed, this is not to suggest that in order 'to balance racist attitudes' we simply 'sho[w] more racism'; a process, which, as Plesske asserts, 'not only banalises the problem, … [but] also does not take into account the qualitative prospective of the insult' (2016: 92–93). Instead, re-approaching race can offer a way of 'looking at things directly and realistically' – an approach that can allow us to 'get some idea about the real at work in social reality' (Zupančič, 2016: 413, 421).

Equally, this approach is not suggesting that racism should be ignored or dismissed but, instead, draws attention to how we can re-approach race as a symbolic-imaginary and how this can help restructure our approach to racism and its (Real) traumatic effects. Indeed, as previously noted, Žižek's (2017b) later work has focused on the importance of the Real as a point of wider political contention and subversion.[7] In what follows, consideration will be given to exploring how Žižek's (1998a, 2002) work on the other offers a unique form of approaching inter-subjective interaction between different racial/ethnic groups. Here, specific consideration will be given to examining how Žižek's (1998a) notion of the other is related to the Real. Žižek explains:

> The Real is not necessarily or always the 'hard real'. It can also have this totally fragile appearance: the Real can be something that transpires or shines through. For example, when you talk with another person and you are charmed by him or her – from time to time you perceive some traumatic,

> mystical, tragic, … dimension in him or her. It is something that is Real, but at the same time totally elusive and fragile.
>
> *(Žižek and Daly, 2004: 69)*

It is to this that we now turn.

Approaching the other

In the UK, the spectacle of race can be identified in the rather shallow displays of cultural diversity predicated on what Yasmin Alibhai-Brown has referred to as 'saris, samosas and steeldrums' (Alibhai-Brown, 2000). Here, race inevitably maintains an unacknowledged spectral presence, influencing the performance of multiculturalism, but all the while being kept at a safe distance. It is this safe distance which underscores Žižek's critique of liberal multiculturalism (outlined in Chapter One), a critique which is echoed in George Orwell's realisation that real class interaction is 'no use' if it involves simply 'clapping a proletarian on the back and telling him that he is as good a man as I am; if I want real contact with him, I have got to make an effort for which very likely I am unprepared' (Orwell cited in Žižek, 2006a: x). What is reflected in Orwell's comments is a clear sense of the Real 'effort' that is required in building a relation with the other.

Žižek's approach to the 'other' is one that works against any presupposed assertion that the individual and society are in some way self-enclosed and/or ontologically complete. As noted in Chapter Two's discussion on the relation between the subject and comedy, analyses of comedy have extended Lacan's notion of the 'mirror phase' by tracing how the subject is constitutively divided and predicated upon a lack-excess dialectic (McGowan, 2017). Put simply, this division occurs when the subject 'enters' the symbolic order and develops an imaginary wholeness; a process that forever 'splits' the subject from the fragmentary Real. This suggests that no identity is ever 'closed' or 'harmonious', but is grounded in a presupposed exclusion (Chow, 2014), and it is this exclusion, which is formulated through the use of language, that forever separates the subject from the world around them. McGowan notes:

> The subject desires as a result of its incompletion, and this desire is identical with lack. Lack defines how we relate to the world, impelling us to seek out what we are missing in the world. The self-identical, non-lacking subject would no longer be a subject and no longer be capable of speaking. Lack is subjectivity.
>
> *(McGowan, 2017: 15)*

Accordingly, if we consider that the Real occupies an 'empty place', an 'impossibility' that forever presents its inscription in the symbolic order, then:

> It is in this sense that the enigmatic Lacanian phrase defining the subject as an 'answer of the Real' is to be understood: we can inscribe, encircle the void

> place of the subject through the failure of his symbolization, because the subject is nothing but the failure of the process of his symbolic representation.
>
> *(Žižek, 2008a: 195)*

Moreover, this 'encircling of the void' is reflected in the subject's relation with the other, so that while:

> I can communicate with the Other, I am 'open' to him (or it), precisely and only insofar as I am already in myself split, branded by 'repression,' i.e., insofar as (to put it in a somewhat naive-pathetic way) I cannot ever truly communicate with myself; the Other is originally the decentered Other Place of my own splitting.
>
> *(Žižek, 1998a: 31)*

Žižek applies this Lacanian reading of the subject in order to consider how any contact with the other 'is propelled by an aversion to one's own vulnerability and lack, which might be mirrored in the other' (O'Dwyer, 2010). As an 'answer of the Real', the subject is forever barred from their 'truth' and it is this truth which 'is look[ed] for in others: what propels me to "communicate" with them is the hope that I will receive from them the truth about myself, about my own desire' (Žižek, 1998a: 31).

It is here possible to trace how this relation to the other, an other perceived as consistent and whole, can be conferred in those racial fantasies which frame the other (McGowan, 2015). In such instances, these fantasies mask the subject's own lack, which is subsequently perceived as 'lost' and, thus, stolen by the other. With regards to racist fantasies, 'whether it be the case of "our" jobs, "our" traditional way of life, "our" wives and children', it is these very properties which 'the other has usurped', forming an 'endlessly self-perpetuating' cycle of racist hatred (Hook, 2008: 146). Alternatively, the other's excess can also be used to replace the subject's lack (McGowan, 2017), as evident in the politically correct subject who 'immerses' themselves in the other's culture.

In both cases, it is through a form of subjective displacement that the subject's relation to/with the other is defined. It is through such displacement that we can view the Real as a constitutive feature of the subject, so that it is in accordance with the Real that racist motivations can be underpinned by a desire to manage the subject's anxieties through certain symbolic discourses, such as open forms of racist rhetoric. These discourses and their fantasmatic support seek 'to answer the question of what society expects from me: for example, "We" must prevent "Them" from stealing "Our" enjoyment' (Wood, 2012: 129). These efforts, however, are a form of excess which seek to achieve an imagined sense of wholeness on behalf of the subject; a wholeness that works to obscure the Real. Indeed, it is through such obfuscation that Real contact with the other is prevented.

Accordingly, under assertions of 'tolerance' and through examples of political correctness, cultural exchange is geared towards avoiding any Real encounter with the other; a vulnerability that is amiable to the subject's desire to abstain from their own inherent lack. For the latter, O'Dwyer notes how 'This avoidance explains the popularity of humanitarian causes, which lies in their inherent paradox, whereby one can "love" from a distance, without getting personally involved' (2010). While the field of fantasy and, specifically, racist fantasies, has been considered in Žižek's (1998a, 2008a, 2008b) examples of the 'Jew' in Nazi Germany as well as in studies on race, racism and postcolonialism (Fanon, 1952; Frosh, 2013; Hook, 2004, 2008), it is those instances which reveal an avoidance to engage with the other that the following discussion will seek to elaborate upon. Here, it is noted that, while professing to build and encourage cultural interaction, the hegemonic power of liberal multiculturalism and political correctness can result in: 1) examples of the other as traumatic; and 2) examples of the other as excessive. Together these two distinctions will be brought together in what Žižek (2010, 2006a) refers to as the 'decaffeinated other'.

That 'traumatic Thing': Trauma and excess in political correctness and the decaffeinated other

By way of elucidating on those 'traumatic' elements which frame the other, Žižek draws upon theological arguments from the Old Testament. Indeed, while Žižek highlights that 'the Old Testament enjoins you to love and respect your neighbor, the reference is not to your imaginary semblable/double, but to the neighbor *qua* traumatic Thing' (Žižek, 2004: 385). Notably, this stands:

> In contrast to the New Age attitude, which ultimately reduces my Other/ Neighbor to my mirror-image or to a means on the path to my self-realization ..., Judaism opens up a tradition in which an alien traumatic kernel forever persists in my Neighbor – the Neighbor remains an inert, impenetrable, enigmatic presence that hystericizes me.
>
> *(Žižek, 2004: 385–386).*

The significance of the other/neighbour as Thing is also drawn upon in Žižek's (2017a) reference to Adam Kotsko's *Creepiness* (2015). Here Žižek notes that '"creepy" is today's name for the uncanny core of a neighbor: every neighbor is ultimately creepy' (2017a: 73). In effective fashion, Žižek's use of Kotsko's work highlights how it is the 'impenetrability of the [other's] desire' which underscore's the subject's traumatic response to *their* acts (2017a: 73). Consequently, it is when this strange neighbour/other gets too close that examples of aggression can be found. As previously touched upon, such aggression is often used to target the other's excessive behaviour which encroaches on the subject. In these cases, it is the other's values, tastes and customs which clash with the 'modern' attributes of the liberal subject (Dean, 2006), resulting in formal attempts to 'liberalize' the illiberal other (Kymlicka, 1996). This is most notable in examples of cultural assimilation, and/or openly opposing certain groups on the grounds that their customs and values bear no semblance to those of Western Europe. In both cases, we see how examples of liberal tolerance are in fact grounded in forms of intolerance. These contradictions are echoed in an 'exemplary case' involving 'the Dutch Rightist populist politician Pim Fortuyn, killed in early May 2002, two weeks before the elections in which he was expected to gain one fifth of the votes' (Žižek, 2018: 178). Notably:

> Fortuyn was a Rightist populist whose personal features and even (most of his) opinions were almost perfectly 'politically correct': he was gay, had good personal relations with many immigrants, with an innate sense of irony… In short, he was a good tolerant liberal with regard to everything except his basic political stance: he opposed fundamentalist immigrants because of *their* hatred towards homosexuality, women's rights, etc.
>
> *(Žižek, 2018: 178 [italics added])*

What the example of Fortuyn highlights is how it is those specific aspects of the 'fundamentalist immigrant' ('their hatred') which helps sustain a 'tolerant' liberalism.

Understanding *that* which constitutes the other's otherness is reflected in Žižek's (2010) notion of the 'decaffeinated other'. Žižek explains: 'What is increasingly emerging as the central human right in late-capitalist societies is the right not to be harassed, which is the right to be kept at a safe distance from others' (2010). Detrimentally, such distance results in 'an experience of the Other deprived of its Otherness – the decaffeinated Other' (Žižek, 2010). This echoes the ways in which race can often act as both spectacle and spectre, most notably, in examples of political correctness, which, while acknowledging race (spectacle), implicitly seek to ignore underlying forms of racism (spectre) by removing those qualities that constitute the other's otherness. Accordingly, although race can be made spectacle – tolerated, celebrated and praised – the spectre of race remains in-visible and, subsequently, unacknowledged. By acknowledging race, political correctness merely regulates and curtails expressions of difference. In doing so, race remains a private difference, making no 'impact on the public sphere' (Sharpe and Boucher, 2010: 36). Here, examples of political correctness, grounded in a toleration of the other, present a path of respecting 'their' difference but always at a distance and never in any Real attempt to acknowledge this difference, so that while 'the other is now integral to "our" imagined community, … at the same time, their otherness, … keeps them distant and indeterminate' (Fortier, 2005: 572). Instead, 'When [they …] com[e] too close, as the plight of refugees and illegal immigrants betrays only too well, the rhetoric of toleration shows its limits' (Aristodemou, 2014: 54).

This limit can be considered in relation to Žižek's (2008a, 2008b) criticisms of capitalism and how we are often compelled to enjoy through purchasing commodities. Paradoxically, this enjoyment is always enacted through a presupposed management and containment of the potential excesses of such enjoyment (instead of alcohol, drink alcohol-free; instead of coffee, drink decaffeinated coffee; have cream, but without the fat). This management of excess is reflected in the 'good Other' who, while remaining 'not too potent or different or indeed authentic so as to pose a real threat to other individuals or to a socially cohesive society' (Malik, 2013: 231), is, nevertheless, 'detoxified' of their (cultural) excess. In such instances, one is able to enjoy the cultural particularities of the ethnic other – their dances, their attire, their communal rituals – while other 'less favourable' aspects of their culture are ignored. As a result, the other is either denigrated and hated (as purported by the far-right, racist subject) or venerated as something to be admired and desired (as seen in the cosmopolitan, multicultural liberal). This management of the other's cultural excess underscores Lentin and Titley's contention that 'the crisis of multiculturalism is not a rejection of culturalism' but, instead, 'a rejection of supposed *cultural excess*, and the compensatory reclamation of power over it' (2011: 17 [italics added]). It is through curtailing, managing and, sometimes, tolerating, this 'cultural excess' that examples of political correctness seek to achieve equality and respect for difference.

Importantly, this approach seeks to refrain from any 'false elevation of the Other' (McLaren, 2001: 628). Instead, we can develop upon the critique of political correctness provided in Chapter One, by highlighting how examples of political correctness reveal two forms of 'managing' the other. In the first instance, the politically correct subject seeks to resolve their lack through excessively drawing from the other's culture to bolster their own 'politically correct' subjectivity, or by masking their own Western guilt by proclaiming the other's cultural misdemeanours as the result of Western-European imperialism/racism. In the second instance, we are left with the politically correct subject patronisingly engaging with the other's lack by offering them certain forms of help that, while ensuring that one has met their politically correct duty, simply encourages the continuation of the other's exploitation. Indeed, these latter forms of management can also, in certain cases, result in a ratified sense of disgust towards the other's beliefs and customs, which are subsequently met with the desire to 'civilize' or, in this instance, 'liberalize', the other. In both cases, we are engaging with forms of fantasy that deliberately seek to avoid any engagement with the Real other or, in the most radical cases, seek to eradicate the other (mass killings, such as genocide, being a clear example).

Encountering the Real other through comedy: A mutual lack in (self-)understanding

In managing and regulating our relations with the other, we can begin to see how political correctness seeks to prevent forms of presupposed harassment by ironing-out the inherent antagonisms and potential impasses that frame our relations with each other. This can be identified in examples of cultural communication, whereby:

> The common ground that allows cultures to talk to each other, to exchange messages, is not some presupposed shared set of universal values, etc., but

> rather its opposite, some shared deadlock; cultures 'communicate' insofar as they can recognize in each other a different answer to the same fundamental 'antagonism,' deadlock, point of failure.
>
> *(Žižek, 1998a: 31)*

Underlying such 'deadlock' is the concern that, traumatically, what we lack is not to be found in the other's enjoyment, but rather a 'fundamental antagonism', which is constitutive of Real cultural exchange. Indeed, it is this inherent failure to communicate – a communication marked by miscommunication – which Lacan's symbolic register seeks to identify (Wood, 2012). In fact, though globalisation creates new opportunities for cross-cultural engagement, such 'opening' can reflect further instances of miscommunication and misunderstanding (Žižek, 2017a). Here, Žižek (2017a) references the comments of Peter Sloterdijk, who, in recognising the dark underside of globalisation, argues for a 'code of discretion'. Žižek extends these thoughts by advocating for the importance of alienation in Western European societies, so that a sense of 'distance is woven into the very social texture of everyday life' (2017a: 74). Such distance allows one not to get 'too close' and not to share the 'inner world' of the other. Whereas Žižek (2017a) is clear to point out that such alienation is *sometimes* beneficial, we can, in line with these thoughts, serve to draw attention to their ability to induce a reflexive short circuit that is amiable to the other as Real.

Accordingly, if we consider, as Žižek does, 'the proverbial African-American from Spike Lee's *Do the Right Thing*, who annoys the whites while he walks around with the boombox turned lou[d]', then we can begin to see how 'It is THIS excessive and intrusive *jouissance* that one should learn to tolerate' (2002: 19 [sic] [emphasis in original]).[8] Rather than viewing these examples as forms of cultural harassment, our toleration of that 'excessive and intrusive *jouissance*' which defines the other can result in forms of cultural communication that takes the possibility of miscommunication as central to human interaction. In fact, this bears a resemblance to how we typically approach love. Indeed, love is never total, nor complete, but instead navigates around those imperfections that fundamentally underscore one's love for their partner. Indeed:

> Lacan's name for this imperfection, for the obstacle which MAKES ME love someone, is *objet petit a*, the pathological tic which makes him/her unique. In authentic love, I love the other not simply as alive, but on account of the very troubling excess of life in him/her. Even the common wisdom is somehow aware of this: as they say, there is something cold in perfect beauty, one admires it, but one falls in love with an IMPERFECT beauty, on account of this very imperfection.
>
> *(Žižek, 2002: 28 [sic] [emphasis in original])*

It is here that we can return to Žižek's notion of the Real and, in particular, to that Imaginary Real which reveals the 'traumatic dimension' of the other (Žižek and

Daly, 2004). That is, if we consider that 'Encountering the Real via the neighbour confronts us with the raw and vulnerable nature of human being, and such an encounter is often avoided in favour of more acceptable and idealistic generalisations of humanity' (O'Dwyer, 2010), then this encounter with the Real is one marked by a path that encourages a form of toleration that neither devalues nor maintains the other's 'otherness' at a distance, but instead seeks an approach of 'coexisting differences' (Žižek, 2006d: 362). Such coexistence is clearly fragile and marked by those cultural faux pas and possible intrusions that inherently frame contact with the other. As a result, while always framed by the symbolic, 'contact with the Real Other is inherently fragile ... the authentic reaching out to the Other can at any moment revert into a violent intrusion into the Other's intimate space...' (Žižek, 2002: 14).

Therefore, it is in view of such fragility that our relations with the other can be redefined. Indeed, if we consider Lacan's notion of *jouissance* – a physical, emotional and psychological pleasure that steers more towards pain – it becomes possible to render a psychoanalytic account of the inherent inconsistencies, impasses and contradictions which frame human interaction (Žižek, 1998a, 2017a). In much the same way that the subject seeks to 'fill' or mask their lack through the other – bearing in mind that for the politically correct subject such lack/excess is ambivalently framed through the subject's desire to excessively patronise the other's lack, or, in other instances, mask their lack through a jealous/aggressive desire towards the other's excess – then it is apparent that what we are dealing with are two modes of *jouissance* (the subject's and the other's), which remain incongruously and antagonistically positioned. Accordingly, by 'project[ing] the core of [their] *jouissance* onto an Other, attributing to this Other full access to a consistent *jouissance*' (Žižek, 2017a: 75), both the politically correct *and* the racist subject reflect a formal semblance in their attempts 'to resolve this deadlock' via forms of fantasy that are either universally humanitarian or openly racist. What belies both accounts is the capacity to achieve an approach that acknowledges the Real other. This is not a celebration of the Real, in the form of some 'sublime' object possessed by the other, but a realisation that:

> the other's *jouissance* is insupportable for us because (and insofar as) we cannot find a proper way to relate to our own *jouissance* – the ultimate incompatibility is not between mine and other's *jouissance*, but between myself and my own *jouissance*, which forever remains an ex-timate intruder.
>
> *(Žižek, 2017a: 75)*

Indeed, this 'acceptance' does not ignore difference, but instead recognises the difference (the 'ex-timate intruder') that is inherent to both the other *and the subject* as well as the discursive structures that frame this relationship. What is shared is a reflexive commonality, which draws attention to the antagonisms both *within* and *between* cultures. This posits a certain form of self-negativity or self-estrangement that can be achieved when 'You imagine looking at yourself with a foreign gaze, through foreign eyes' (Žižek, 2013a: 136). It is through this reflexive 'capacity to be surprised, not by others, but by ourselves seeing how what we are doing is strange' (Žižek, 2013a: 136) that we can begin to move towards a more fundamental acknowledgment that 'the privileged way to reach a Neighbour is not that of empathy, of trying to understand them, but a disrespectful laughter which makes fun both of them and of us in our mutual lack of (self-)understanding (inclusive of "racist" jokes)' (Žižek, 2017a: 79).

Racist jokes: 'something to be circumvented, alluded to, played with, exploited, manipulated, made fun of'

This chapter has sought to trace how Žižek's (1998a, 1998b, 2002) conception of the Real serves as a formative feature of the relations between subject and other and, more specifically, as a decisive part of cultural communication: of being with, relating to and knowing the other. While remaining aware of the concern that 'the Real should not be identified exclusively as an explicit force of negation', we can instead view it as a disruptive and fragmentary feature within the symbolic which becomes apparent when we consider how the Real 'plays a more implicit and evanescent role in the construction of our everyday forms of social reality' (Žižek and Daly, 2004: 8). By way of conceiving this Real as fundamental to a critique of political correctness, it is important 'to recall the constituted, provisional and historically contingent nature of every social order' (Edkins, 2003: 14), including the various contingencies which mask and structure our formalisations of race as well as universal forms of abstract management, such as political correctness. While for Edkins, such a 'position' is echoed in what 'Žižek calls "traversing the fantasy", "tarrying with the negative" or fidelity to the ontological crack in the universe', it is of greater importance that we recognise that this position '*is uncomfortable*' (2003: 14 [italics added]). We should also be aware that 'subversion cannot be guaranteed' (Yao, 2012: 3), as Yao explains:

> we cannot say, … that a Chinese man making a racist joke about Chinese people necessarily neutralizes the racist premise of the joke. Such a guarantee is impossible because the premise of the joke is not held entirely within its content, but also lies outside in the concrete forms of social, political and economic injustice.
>
> *(2012: 2)*

Turning towards the joke's form, it is argued that such interaction is prescribed by an uncomfortableness that can provide an important site of making Real contact with the other and can help subvert and redefine the universal significance of political correctness. In fact, such examples are echoed in Weaver's analysis of the black US comedian Richard Pryor, who reused racial categories in order to 'provide a key site of reversal and resistance' (2010: 38).

To this extent, Chow (2014) has detailed how laughter traces those fissures which characterise the symbolic. Yet, 'in doing so, the joke approaches the void of the Real' and, as a result, 'joking is a strange and risky social behaviour' (Chow, 2014: 229). Nonetheless, while aware of such risk, it is also apparent that if the subject's relation to the other is framed via an excessive enjoyment, then it is through reflexively acknowledging the effects of this enjoyment that the subject can more accurately approach the Real other. Certainly, this does not ignore the importance of fantasy. In fact, if 'the Real [... is] the monstrous outside, the "Thing", which we cannot ever truly approach but can only ever protect ourselves against through the formations of fantasy' (Noys, 2010), then such fantasies are a formative part of those excessive elements that frame the subject's relation to the other. Accordingly, it is here that Mitchell's (2012) race as symbolic-imaginary recalls the underlying significance of approaching racist fantasies that undermine or reorder our approach to racism. What is significant is that, in accordance with these fantasies, we 'recognize [... the Real] as the projection of our own excesses, as our own refusal to admit the negativity at the heart of our existence' (Noys, 2010).

Such contact with the other prefigures a sense of failure, geared around the traumatic obstacles (*objet a*) which underscore our cultural relationships. In fact, while referring to Lacan's notion, 'there is no sexual relationship', Žižek (2015) outlines how such a statement does not mean that every sexual relationship is doomed to failure. Instead, it is the very imperfections and the idiosyncrasies that are referred to in Lacanian terms as the *object petit a* which provide the 'very obstacle [which] can be turned into a comic resource, [and] can function as something to be circumvented, alluded to, played with, exploited, manipulated, made fun of ... in short, sexualized' (Žižek, 2015: 306). Accordingly, while 'Sexuality is here an exploit which thrives on its own ultimate failure' (Žižek, 2015: 306), the same can also be said of those jokes and comic sequences which perform the failure(s) at the heart of our social interactions.

Moreover, in accordance with Hsiao (2010), comedy can trace that paradoxical path between approaching something that is visible via its invisibility. If we consider that in various comedy performances, certain 'jokes' and comic sequences may deliberately draw upon racial stereotypes for comic effect, then it is also apparent that the comic performance of 'race' – that is, it's spectacle – can be used to deliberately acknowledge and draw attention to the spectre of race. In other words, through its absent-presence, the spectre of race can be approached via the mode of the comic spectacle.

Indeed, what has been outlined in the above discussion is a path that seeks to re-approach race via the effects of racism. In part, this requires conceiving race as 'the intricate complexion of love and hate, alterity and enmity that make up the phenomenon of racism' (Mitchell, 2012: 37). Unfortunately, such 'complexion' is either ignored, obfuscated or overlooked in examples of political correctness, which, while performing a sense of racial tolerance, support pervasive forms of intolerance by obfuscating the significance of race through private regulation (tolerating the other's difference, but maintaining a difference to such difference). By way of drawing attention to those instances of human (mis)communication, the following chapter will serve to outline how comedy's Real subversion can help to redefine our relations to political correctness and the other.

Notes

1 See also Weaver (2010).
2 See also Žižek (2000).
3 This is echoed by Kingsbury, who follows this argument by considering how the body's relation with the symbolic emphasises 'The tensions between the ways in which the symbolic order colonizes or "mortifies" … the bodies and psyches of living beings and the disturbances of the real *qua* drive that threaten to dissolve people's sense of reality' (2017: 3).
4 See also Selznick and Steinberg (1969).
5 See also Žižek (1998b).
6 In this quotation, Hsiao (2010) is referring explicitly to the performance of blackface minstrelsy.
7 This is extended in the work of Dean (2006) and McMillan (2013).
8 The character Žižek refers to in this example is Radio Raheem (Bill Nunn).

References

Ali G Indahouse. 2002. Film. Universal Pictures.

Alibhai-Brown, Y. 2000. *After Multiculturalism*. London: Foreign Policy Centre.

Alonso, P. 2016. Sacha Baron Cohen and *Da Ali G Show*: A critique on identity in times of satiric infotainment. *The Journal of Popular Culture*, 49 (3), 582–603.

Aristodemou, M. 2014. A constant craving for fresh brains and a taste for decaffeinated neighbours. *The European Journal of International Law*, 25 (1), 35–58.

BBC. 2002. Is Ali G Racist? [Online]. *BBC News*. Available from: http://news.bbc.co.uk/1/hi/talking_point/1885312.stm [Accessed 1 March 2019].

BBC. 2019. Liam Neeson says he's 'not racist' after controversial interview [online]. *BBC News*. Available from: www.bbc.co.uk/news/entertainment-arts-47133868 [Accessed 1 October 2019].

Bebber, B. 2014. *Till Death Us Do Part*: Political satire and social realism in the 1960s and 1970s. *Historical Journal of Film, Radio and Television*, 34 (2), 253–274.

Boakye, J. 2019. Smooth, angry, cool, powerful: how we talk about blackness [online]. *The Guardian*. Available from: www.theguardian.com/books/2019/apr/13/smooth-angry-cool-powerful-how-we-talk-about-blackness [Accessed 20 January 2020].

Brockes, E. 2016. Whether it's Ali G or Tina Fey, ironic racism just isn't funny anymore [online]. *The Guardian*. Available from: www.theguardian.com/commentisfree/2016/mar/03/sacha-baron-cohen-ali-g-tina-fey-amy-poehler-ironic-racism [Accessed 1 March 2019].

Brown, R. 1995. *Prejudice: Its Social Psychology*. Oxford: Blackwell.

Buchanan, R. T. 2014. Former Monty Python John Cleese: Political correctness is 'condescending' [online]. *Independent*. Available from: www.independent.co.uk/news/people/news/former-monty-python-john-cleese-political-correctness-is-condescending-9891121.html [Accessed 19 August 2018].

Butler, J. 1999. *Gender Trouble: Feminism and the Subversion of Identity*. New York, NY: Routledge.

Campbell, M. 2017. The mocking mockumentary and the ethics of irony. *Taboo: The Journal of Culture and Education*, 11 (1), 53–62.

Chow, B. 2014. The tickling object: On Žižek and comedy. In: B. Chow and A. Mangold, eds. *Žižek and Performance*. Basingstoke: Palgrave Macmillan, 224–252.

Curry and Chips. 1969. TV Series. ITV.

Dean, J. 2006. *Žižek's Politics*. New York, NY: Routledge.

Do the Right Thing. 1989. Film. Universal Pictures.

Edkins, J. 2003. *Trauma and the Memory of Politics*. Cambridge: Cambridge University Press.

Elsworth, C. 2006. The joke is on the racists, says relaxed Borat [online]. *Telegraph*. Available from: www.telegraph.co.uk/news/uknews/1534364/The-joke-is-on-the-racists-says-relaxed-Borat.html [Accessed 1 March 2019].

Fanon, F. 1952. *Black Skin, White Masks*. London: Pluto Press.

Fawlty Towers. 1975–1979. TV Series. BBC Two.

Flisfeder, M. and Burnham, C. 2017. Love and sex in the age of capitalist realism: On Spike Jonze's Her. *Cinema Journal*, 57 (1), 25–45.

Flisfeder, M. and Willis, L.-P. 2014. Introduction: Žižek and media studies, beyond Lacan. In: M. Flisfeder and L.-P. Willis, eds. *Žižek and Media Studies: A Reader*. New York, NY: Palgrave Macmillan, 1–14.

Fortier, A.-M. 2005. Pride politics and multiculturalist citizenship. *Ethnic and Racial Studies*, 28 (3), 559–578.

Frosh, S. 2013. Psychoanalysis, colonialism, racism. *Journal of Theoretical and Philosophical Psychology*, 33 (3), 141–154.

Gibson, J. 2000. Comics find Ali G is an alibi for racism [online]. *The Guardian*. Available from: www.theguardian.com/uk/2000/jan/11/race.janinegibson [Accessed 1 March 2019].

Gilroy, P. 2004. *After Empire: Melancholia or Convivial Culture?* Abingdon: Routledge.

Hook, D. 2004. Racism as abjection: A psychoanalytic conceptualisation for a post-apartheid South Africa. *South African Journal of Psychology*, 34 (4), 672–703.

Hook, D. 2008. The 'Real' of racializing embodiment. *Journal of Community & Applied Social Psychology*, 18, 140–152.

Horton, H. 2019. Whoopi Goldberg insists friend Liam Neeson is 'not a bigot' [online]. *Telegraph*. Available from: www.telegraph.co.uk/news/2019/02/06/whoopi-goldberg-defends-friend-liam-neeson-insists-not-bigot/ [Accessed 1 October 2019].

Hsiao, L.-C. 2010. Color (un)conscious: Psychoanalysis, resistance, and the specter/spectacle of race. *Concentric: Literary and Cultural Studies*, 36 (1), 159–187.

Kamm, J. and Neumann, B. 2016. Introduction: The aesthetics and politics of British TV comedy. In: J. Kamm and B. Neumann, eds. *British TV Comedies: Cultural Concepts, Contexts and Controversies*. Basingstoke: Palgrave Macmillan, 1–22.

Kapoor, I. 2018. Žižek, antagonism and politics now: Three recent controversies. *The International Journal of Žižek Studies*, 12 (1), 1–31.

Keating, A. 1995. Interrogating 'whiteness,' (de)constructing 'race'. *College English*, 57 (8), 901–918.

Kingsbury, P. 2017. Uneasiness in culture, or negotiating the sublime distances towards the big Other. *Geography Compass*, 11 (6), 1–11.

Kotsko, A. 2015. *Creepiness*. Alresford: Zero Books.

Kymlicka, W. 1996. *Multicultural Citizenship: A Liberal Theory of Minority Rights*. Oxford: Clarendon Press.

Lane, C. 1997. The psychoanalysis of race: An introduction. *Discourse*, 19 (2), 3–20.

Lentin, A. 2018. Beyond denial: 'Not racism' as racist violence. *Continuum*, 32 (4), 400–414.

Lentin, A. and Titley, G. 2011. *The Crisis of Multiculturalism: Racism in a Neoliberal Age*. London: Zed Books.

Littlewood, J. and Pickering, M. 1998. Heard the one about the white middle-class heterosexual father-in-law? Gender, ethnicity and political correctness in comedy.

In: S. Wagg, ed. *Because I Tell a Joke or Two: Comedy, Politics and Social Difference*. London: Routledge, 291–312.

Lockyer, S. and Pickering, M. 2008. You must be joking: The sociological critique of humour and comic media. *Sociology Compass*, 2/3, 808–820.

Love Thy Neighbour. 1972–1976. TV Series. ITV.

Malik, S. 2013. 'Creative diversity': UK public service broadcasting after multiculturalism. *Popular Communication*, 11 (3), 227–241.

McGowan, T. 2007. The temporality of the Real: The path to politics in *The Constant Gardener*. *Film-Philosophy*, 11 (3), 52–73.

McGowan, T. 2015. *Psychoanalytic Film Theory and The Rules of the Game*. New York, NY: Bloomsbury.

McGowan, T. 2017. *Only a Joke Can Save Us: A Theory of Comedy*. Evanston, IL: Northwestern University Press.

McLaren, P. 2001. Slavoj Žižek's naked politics: Opting for the impossible, a secondary elaboration. *JAC*, 21 (3), 613–647.

McMillan, C. 2013. *Žižek and Communist Strategy: On the Disavowed Foundations of Global Capitalism*. Edinburgh: Edinburgh University Press.

Medhurst, A. and Tuck, L. 1996. Situation comedy and stereotyping. In: J. Corner and S. Harvey, eds. *Television Times: A Reader*. London: Arnold, 111–116.

Michallon, C. 2019. Liam Neeson interview: Rape, race and how I learnt revenge doesn't work [online]. *Independent*. Available from: www.independent.co.uk/arts-entertainment/films/features/liam-neeson-interview-rape-race-black-man-revenge-taken-cold-pursuit-a8760896.html [Accessed: 1 October 2019].

Mitchell, W. J. T. 2011. Playing the race card with Lacan. *Journal of Visual Culture*, 10 (3), 405–409.

Mitchell, W. J. T. 2012. *Seeing Through Race*. Cambridge, MA: Harvard University Press.

Morrison, T. 1992. *Playing in the Dark: Whiteness and the Literary Imagination*. Cambridge, MA: Harvard University Press.

Myers, T. 2003. *Slavoj Žižek*. Abingdon: Routledge.

Nielsen, A. L. 1988. *Reading Race: White American Poets and the Racial Discourse in the Twentieth Century*. Athens, GA: University of Georgia Press.

Norris, V. 2014. *British Television Animation, 1997–2010: Drawing Comic Tradition*. Basingstoke: Palgrave Macmillan.

Noys, B. 2010. The horror of the Real: Žižek's modern gothic. *The International Journal of Žižek Studies*, 4 (4). Available from: http://zizekstudies.org/index.php/IJZS/issue/view/20 [Accessed 30 November 2020].

O'Dwyer, K. 2010. Žižek on love [online]. Available from: https://philosophynow.org/issues/77/Žižek_on_Love [Accessed 10 March 2019].

Olusoga, D. 2019. What does Liam Neeson's 'primal urge' really tell us about racism [online]. *The Guardian*. Available from: www.theguardian.com/commentisfree/2019/feb/09/what-does-liam-neeson-primal-urge-tell-us-about-racism [Accessed 20 January 2020].

Plesske, N. 2016. 'Sambo' and 'snowflake': Race and race relations in *Love Thy Neighbour*. In: J. Kamm and B. Neumann, eds. *British TV Comedies: Cultural Concepts, Contexts and Controversies*. Basingstoke: Palgrave Macmillan, 83–98.

Quirk, S. 2018. *The Politics of British Stand-Up Comedy: The New Alternative*. Gewerbestrasse, Switzerland: Palgrave Macmillan.

Salter, L. 2016. Populism as a fantasmatic rupture in the post-political order: Integrating Laclau with Glynos and Stavrakakis, Kōtuitui. *New Zealand Journal of Social Sciences Online*, 11 (2), 116–132.

Saunders, R. A. 2007. In defence of Kazakshilik: Kazakhstan's war on Sacha Baron Cohen. *Identities: Global Studies in Culture and Power*, 14 (3), 225–255.

Selznick, G. J. and Steinberg, S. 1969. *The Tenacity of Prejudice: Anti-Semitism in Contemporary America*. New York, NJ: Harper and Row.

Sharpe, M. and Boucher, G. 2010. *Žižek and Politics: A Critical Introduction*. Edinburgh: Edinburgh University Press.

Swaim, B. 2016. Donald Trump tries to kill political correctness – and ends up saving it [online]. *Washington Post*. Available from: www.washingtonpost.com/opinions/donald-trump-has-made-political-correctness-credible-again/2016/11/01/0f397c0c-9fb1-11e6-a44d-cc2898cfab06_story.html?utm_term=.441518d5bfc9 [Accessed 20 January 2020].

Taken. 2008. Film. 20th Century Fox; EuropaCorp International.

Taken 2. 2012. Film. EuropaCorp.

Taken 3. 2014. Film. EuropaCorp; 20th Century Fox.

Taylor, A. 2009. *Examined Life: Excursions with Contemporary Thinkers*. New York, NY: The New York Press.

Taylor, P. A. 2010. *Žižek and the Media*. Cambridge: Polity.

The Independent. 2019. Liam Neeson interview: Listen to audio of actor recounting wanting to kill a 'black bastard' for raping someone close to him [online]. Available from: www.independent.co.uk/arts-entertainment/liam-neeson-audio-interview-kill-black-bastard-rape-cosh-recording-tape-cold-pursuit-a8763111.html [Accessed 20 January 2020].

Vogt, E. 2007. Exception in Žižek's thought. *Diacritics*, 37 (2–3), 61–77.

Waxman, S. 2007. Equal-opportunity offender plays anti-Semitism for laughs [online]. *NY Times*. Available from: www.nytimes.com/2006/09/07/movies/07bora.html [Accessed 1 March 2019].

Weaver, S. 2010. The 'Other' laughs back: Humour and resistance in anti-racist comedy. *Sociology*, 44 (1), 31–48.

Weaver, S. 2011. Liquid racism and the ambiguity of Ali G. *European Journal of Cultural Studies*, 14 (3), 249–264.

Wood, K. 2012. *Žižek: A Reader's Guide*. Chichester: Wiley-Blackwell.

Yao, D. 2012. Learning to tickle: How to transmit knowledge as if re-telling a joke. *The International Journal of Žižek Studies*, 6 (2), 1–12.

Young, I. M. 1990a. *Justice and the Politics of Difference*. Princeton, NJ: Princeton University Press.

Young, I. M. 1990b. Abjection and oppression: Dynamics of unconscious racism, sexism and homophobia. In: A. B. Dallery and C. E. Scott, eds. *Crises in Continental Philosophy*. New York, NY: State University of New York Press, 201–214.

Žižek, S. 1996. Sex in the age of virtual reality. *Science as Culture*, 4 (4), 506–525.

Žižek, S. 1997. Multiculturalism, or, the cultural logic of multinational capitalism. *New Left Review*, 1 (225), 28–51.

Žižek, S. 1998a. *Tarrying with the Negative: Kant, Hegel, and the Critique of Ideology*. Durham, NC: Duke University Press.

Žižek, S. 1998b. Love thy neighbour? No, thanks! In: C. Lane, ed. *The Psychoanalysis of Race*. New York, NY: Columbia University Press.

Žižek, S. 2000. Class struggle or postmodernism? Yes, please! In: J. Butler, E. Laclau and S. Žižek, eds. *Contingency, Hegemony, Universality: Contemporary Dialogues on the Left*. London: Verso, 90–135.

Žižek, S. 2002. The only good neighbor is a dead neighbor. *Identities: Journal for Politics, Gender and Culture*, 2 (2), 9–31.

Žižek, S. 2004. The structure of domination today: A Lacanian view. *Studies in Eastern European Thought*, 56, 383–403.

Žižek, S. 2005a. *The Metastases of Enjoyment: Six Essays on Women and Causality*. London: Verso.
Žižek, S. 2005b. The Christian-Hegelian comedy [online]. *Cabinet Magazine*. Available from: www.cabinetmagazine.org/issues/17/Žižek.php [Accessed 10 March 2019].
Žižek, S. 2006a. Preface to the paperback edition: The big other between violence and civility. In: R. Butler and S. Stephens, eds. *Slavoj Žižek: The Universal Exception*. London: Continuum, vii–xxxii.
Žižek, S. 2006b. Why we all love to hate Haider. In: R. Butler and S. Stephens, eds. *Slavoj Žižek: The Universal Exception*. London: Continuum, 33–41.
Žižek, S. 2006c. A leftist plea for Eurocentricism. In: R. Butler and S. Stephens, eds. *Slavoj Žižek: The Universal Exception*. London: Continuum, 183–208.
Žižek, S. 2006d. *The Parallax View*. Cambridge, MA: The MIT Press.
Žižek, S. 2008a. *The Sublime Object of Ideology*. London: Verso.
Žižek, S. 2008b. *The Plague of Fantasies*. London: Verso.
Žižek, S. 2010. Liberal multiculturalism hides an old barbarism with a human face [online]. *The Guardian*. Available from: www.theguardian.com/commentisfree/2010/oct/03/immigration-policy-roma-rightwing-europe [Accessed 4 March 2019].
Žižek, S. 2012a. *Less Than Nothing: Hegel and the Shadow of Dialectical Materialism*. London: Verso.
Žižek, S. 2012b. Introduction: The spectre of ideology. In: S. Žižek, ed. *Mapping Ideology*. London: Verso, 1–33.
Žižek, S. 2013a. *Demanding the Impossible*. Cambridge: Polity.
Žižek, S. 2013b. The role of chimney sweepers in sexual identity. *International Journal of Zizek Studies*, 7 (2), 1–9.
Žižek, S. 2015. *Absolute Recoil: Towards a New Foundation of Dialectical Materialism*. London: Verso.
Žižek, S. 2016. *Disparities*. London: Bloomsbury.
Žižek, S. 2017a. *Against the Double Blackmail: Refugees, Terror and Other Troubles with the Neighbour*. London: Penguin.
Žižek, S. 2017b. *Incontinence of the Void: Economico-Philosophical Spandrels*. Cambridge, MA: MIT Press.
Žižek, S. 2018. *Like a Thief in Broad Daylight: Power in the Era of Post-Humanity*. London: Allen Lane.
Žižek, S. and Daly, G. 2004. *Conversations with Žižek*. Cambridge: Polity Press.
Zupančič, A. 2008. *The Odd One In: On Comedy*. Cambridge, MA: MIT Press.
Zupančič, A. 2016. You'd have to be stupid not to see that. *Parallax*, 22 (4), 413–425.

4

COMEDY'S REAL SUBVERSION

Subversive comedy

Let's be clear: the argument that has been traced thus far is not one that simply calls for more 'open racism'. Instead, it was suggested in the preceding chapter that our approach to racism can be reconsidered when we examine how examples of 'race', such as racial stereotypes, are marked by the Real; an effect made visible in social interactions and comic performances. Significantly, the purpose here is not to deride comedy as a form that is unhelpful for tackling racism, but instead to highlight how it can be used to approach 'racism' in an alternative and critical fashion. As previously detailed, if Real contact with the other is to be made, if a shared solidarity is to be achieved, then making such contact through shared obscenities may offer a unique form of social interaction, pertinent to the social efficacy that is achieved when we share a good joke (Yao, 2012).

More broadly, it is argued that this approach fits within the coordinates afforded by analyses that seek to explore the dynamics underpinning cultural diversity in global, neoliberal societies (Martín-Lucas and Ruthven, 2017). As Gilroy asserts, 'We have been waiting for a more sophisticated and political understanding of cultural change, influence, and adaptation that can defend and explain the spontaneous tolerance and openness evident in the underworld of Britain's convivial culture' (2004: 144). To this end, Gilroy (2004) highlights how, far outside the official forms of multiculturalism professed and administered by UK governments and politicians, there exists an everyday form of multiculturalism – a convivial form. Key to this development, however, is ensuring that such conviviality is used to counter the UK's postcolonial melancholia; a melancholia forged from the UK's inability to fully mourn the loss of its imperial past and world-power status. What is important in Gilroy's (2004) approach, therefore, is that instead of laughing at immigrants and racial others, the UK directs its laughter at its own convivial diversity. It is in detailing this approach that Gilroy (2004) turns to the fictional character, 'Ali G'. In accordance with the discussion of Ali G in Chapter Three, Gilroy highlights how Ali G's 'unfixed' and 'unstable' cultural construction:

> might also have helped to break laughter's complicity with postcolonial melancholia and to locate new sources of comedy in a remade relationship with our heterogeneous selves, working through the aftereffects of empire in a self-consciously multicultural nation. … It helps instead to cultivate the everyday, ordinary virtue involved in managing healthier relationships with otherness that are not deformed by fear, anxiety, and violence.
>
> *(2004: 149)*

While agreeing with Gilroy's (2004) concern that healthy, culturally heterogenous relationships should not be marked by violence, there remains the potential to examine how such heterogeneity can be used to expose underlying contentions in multicultural discourses. In fact, it is here that 'By playing the fool, Baron Cohen's characters, acting as journalists, show how multiculturalism's political correctness is deeply related to existing bigotries' (Alonso, 2016: 589).

Given this, it is through comedy, humour and the telling of jokes that such risky forms of cultural interaction can be performed. Indeed, Weaver highlights how:

> Jokes require ambiguity or incongruity as content, and, as a rhetorical device that is similar to metaphor, have the inbuilt ability to have an impact on truth perceptions (and the perception of ambivalence), all paradoxically in a non-serious discursive realm.
>
> *(2010: 35)*

Echoing Freud (2003), such ambiguity, incongruity and ambivalence is what provides comedy a unique significance in allowing what is forbidden to be expressed. Yet, it is this non-seriousness, embedded within certain discursive figurations, which serves to limit the potential subversion of comedy, eliciting a sense of exclusivity that can just as easily exclude certain individuals and groups as it can include them. Chow explains that while:

> Laughing together can be therapeutic, even healing. … it can have effects that are socially and politically damaging: consider the phenomenon of the Working Men's Club comic in the United Kingdom (Bernard Manning, Roy 'Chubby' Brown), known for peppering their material with jokes [that] tak[e] as their target women, ethnic minorities, immigrants, LGBTQ individuals – in other words, anyone outside of their mainly male, white, working-class audiences. These performances create communities of laughter, but these communities are not open and universal but closed and exclusive.
>
> *(2014: 231)*

Such forms of subversive expression, as detailed in Chapter Three, should not be seen as opportunities to promote and express racist stereotypes – a process that would simply echo 'not-racist' assertions (Lentin, 2018). Furthermore, according to Pérez:

> While one can argue that discussing racial topics while trying to challenge traditional racist tropes is not racist in the conventional sense, race-based humor often teaches the audience how to think about race while reifying and relying on racial stereotypes.
>
> *(2013: 483)*

Subsequently, while many comedians assert that comedy provides a way of transgressing and provoking social norms and values (Friedman, 2014; Jeffries, 2014; O'Hara, 2016), it is important that due consideration is afforded to which norms and values are being provoked and, specifically, to what purpose.

Equally, it was highlighted in the previous chapter how 'explicitly' acknowledging and promoting one's 'not racist' credentials can often allow for an implicitly racist assertion to be made. In a certain way, 'I am not racist, but…' provides a symbolic gesture that subsequently permits the evocation of racist claims. These gestures can take on a universal significance, in that their universality is predicated on excluding those who do 'see' race and, when making 'racial' claims, are left with the accusation of unnecessarily asserting racial distinctions. Consequently, while 'the workings of race often operate at the level of the unconscious, as evinced in the spectacle of racial difference which brings to the fore the constitutive inconsistency of the socio-symbolic order', it is the, 'I am not a racist, but…' clarification, which reveals how 'the unspeakable about race … is lost in the spotlight' (Hsiao, 2010: 184).

Moreover, it is important that comedy, humour and the telling of jokes do not fall foul of regulatory controls, whereupon comedians become managed and informed on what they can and can't say (BBC, 2018; Kisin, 2018; Loughrey, 2018). While this speaks to those forms of curtailment that have been prescribed to political correctness, Chapters One to Three have endeavoured to expose how analyses of comedy and racist humour cannot be removed from broader criticisms of multiculturalism and its administering of political correctness.

Accordingly, by turning to the explicitness of racist jokes, one is not assuming or even resigning oneself to a simple cynicism: 'I know this joke is racist, but, nevertheless, let me have my racism'. Indeed, such examples point to the easy manipulation of a cynical attitude to help support racist assertions while also revealing a certain 'insensitivity to reflection' (Žižek, 1999). Instead, what the previous chapters have drawn attention to is how a certain negativity, constitutive of both the subject (the lack at the heart of the subject) and reality (the parallax gap), can be brought to bear through the reflexive short circuit that is prescribed by the parallax view. Acknowledging this reflexive negativity is not meant to encourage a negative response or attitude, but instead seeks to induce a shift, a *change*, in how one traverses and encounters this negativity (Zupančič, 2003). What is important is that such reflexivity is acknowledged as part of the comic sequence. This is not a coincidence of 'two' or a 'distancing' of the self from the social, but the non-coincidence of the One – a reflexive short circuiting that comically acknowledges its self-division, its own inherent lack or 'gap'.

Integral to this latter assertion is the transiting of the 'gap' which becomes visible through the minimal difference that is afforded by a parallax view, and which, in the case of comedy, presents the essential non-coincidence of the One with itself. It is this non-coincidence which is shared by subjects both in and through their social interactions (Žižek, 2002, 2010, 2017b). In addition, this is not a heightened form of 'reflexivity' akin to the self-management that is now required as part of our 'risk society' (Beck, 2005; Žižek, 1999). Rather, this is a form of reflexivity that points to the inherent 'gaps' and tensions that underscore our symbolic order; a reflexivity guided by a self-separation in the subject *and* the big Other (Verhaeghe, 2018). It is in this way that we become aware that while the big Other does (not) exist, its inherent ambiguities point to an unstable grounding for the subject.

This ambiguity is echoed in critical scholarship on stand-up comedy. In their analysis of the British comedian Stewart Lee, Berlant and Ngai (2017) highlighted how one particular joke served to walk a 'risky' path between racism and anti-racism. While acknowledging that Lee's racist stereotyping could have very easily have been seen as funny *because* of its racist stereotyping, Berlant and Ngai assert that Lee must have also been aware 'that there is no way to make his antiracist humor at a safe distance from racist humor' (2017: 246). If we consider that the above critique has sought to admonish political correctness for its 'safe-guarded' approach to race relations – relations that undermine any Real relationship – then Berlant and Ngai's consideration that there is no 'safe distance' between anti-racist and racist humour bears a clear semblance to the risky, complicated and excessive elements which frame the subject's contact with both itself and the other (Žižek, 2002, 2004). Furthermore, it is this inherent ambiguity – the lack of any safe distance – which humour and comedy can expose.

In the case of race, it is this desire to provide a 'safe space' which emphasises how the spectacle of race is frequently haunted by its spectre, which remains unacknowledged and ignored (Hsiao, 2010). For false comedy, these contradictions are continually ignored – both in racist jokes and comic performances that 'spectacularise' racial stereotypes for cheap, comic effect, as well as in those examples where the rhetoric of political correctness controls, regulates and, ultimately, obfuscates the very Real effects of racism through false forms of cultural tolerance. In fact, it is this latter path that paradoxically presents a far more pervasive form of ignorance: a spectacularising of race and its distinguishing features – via forms of self-awareness and displays of cosmopolitan capital – while also ignoring or obfuscating the spectral presence of race in all its traumatic significance (one shouldn't cause offence to or be harassed by the other).

More importantly, if we consider that the use of humour 'is to reveal again and again how the symbolic is at once an impossible (indeterminate) yet necessary dimension' (Kunkle, 2008), and that the Real is that which casts a shadow over any intended effort to approach it (Moolenaar, 2004), in a similar way we can observe how the spectre of race provides a shadow that symbolically, yet indeterminately, frames the racist joke. Rather than being ignored, such indeterminate framing highlights how the spectre of race can – via the telling of a racist joke and the lack of any 'safe distance' – deliberately 'disrupt our orientations in the Symbolic by revealing the gap, the Real at its core' (Kunkle, 2008). This is revealed not in any positive sense, but in the acknowledgment of that obscene element that establishes the intersubjective exchange between the subject and the other – a minimal 'symbolic pact' (Žižek, 2002). It is in this way that a racist joke can be reused in a non-racist, subversive way.

Therefore, in order to achieve such subversion, first, we require an approach that does not refrain from those excessive elements which allow us to confront the Real; and, second, we cannot approach the other without being aware of the reflexivity that is required when approaching the Real of *their* as well as *our* otherness. By way of achieving this reflexivity, the following sections will provide a summative, yet critical, outline of comedy's Real subversion.

Vulgarity in action: Political correctness, the symbolic Law and the superego

In short, the potential for failure and affiliation which underscores social interaction stands opposed to the delimited and controlled way that political correctness seeks to avoid racial harassment and offence by managing the individual and by controlling 'language' via universal forms of 'correct' behaviour. When used alongside Zupančič's (2008) comedy as concrete universal, Žižek's (2006a) understanding of parallax can offer a path to critiquing the symbolic foundations on which political correctness relies; a process that can help reveal its vulgar underside. Here, the adjective 'vulgar' is, in this instance, deliberately used in order to draw attention to political correctness as an abstract form – indeed, as an 'immaterial' power, grounded in its own vulgar obscenity.

By way of exploring this immateriality we can, briefly, turn to Franz Kafka's *The Trial* and its protagonist, 'K.', who is arrested for a crime he does not know he's committed. Here, Buk-Swienty offers a Lacanian interpretation of K.'s predicament:

> The details concerning K.'s trial are never explained to him or to the reader. His case remains nothing but an effect ostensibly without cause. The Law seems as nothing but a certain will enacted from an indeterminate place. In other words, the Law in *The Trial* remains intangible. An immaterial materiality. Immaterial because in the place where the Law should be anchored, that is the texts of the 'Law books', there is vulgarity. Thus vulgarity is produced when an attempt to reduce the Law to materiality is made. Material because despite the fact that the Law is not stabilized as meaning in text, it exerts

material presence through, for example, symbolic figures. Figures such as the guards that 'arrest' K., the magistrates that supervise his case, and ultimately the henchmen that kill him in the final chapter.

(2016)[1]

Revealing this vulgarity presents an effective means for approaching Zupančič's (2008) concrete universal and how, when concretised in the 'Law books', the vulgar underside (its own inherent inconsistencies) is laid bare. Recognising this vulgar underside remains crucial to Žižek's (2008a) understanding of power and his move away from analyses which consider power as residing in discursive forms of ideological manipulation. That is, while not ignoring the importance of power's discursive significance – as it pertains to the functioning of the symbolic order/symbolic Law – it is, for Žižek (2005, 2008a, 2008b), notable that such power resides in a libidinal economy grounded in enjoyment. That is, alongside the symbolic Law is the superego injunction: 'Enjoy!' It is our enjoyment which 'is regulated and governed by a certain phantasmatic formation that domesticates enjoyment by commanding, directing, forbidding it', and which, as noted by Contu, 'enables us to explain what, in many discursive studies, is simply seen as a paradox' (2008: 376). Here, Žižek elaborates:

> In so far as the superego designates the intrusion of enjoyment into the field of ideology, we can also say that the opposition of symbolic Law and superego points towards the tension between ideological meaning and enjoyment: *symbolic Law guarantees meaning, whereas superego provides enjoyment which serves as the unacknowledged support of meaning.*
>
> *(2005: 56–57 [italics added])*

This paradoxical opposition between the Law and the superego corresponds with a number of notable examples drawn from popular culture, such as the infamous scene from *Casablanca* (1942) where the audience are left wondering whether Isla (Ingrid Bergman) and Rick (Humphrey Bogart) sleep together. While the act is never shown, the audience are subject to a cut-away shot of a lighthouse, which then returns to Rick smoking at the window. Žižek (2005) highlights how, at the level of the symbolic Law, the letter of the law is followed and adhered to (bearing in mind that *Casablanca* was produced during the period of the Hays Code, the sex scene is not explicitly shown). At the same time, however, this symbolic Law is underscored by the superego's preferment to 'Enjoy!'; that is, to enjoy our imaginations as they work against this Law or, in the company of like-minded companions, to share in the Law's hidden disavowal (encouraging us to believe that the forlorn lovers did in fact have sex) (Sharpe and Turner, 2018).

What remains important in the opposition between the symbolic Law and the superego is that 'The law itself needs its obscene supplement, it is sustained by it' (Žižek, 2015: 6). Moreover, this sustenance is continued through our own investment: 'the more we submit ourselves to the superego imperative, the greater its pressure, the more we feel guilty' (Žižek, 2005: 67). Evidence of this guilt underscores the ideological power of political correctness and its obfuscation of politically incorrect motifs. Indeed, as the above discussion has argued, while examples of political incorrectness, such as racist jokes, are openly disavowed, they maintain a certain unseen presence that upholds their operation. This presence is upheld through an 'official moralism [... that] functions by making us feel guilty all the time' (Žižek, 2018b). In such instances, politically correct prohibitions present rules and codes of behaviour, which, if they are truly successful, would require their own violation (Žižek, 1999).

This is apparent in Žižek's (2018a, 2018b) examples on recent developments in women's emancipation, such as the #MeToo movement, and the drive towards preventing sexual harassment and other forms of sexual violence. In many ways, these preventions can end up relying upon their own subtle forms of violence. Key here is that the ambiguity of meeting a sexual partner becomes lost in the regularities of the symbolic Law, so that recent attempts to codify and regulate the act of sexual seduction 'can also put a woman into a humiliating position' (Žižek, 2018b). Žižek notes how attempts to ensure a 'safe', non-offensive scenario of attempted seduction can result in occasions where:

> A woman who, to put it bluntly (and why not?), passionately wants to get laid by a man ... has to perform the equivalent of publicly stating, 'Please fuck me!' Are there not more subtle (but nonetheless unambiguously clear) ways to do this?
>
> *(2018b)*

The point being made in this example is that the regulation demanded by political correctness (the symbolic Law) can often result in open forms of acknowledgment which require a more obvious, and less subtle, approach – an approach that can lead to, and, result in, examples of shame and embarrassment.

An example of this can be found in the dark comedy *Dead to Me* (2019–present). Here, the character Jen (Christina Applegate), whose husband has recently been killed in a hit-and-run, attends a retreat for bereaved spouses. At a karaoke event organised by the retreat, Jen nervously approaches Jason (Steve Howey) with the intended desire to 'fuck him' (before approaching Jason, Jen exclaims to her friend: 'I'm going to try and fuck that guy'). Clearly nervous and hoping to apologise for a previous offence that she made earlier in the day, Jen remarks that the offence was in fact 'a lame attempt to try and flirt with' Jason. Upon hearing this, Jason remarks that he is flattered that Jen would like to flirt him, before stating: 'You're beautiful'. Happily shocked by the remark, Jen takes a breath and awkwardly whispers: 'Do you wanna fuck?' The following ensues:

JASON: What did you say?
JEN: Umm... do you... (*Jen, again, mouths the following, which is barely audible*) wanna fuck?

JASON: I'm sorry I can't hear you.

JEN: (*clearly embarrassed*) I'm sorry... umm... would you like to dance?

JASON: (*smiling*) Oh sure, yeah. Because for a second, I thought that you were asking me if I wanted to fuck.

This short scene effectively demonstrates the underlying impasses and awkward encounters that inevitably proceed when one takes a more 'open' approach to, in this instance, heterosexual seduction. Notably, as is clear in the above example, such forms of open expression, which may in fact reveal the positive assertion of female empowerment, can just as easily work to maintain latent forms of patriarchal power and enjoyment. In the scene, Jen feels guilty (as evident in the whispered assertions) about asking Jason to sleep with her, and while Jason knew all along and clearly enjoyed the fact that Jen wanted to fuck him, he just needed her to embarrassingly re-declare it.

To this end, while examples of political correctness can result in pervasive forms of guilt, in other instances, its derision can encourage a sense of enjoyment that relishes in its open denouncement, perhaps best expressed in the often-cited statement: 'political correctness gone mad!' This echoes Žižek's account of the bureaucracy inflicted by the Soviet Union, whereby 'the enjoyment of the very stupidity of the System – a relish in the emptiness of the official ritual, in the worn-out stylistic figures of the predominating ideological discourse' was frequently performed (2005: 64). Equally, we can begin to see how such forms of enjoyment underscore examples of cynicism which seek to comically reveal and perform the stupidity of political correctness (all the while maintaining its hegemonic authority).

To return to our discussion on the superego, it can be suggested that the ideological efficiency of political correctness stems, in part, from its ability to institute a 'solidarity-in-guilt' – a space which is established when one shares or hears a 'dirty' joke. In such instances, it is the superego which remains fetishistically disavowed, as evident in forms of '"progressive" cultural critique' whereby the 'fetishizing elevation of an author (typical candidates: Alfred Hitchcock, Jane Austen, Virginia Wolf....) all of whose "politically incorrect" misdeeds are pardoned in advance or reinterpreted as subversive-progressive in an unheard-of, hidden way' (Žižek, 2005: 58). Here, 'The community's enjoyment is provided by this very collective disavowal – for example, by our insistence on the "progressive" character of Hitchcock, which suspends the symbolic efficiency of what obviously does not enter this frame' (Žižek, 2005: 58). Therefore, whereas what is ignored, obfuscated or kept hidden can help to sustain a group's cohesion and identity, we can identify moments where such forms of disavowal are openly acknowledged and, perhaps, even naively, undermined. Žižek notes:

> one should reread Hans Christian Andersen's 'The Emperor's New Clothes' along these lines: of course everybody knew that the emperor was naked, yet

> it was precisely the disavowal of this fact that held the subject together – by stating this reality, the unfortunate child effectively dissolved the social link.
>
> *(2005: 58)*

The open acknowledgment of what is disavowed can posit a decidedly subversive effect. Staying with the image of the child who acknowledges the Emperor's nakedness, one is reminded of the various, and still ongoing, climate protests that took place in 2018/19 and which were, in part, orchestrated around the actions of Greta Thunberg, a Swedish schoolgirl who initiated the international 'School Strike for Climate' movement. What is significant is that Thunberg's 'demands' – originally a demand for Swedish and later European governments to reduce their carbon emissions in accordance with the results of climate change research – are made in the face of what most of us acknowledge, but clearly disavow: 'I know very well that climate change is occurring, but nevertheless…'. Thunberg's actions, and the global climate change protests that began in her wake, are clearly subversive in that they openly challenge examples of cynicism towards the effects of climate change.

This subversion can also be identified in examples of comedy. Yet, it is here that the contours of this subversion, especially in the case of racist comedy, need to be carefully drawn. Indeed, as Kamm and Neumann highlight:

> In a situation of generically framed incongruity, the violation of standard expectations can be enjoyable precisely because it offers recipients a temporary respite from the rigid norms of everyday life, allowing them to playfully adopt alternative, distancing and critical attitudes.
>
> *(2016: 5)*

In such cases, it is easy to see how such 'temporary respite' can, in the shadow of Bakhtin's (1984) carnivalesque and Critchley's (2002) cynicism, offer a form of ironic distance which only 'hints at repressed realities and possibly tabooed desires' (Kamm and Neumann, 2016: 5). Such forms of comic respite and their comic violation secure symbolic authority through its inherent transgression. To this extent, it is argued that a more subversive significance can be found when we consider the potential failure of the symbolic order through its *performed* disavowal.

Comedy and *objet a*: Finding sense in nonsense, finding ease in uneasiness

Indeed, we can approach this potential for failure by examining the symbolic order's fictional form. That is, 'The symbolic order can function only by maintaining a minimal distance towards reality, on account of which it ultimately has the status of a fiction' (Žižek, 2005: 76). Here Žižek draws attention to the fact that when we get what we truly desire, 'when our words realize themselves "to the letter"' (2005: 76), we are often reduced to examples of anxiety, shame and embarrassment (as evident in the above scene from *Dead to Me*). As a result, for the symbolic order to function, it must not be taken *too literally* and, as a consequence, the subject must maintain a minimal distance to reality through examples of (un)acknowledged creative fiction. Following Žižek, we can think of numerous 'creative fictions', drawn from polite conversation, which are not to be taken literally.[2] It is under conditions of 'hyperreality', however, that our symbolic fictions begin to be undermined (Baudrillard, 1994; Flisfeder, 2017). Žižek notes:

> In the 'society of spectacle', the overgrowth of imaginary 'realistic presentations leaves less and less space open for this symbolic fiction. What gets lost with media realism, from toys to videos, is the experience of 'less is more': when you listen to an opera on CD, the very fact that 'you don't see anything' enable you to fill out this void with creative fiction. In contrast, there is always something vulgar about an opera on video, due to the very fact that 'you can see everything'
>
> *(2005: 76)*

The issue here is that reality, and our relation to reality, can only constitute itself when our symbolic fictions and imaginary constructions work on a minimal difference *to* reality itself (Žižek, 2006a). It is in this way that when such difference is dissolved, when one receives what they desire, a traumatic response on behalf of the individual can ensue. Receiving such desire is amiable to gaining an overproximity to the *objet a*. Crucially, what occurs here is that 'The void filled out by creative symbolic fiction is the *objet a*, the object-cause of desire, the empty frame that provides the space for the articulation of desire' (Žižek, 2005: 76). In this sense, the subject is not externalised, and thus *distanced* from reality, as per the criticisms afforded to both Critchley (2002) and Heller (2005) (see Chapter Two), but instead 'reality itself is constituted by means of the withdrawal of *objet a*: we can relate to "normal" reality only in so far as *jouissance* is evacuated from it, in so far as the object-cause of desire [*objet a*] is missing from it' (Žižek, 2005: 76).

As a result, it is in the absence of the *objet a* that reality and the subject are constituted through a minimal difference:

> The necessary consequence of *a's* overproximity to reality, which suffocates the activity of symbolic fiction, is therefore a 'de-realization' of reality itself: reality is no longer structured by symbolic fictions; fantasies which regulate the imaginary overgrowth get a direct hold on it.
>
> *(Žižek, 2005: 76)*

What is important here is the 'direct hold' that our imagined fantasies can achieve on reality and, as a consequence, the impact upon the subject when this 'hold' is directly experienced. These fantasies are laid bare when we acknowledge that:

> each of us has some private ritual, phrase (nicknames, etc.) or gesture, used only within the most intimate circle of our closest friends or relatives; when

> these rituals are rendered public, the effect is necessarily one of extreme embarrassment and shame – we want to sink into the ground...
>
> *(Žižek, 2005: 85)*

It is this 'private' kernel which 'is irreducibly decentred with regard to the symbolic texture which defines the subject's identity' (Žižek, 2005: 77), and it is this externality, an ex-timate kernel (the *objet a*), that is decentred from the subject but whose extraction provides the subject a relative difference in which to achieve a sense of consistency within the symbolic order.

Key to this, however, is the fact that this *objet a*, while remaining crucial to the subject, is nonetheless an immaterial phenomenon which remains integral to the subject's being (its significance can often be arbitrary). There is, therefore, a certain 'sense*lessness*' which underscores the (un-)importance of the *objet a*. Indeed, while the *objet a* can take many forms, its importance resides in the fact that it's *appearance*, or lack of, gives the allusion to some*thing* that needs to be explained, understood, obtained and/or found.[3] It is in this respect that we can consider this 'strange object' (*objet a*) alongside Heller's concern that 'Jokes are serious, since there *must be sense in senselessness*' (2005: 135 [italics added]). In other words, while 'We laugh at senselessness, ... it is the sense of the senseless that gives us pleasure, and this is something serious' (Heller, 2005: 135). This 'sense of the senseless' can be considered in relation to the *objet a*, so that when we materialise that 'ritual, phrase or gesture' which is meant to be kept hidden, when we render its absent-presence *present*, we are effectively drawing attention to that aspect of 'sense' which is brought to bear in nonsense. According to Heller, 'Without the sense in nonsense there is no joke', a statement she follows with the question: 'What are we laughing at?' (2005: 136). While for Heller, we are laughing 'At a story which ridicules the simplicity of our one-track expectations; that is, at *ourselves*' (2005: 136 [italics added]), this understanding can be provided a decidedly Lacanian reflection when we consider that it is the 'split' or the 'gap' itself, both in the subject and the symbolic order, which is laid bare in the ridiculing of the 'one-track expectation'. Or, in Lacanian terminology, the over-proximity which is achieved when the *objet a* (that ex-timate kernel) is acknowledged through the joke's ridicule. Importantly, this acknowledgment is not achieved with the intrusion of an outside form, but, from a parallaxical perspective, such acknowledgment presents a short circuit that induces us to laugh at ourselves (our own phantasmatic/symbolic formations, *objet a*) and at the excessive repetition of the same. To this end, it is in openly identifying with the *objet a*, and its own 'excessive instability' and 'impossibility' (Vogt, 2007: 62–63), that comedy can induce a certain subversive recognition.

This subversion can be recognised in examples of 'trauma'. Here Heller notes how, 'in laughing at a person who holds much political and martial power, one can gain or practice moral power', so that 'The convicted can laugh in the face of his judge, the person awaiting execution, in the face of his executioner' (2005: 26–27). This is supported with the following example:

> A woman once told me that in a concentration camp, an SS soldier commanded her to kneel down, for he was going to shoot her. When, instead of pleading for her life, she started to laugh in the man's face, he became so embarrassed that he suddenly walked away.
>
> *(Heller, 2005: 26–27)*

Indeed, what is *it* in this moment that, in the case of the woman's laughter, subversively re-orientated the situation, causing embarrassment for the SS officer? Was *it* the open acknowledgment of the enjoyment that the officer obtained in humiliating the woman? Or was *it* the woman's pervasive laughter, a signal that she may in fact enjoy the humiliation? In either instance, what we see is the open acknowledgment of a certain gesture that bears no relation to the situation described, but which, in all its incongruity, seems to be the right form of response (amidst the horrors of the holocaust, the only response left would be to laugh). It is in this regard that Heller's (2005) example bears a resemblance to Žižek's (1999) contention that the best holocaust movies are comedies – an argument predicated on the concern that the audience's laughter can elicit the uncomfortable acknowledgment of laughter's hideous underside. A similarly comic theme can be identified in Kurt Vonnegut's 'anti-war' novel, *Slaughterhouse Five* (2009).

As noted in the above examples, this process is not specific to comedy. Rather, what comedy can induce is a certain excessive over-identification, similar to Heller's over-identification with the social a priori. To draw upon a non-comedy example, it is this excess which is noted in Žižek's account of the character Kurtz in *Apocalypse Now*:

> the figure of Kurtz … is … not … a remainder of some barbaric past, but … the necessary outcome of the modern Western power itself. Kurtz was the perfect soldier – as such, through his over-identification with the military power system, he turned into the excess which the system has to eliminate. The ultimate horizon of *Apocalypse Now* is this insight into how Power generates its own excess, which it has to annihilate in an operation which has to imitate what it fights.
>
> *(2006a: 370)*

What remains crucial in this analysis is the over-identification that Žižek (2006a) prescribes to Kurtz; an over-identification which openly demonstrates the 'obscene' agency of the superego – its excessive violence and its need to be 'removed' (in the film, the mission to kill Kurtz is 'off record'). To this end, and while well aware that *Apocalypse Now* and the original story from which it is based on, Joseph Conrad's *Heart of Darkness* (2008), are not comedies, there is, nonetheless, a certain comic form to Kurtz's digression: that of a man who believes himself to be a native deity, a comical re-enactment of the arrogant and tyrannical embodiment of European colonialism/US military aggression in all its excessive ridiculousness. By over-identifying with this excess, we see, in Kurtz, the absurdity of those systems grounded in colonial and military power. Echoing the excess of Kurtz, we can perhaps go further and see a similar process at play in political correctness and how its own excessive and 'self-destructive deadlock' can be identified in its desire to manage, regulate and formalise all aspects of social interaction (Žižek, 2018a: 226).

Accordingly, what Heller (2005) and Žižek (1991, 2005) both draw attention to is that excessive element which cannot be represented unless achieved through a symbolic fiction or, for present purposes, comic form. While the effects of comedy's excess have been considered in McGowan's (2016, 2017) work on comedy, and in his comparison of both Charlie Chaplin and Buster Keaton, we can extend this line of inquiry in order to consider those comic moments which serve to perform this excessive element as part of the comic sequence. Drawing attention to this excess, via comedy, can help direct attention to the efficiency of the obscene underside which marks the superego (Žižek, 2005).

Certainly, as has been highlighted in previous chapters, in the case of racist humour, the open acknowledgment of forms of excessive racist humour can work to support racist assertions. Indeed, Billig notes that:

> Under the cover of the joking situation, prejudiced thoughts can be expressed and socially enjoyed. In this way, the downgrading of outsiders escapes the censure that would inevitably accompany the expression of 'serious' prejudice in many contemporary discursive situations. The joking context creates a temporary situation which seems to permit laughter at exaggeratedly stereotyped unreal members of the outgroup, as jokers celebrate the funniness of their joking and deny their own racism.
>
> *(2005: 33)*

Yet, in accordance with Billig (2005), we can subsequently consider how examples of politically incorrect humour may just as easily serve as the superego's obscene underside. As a result:

> Superego demands obedience and enjoyment, transgression and compliance, staining everything with its obscene excess. If the official rules demand racial tolerance, superego demands our vigilance in the face of irremedial racist guilt. At the same time, the truth of racist guilt, the racism that persists and flourishes through and in the face of official tolerance, creates racist solidarities – our racist jokes become transgressive, permission to break the rules, submission to the injunction 'Enjoy!'
>
> *(Dean, 2006: 156–157)*

How we relate to this 'obscene excess' continues to be a salient feature in work that has considered the political mobilisation of Žižek's philosophical outlook (Dean, 2006; McMillan, 2013; Sharpe and Boucher, 2010). With regard to comedy it is posited that a political significance can be maintained when, despite

Dean's (2006) apprehensions, it subversively performs an over-identification with the superego imperative, drawing attention to the inherent inconsistencies of the symbolic order. Indeed, by over-identifying with the fantasies that seek to mask the Real, we can more fully identify with those aspects of society that are subsequently disavowed as part of its functioning. As Stavrakakis asserts, 'Every critical discourse, as the critique of ideology, has to go through fantasy and detect in the projection of the symptom the lack, the split of our social reality' (2016). Certainly, there is the possibility that one subscribes to this fantasy in its entirety and subsequently fails to identify those symptoms which our ideological fantasies seek to obfuscate, but it is at this point that comedy can play its subversive role: bringing to light that which is both asserted by the symbolic Law as well as that which it keeps hidden (superego). Central to this claim is the acknowledgment of, or the over-identification with, the *lack* at the heart of the symbolic Law. It is in this way that comedy can expose its 'unique capacity for showing us that our enjoyment consists not in overcoming lack or realizing our desire but in enjoying that lack' (McGowan, 2017: 46). Moreover, it is in enjoying this lack that one can obtain a parallax shift (an ontological shift) that presents what was hidden, but is now acknowledged. This enjoyment of the lack is one which follows a process of negation, and which bears a resemblance to Zupančič's analysis of Maurice Blanchot's short essay, *The Apocalypse is Disappointing* (1997). Here, Zupančič notes how:

> In its minimal form his [Blanchot's] argument runs like this: the threat of the Bomb and its destructive potential made appear, for the first time, the idea of a whole (of the world) – a whole, precisely, that can be lost, or disappear forever. We can lose it all; but the idea of the whole (of an all that can be lost) only appears through a negation; it only constitutes a whole in the perspective of being potentially lost. In other words, there is no (existing) totality, no 'whole of the world,' which could be eventually (actually) lost in an atomic apocalypse; it is, paradoxically, only the perspective of this very (potential) loss which constitutes it, or makes it appear, as such a totality or whole.
>
> *(2017/18: 17–18)*

What is apparent in this example is that it is through such negation – the total destruction of the world – that the idea of a world worth saving comes to fruition. In the same way, it is when one 'over-identifies' with such an idea – the world's annihilation – that what was once taken for granted (the everyday, routine existence of the world) now becomes visible.

It is this process of negation which underscores 'a strategy of *overidentification*, which takes into account the fact that the obscene superego *qua* basis and support of the public Law is operative only in so far as it remains unacknowledged, hidden from the public eye' (Žižek, 2005: 71). Here, Žižek questions: 'What if, instead of critical dissection and irony which reveal their impotence in the face of racism's phantasmic kernel, we proceed *a contrario* and identify publicly with the obscene superego?' (2005: 71). What remain central to this subversive process are the limits it can expose. Accordingly, by comically over-identifying with political correctness, we walk a path of deliberately performing its own internal limits and its own excessive surplus. This is marked not by an intrusion from 'outside' but from the lack and/or division *within* this form (the One) itself. This 'internal' subversion can expose the 'obscene excess' which, in the comic performance, obtains a subversive potential via the 'minimal difference' that is achieved towards the superego's injunction. That is, in a parallaxical approach, this minimal difference presents a realisation of the 'gap' within the self-division of the One. In doing so, it can be considered along the same lines that one 'approaches' the Real (Žižek, 2017a).

Indeed, in this light, the adoption of a racist joke is not simply an attempt to deliberately enjoy the subversion of political correctness: this is not a simple recourse to 'Enjoy!' the guilt that one can achieve through being 'subversive' – rather, it is to draw attention to the minimal difference which is achieved in comedy through what Lacan refers to as a 'traversing of the fantasy'. Equally, this is not a form of scepticism on behalf of the subject, akin to cynical distance, but a realisation of what was there, but was not acknowledged; of what was expected to be different, but was actually the same; of what is known, but which can only be ambiguously understood. It is therefore an acknowledgment of the Real (and the superego) as 'a borderline experience, an experience of in-between-ness, created by the confrontation with unexpected and absurd situations, which attract and fascinate by generating a feeling of pleasurable uneasiness' (Kamm and Neumann, 2016: 5). This uneasiness does not need to be monopolised by feelings of guilt (superego), but can instead form a constitutive part of encountering the other.

It is in this sense that certain 'jokes' can 'break against the enforced proprieties and casual hypocrisies of "liberal tolerance," … demonstrat[ing] a brave sense of ease about the ordinary, "unpleasant" stuff that lies at the base of all of our dreams and thoughts' (Sayeau, 2013). To this end, it is not just that which lies at the base of our dreams and thoughts, but that which remains inherent to the other and which, in a way that steers clear of any regulated path, requires an acknowledgment of the ambiguities that underscore relations with the other. The path that is being traced here is one that follows the psychoanalytic process:

> The final stage of the psychoanalytic cure is reached when the subject recognizes himself, his own motivations, in the censured chapters of his self-expression, and is able to narrate the totality of his life story. In a first approach, psychoanalysis thus proceeds along the path of causal explanation: it brings to light the causal chain which, unbeknownst to the subject, produced the symptom. However – and herein resides the proper notion of self-reflection – *this very explanation of the causal chain cancels its efficacy*. And adequate interpretation does not only lead to the 'true knowledge' of the symptom, it simultaneously involves the symptoms' dissolution, and thereby

> the 'reconciliation' of the subject with himself – the act of knowing is in itself an act of liberation from unconscious coercion.
>
> *(Žižek, 2005: 25)*

Such self-expression, constitutive of the 'reconciliation' that one achieves, is not a solely individual process, but rather one that is shared between, in the above example, the analyst and analysand. As will be discussed below, it is in this way that our own 'liberation' from political correctness can stem primarily from that which it seeks to manage – relations with the other.

The 'trouble' with jokes

Central to the above discussion is the underlying contention that, in the case of racist jokes, we can begin to consider how racism's (Real) (im)material power can be re-approached by acknowledging, and in the process, reducing, racism to its vulgar materiality (it's superego incentive). To recite an earlier quote from Žižek regarding the *objet a*, racial stereotypes 'can be turned into a comic resource', and, as is evident in the case of human seduction, 'can function as something to be circumvented, alluded to, played with, exploited, manipulated, [and] made fun of' (Žižek, 2015: 306). Such a resource is deliberately precarious and consequently steers between the fragile possibility of achieving consensus or dissensus, yet it is this possibility which Chow reflects upon when he notes that, 'In the midst of the pleasurable *sensus communis* of laughing together is the possibility of dissensus; in this way, performance comedy demonstrates the precariousness of our identifications and our ways of being together' (2014: 231). This is echoed by Berlant and Ngai who argue that while 'Comedy theory has tended to foreground detachment', it is its ability to encourage 'proximity' – a proximity which in this case can be perceived as a proximity to the Real (of the other) – which 'deserves particular attention' (2017: 248). They continue:

> In the comedic scene things are always closer to each other than they appear. They are near each other in a way that prompts a disturbance in the air. People can enjoy that disturbance, and one thing they can enjoy in it is that it feels automatic, spontaneous, freed-up. Pressed a little, the enjoyment is not always, hardly ever, unmixed; but in the moment, the feeling of freedom exists with its costliness.
>
> *(Berlant and Ngai, 2017: 248)*

This sense of antagonism and disturbance, which neatly captures the precarity of social interaction, not only underscores our relations with the other but, more importantly, frames our approach to comedy as that which can help us 'touch the Real' through the potential success/failure of human affiliation.

Certainly, as previously noted, 'The reinvention of racist humour as a lens to illuminate the tensions in our multi-cultural society is at best a risky practice'

(Peters and Becker, 2010: 197). The argument traced above is well aware of these risks, but what it hopes to draw attention to is the ambiguity that inevitably structures subject-other relations; relations that can succumb to examples of racism, but which also offer an alternative form for re-approaching the ambiguity that structures these relations. In fact, with regards to class, Raisborough et al. outline how 'contemporary theorists of class-making … need to pick up on class unease, benevolence and sympathy as mechanisms for class-making' (2012: 262–263). If we consider this in relation to examples of race, then exploring those instances where race is 'made' – and by this we are referring to both its symbolic and imaginary significance – requires a consideration of those examples where 'unease, benevolence and sympathy' occur as part of Real social interactions as well as the contingency which underscores our socio-symbolic orders.

Therefore, by acknowledging that 'humour can work subversively, as it produces "a consciousness of contingency"', from which 'the world is exposed as not naturally given or necessary but possible to reimagine' (Sigurdson, 2013: 237), we can begin to see how one of the functions of jokes is to deliberately 'trouble the social-symbolic order and hold out the possibility of escape from it' (Chow, 2014: 229). Such 'escape' can occur through a parallax shift which both reveals, and subsequently distorts, our initial interpretations. For example, consider Chow's Žižekian deconstruction of a joke:

> The reader (or audience), must stumble over the joke, which in turn often provokes discomfort. Our (stupid) first impression is that the joke is a meaningless distraction. Our second impression, the antithesis of the first, is the ingenious and informed interpretation that actually, there is a serious message behind these jokes, that their content actually reveals something philosophically profound. But in Žižek's dialectical thinking, we must always return to the appearance, to our stupid first impression: actually, the joke *is* meaningless, but by being meaningless it demonstrates the contingent and incomplete nature of our symbolic universe(s).
>
> *(2014: 232)*

Here, 'Žižek's dialectical thinking' can be reconsidered as an example of parallax, one in which our 'stumbling' and 'discomfort' are not viewed as meaningless or entirely 'stupid', but as fundamental to our social interactions. Moreover, Zupančič's (2008) contention that comedy occurs through a concrete universality can help bridge our parallaxical reorientation to/with the symbolic order. What remains implicit to this line of inquiry, however, is the underlying concern that identifying the inconsistencies of the symbolic requires us to identity those ambiguities (or vulgar underside) which maintain it.

As previously noted, such ambiguity forms a central feature of jokes regarding race and the use of racial stereotypes (Perez, 2013; Weaver, 2010, 2011). In fact, 'As both an aesthetic mode and a form of life, [… comedy's] action just as likely produces anxiety: risking transgression, flirting with displeasure, or just confusing things in a way that both intensifies and impedes the pleasure' (Berlant and Ngai, 2017: 233). This is echoed in Weaver's analysis of British comedian Lenny Henry, which notes that Henry's use of racial stereotypes, while identifying their 'absurdity', nevertheless 'do not remove the polysemic potential in the discourse … Thus the rhetorical potential is ambiguous' (2010: 40). Similarly, if we consider that our previous critique of political correctness, with its over-focus on cultural tolerance, 'does not stop discrimination, it merely changes its face, making it more subtle, so subtle that it becomes confined to small acts of confrontation or omission that ultimately add up to continuous affronts about ones colour or difference (accent, lifestyle, way of dressing)' (Rudge et al., 2012: 41), then, again, what we are dealing with here is an underlying sense of ambiguity which, under the rhetoric of political correctness, remains, on the one hand, ignored, and, on the other, superficially admonished. By way of approaching this ambiguity, we can return to the Real:

> Contrary to what some people think, the Lacanian notion that the Real is impossible doesn't mean simply that you cannot do anything about the Real. The fundamental wager, or hope, of psychoanalysis is that with the symbolic you can intervene in the Real. … So the basic wager of psychoanalysis is that you can do things with words; real things that enable you to change modes of enjoyment and so on.
>
> *(Žižek and Daly, 2004: 150)*

With regards to racism, the basic wager being made in this analysis is that we can approach racism through symbolically intervening in its Real effects. One way this can be achieved is by highlighting, or comically performing, the Real of racism as it is symbolically framed in examples of political correctness. That is, its ontological inconsistency can be identified in those inconsistencies and incongruities that inherently frame our relation to political correctness.

Joking and the Real

In order to examine that shared 'space' which is inhabited when we tell a joke, we can consider Žižek's contention that 'A much more effective experience of universal humanity, i.e., of the meaninglessness of the conflict we are engaged in, can take the shape of a simple exchange of gazes which tells everything' (2002: 11). He notes that:

> During one of the anti-apartheid demonstrations in the old South Africa, when a troop of white policemen was dispersing and pursuing black demonstrators, a policeman was running after a black lady, a rubber truncheon in his hand. Unexpectedly, the lady lost one of her shoes; automatically obeying his good manners, the policeman picked up the shoe and gave it to her; at this moment, they exchanged glances and both became aware of the inanity of

> their situation – after such a gesture of politeness, i.e. after handling her the lost shoe and waiting for her to put it on again, it was simply IMPOSSIBLE for him to continue to run after her and to hit her with the truncheon; so, after politely nodding at her, the policeman turned around and walked away... The moral of this story is NOT that the policeman suddenly discovered his innate goodness, i.e. we are NOT dealing here with the case of natural goodness winning over the racist ideological training; on the contrary, in all probability, the policeman was – as to his psychological stance – a standard racist. What triumphed here was simply his superficial training in politeness.
>
> *(Žižek, 2002: 11 [emphasis in original])*

While Žižek (2018a) has extended this example of politeness in later analyses, we can use the aforementioned scene to help illustrate a specific 'concrete' moment from which the universal vulgarity of apartheid in South Africa and its implicit inanity were undermined in a concrete moment of Real contact. Moreover, it is perhaps possible to perceive a sense of comedy in the above example and not in a way that undermines the wider racial significance of a white policeman chasing a black anti-apartheid protestor. One can imagine the sense of parallax, the shift in perspective, that occurs when, looking at each other, both subjects are left asking (and chuckling): 'What on earth are we doing?' It is in this regard that Žižek offers the following assertion: 'in order to transform this magic moment of the suspension of symbolic barriers into a more substantial achievement, something more is needed – like, for example, the sharing of obscene jokes' (2002: 11–12).

It is here that we can begin to determine how comedy resides in an intimate space between the joke-teller and the listener/audience. In similar fashion to 'making a pass', it is in this 'potentially dangerous moment, [that] one exposes oneself, intruding into another person's intimate space' (Žižek, 2018b). If we compare this to 'flirting' (notably, the act of flirting is one closely related to comedy and humour), then there is an inherent 'ambiguity of the sexual encounter [that] is inevitably prone to misinterpretation' (Grant, 1994: 84). Here, Grant (1994) draws attention to Paglia's assertion that, when one partakes in a date, 'Sex is hovering in the air' (Paglia, 1993 cited in Grant, 1994: 84–85). In comedy, the same implicit possibility of misinterpretation – indeed, the possibility of causing offence – is always 'hovering in the air'.

This possibility for misinterpretation is echoed in Dahlgren's assertion that 'the looseness, open-endedness of everyday talk, its creativity, potential for empathy and affective elements, are indispensable for the vitality of democratic politics' (2002: 11 cited in Das and Graefer, 2017: 12). In fact, with such potentiality being marked by the inherent lack/excess in communication, it is apparent that in any situation we can always say too much or even too little (Žižek, 2005). As a consequence:

> Foregrounding the breakdown of communication and crisis in understanding comedy lays bare the many pitfalls and challenges inherent in seemingly

> ordinary, logical and economically structured conversation. But communicative failure, nonsense and misunderstanding also have a pleasurable and creatively liberating potential for they temporarily release viewers from the self-imposed obligation of communicating effectively and grant the (childish) pleasure of suspending everyday rules.
>
> *(Kamm and Neumann, 2016: 4)*

To this end, when approaching the other through comedy, there is always the possibility of ambiguity, miscommunication and, possibly, violence, which remains inherent to comedy's form. Accepting such 'failure', however, does not necessarily offer a pessimistic account, fuelled by the assertion that all comedy should offend. Rather, it more appropriately draws attention to those moments where comedy can have the obverse effect, when sharing a joke or performing a comedy sequence can achieve contact with the Real other.

In addition, it is here that we can trace a different approach to the notion of 'surprise' in comedy. As reflected in the policeman-protestor example, the subtle change in the policeman reveals a certain *stutter* in the scene described: a jolt or a skip that, rather than including something 'new', denotes a certain hesitation in the symbolic order. Bonic notes:

> The reason we laugh is because we are surprised by something, an 'odd' element that suddenly appears (often a double, or in some ways illogical). We are not surprised because we see something new (nor even see with new eyes, as the cliché goes).
>
> *(2011: 106)*

It is in this appearance of a 'double' that we get the *punch*line. In these instances, we are dealing with a *stutter* that parallaxically draws attention to the division of the One and its inherent inconsistency. This steers away from simply focusing on and admiring the 'shock' which can be induced when telling a risky joke, as evident in those affects which become enamored with the desire to conjure 'shock value'. Instead, when I tell a joke (obviously aware of the punchline), or when a joke is told to me, we inevitably encounter an encroachment of the subject onto the other and, when hearing a joke, the encroachment of the other onto the subject. While this draws attention to the formal features of the joke, in the case of the comic sequence, it is this stutter – this encroachment – which is extended over a temporal frame. In so doing, comedy and the sharing of obscene jokes can identify and approach the (potential) antagonisms that underscore human interaction through the vulgarity of sharing an obscene joke.

In what follows, closer attention will be paid to exploring how these antagonisms can help constitute comedy's Real subversion. Achieving this, however, will require a consideration of the symbolic order, the big Other and the universal, with specific attention being given to how these three notions can be brought together through a shared sense of 'lack'.

Subversion and the symbolic order: Inducing a shift in perspective

In accordance with our previous discussion of both the Real and parallax, we can begin to see how it is through both terms – the parallax Real – that a 'minimal difference that cuts across and divides the same object among the various different perspectives' (Flisfeder, 2012: 147) can be observed. It is this minimal difference which is brought to bear in the stutter of the symbolic order. Grounded in their use of Hegel, both Žižek and Zupančič reveal how 'a genuine shift in our original perspective can provide us with new forms of philosophical (in)sight' from which 'a decisive shift in our observational position can grant us an alternative perspective on what we, as cultural subjects, perceive as our ontological reality' (Mangold, 2014: 7). Indeed, if true comedy reflects the universal expressed in the concrete, then such expression suggests a fundamental shift in the universal itself, which is conducive to an underlying shift in the symbolic order/big Other. Moreover, it is through Zupančič's (2008) consideration of true comedy, as a reflection of the concrete universal, that this shift can be performed.

Accordingly, while false comedy 'may amuse us, make us laugh, even disturb us by disclosing the "truths" of ideology, human existence, etc.', it inevitably leaves these truths 'fundamentally unchanged' (Bonic, 2011: 97). Instead, for Zupančič (2008), and here we can draw a direct link between Zupančič (2008) and Hegel's (1998) *Phenomenology of Spirit*:

> Comedy, … does not just augur a shift from the perspective of universal values to that of limited and imperfect individuals in their concrete materiality, as if it were a turn away from universal values. Rather, for Hegel, comedy lays bare the limitations and imperfections of the abstract universal itself – and thus brings to light the manifold concrete, dramatic perils to which our deepest values are exposed in the extraordinary and surprising lives of individual human beings.
>
> *(Kottman, 2009: 18)*

Through Zupančič's (2008) 'short circuit' we see how true comedy can permit us to self-identify with the abstract, universal, socio-symbolic constructions and fantasies which constitute our material existence. It is in this way that the 'gap' in the universal can serve as a modality of the Real (McMillan, 2013). This is reflected in the notion of anamorphosis in Lacan and Žižek's interpretation of the skull in Holbein's *The Ambassadors* (1533) and which is continued in Žižek's (1991) 'looking awry'. It is this sense of anamorphosis which is exposed through comedy.

Key to this anamorphic parallax shift is its ability to highlight the tensions which become visible the moment we perceive a shift in our perspective and see, not two separate objects, but *the same object approached through its own non-coincidence*. For Zupančič (2008) such non-coincidence points to the ontological 'gap' inherent within reality and, more importantly, to the 'gap' which makes comedy possible. In the case of identity and, in particular, racial identities, this can offer a unique approach. That is, what parallax advises us to bear in mind are the tensions and antagonisms inherent to identity, not necessarily in a pejorative sense, but as something that is acknowledged and approached through examples of comedy.

Accordingly, through comedy, we can draw attention to that 'fragile space of exchange and circulation' which occurs as part of cultural communication (Žižek, 2006a: 8). One should not refrain from or ignore such negativity, but consider it as an approach to the Real. Importantly, as previously noted, the Real is indirectly configured within the symbolic order, so that while any symbolic act seeks to prohibit the Real, such prohibition inevitably 'occults the inherent deadlock of the Real' (Žižek, 1998: 129 [italics removed]). It is in acknowledging this deadlock that 'one can "touch the real" only by applying oneself to its symbolization, up to the very failure of this endeavor' (Žižek, 1998: 129). Therefore, by acknowledging the inherent deadlocks that occur in interactions across a whole range of social situations (and, again, this is not meant in a pejorative sense), we can better appreciate 'the potential (and potential failure) of affiliation with others' (Chow, 2014: 231). It is through the Real, 'In all its brutal immediacy', that we can begin to consider how 'the negative can have a deeply symbolic effect' (Zupančič, 2017/18: 27) that, in a form of reflexivity, can parallaxically render our own sense of 'lack' – indeed, our own strangeness.

In fact, if we consider this in view of Žižek's (1998, 2002) work on the other, then we can recognise that it is not the other which prevents 'me' from achieving 'my' full identity but, on the contrary, it is any full identity, any complete understanding of 'me', which is always blocked, thwarted and impossible. Externalising these frustrations onto the other works to obfuscate this recognition. This can boil over into open racist hostility, fuelled by racist fantasies of how the other steals/blocks the subject's full identity, as well as patronisingly positioning the other through forms of shallow humanitarianism. Instead, it has been argued that such hatred can be radically redefined as drawing attention to the subject's own sense of strangeness: that, in short, we are strangers to ourselves (Žižek, 2017b). This reflexive short circuit provides a coincidence between our own lack and excess, which not only constitutes, but also traumatically defines, our subjectivity (McGowan, 2017). In fact, 'Though comedy itself has an ambivalent political valence', for McGowan, 'grasping its structure points us in the direction of a traumatic equality' (2017: 16). It is this 'traumatic equality' which avers that strange sense of strangeness which characterises our relations with the other *and ourselves*. In this instance, it is parallax that can help support a form of reflexivity which allows us to acknowledge our own strangeness; a strangeness which is itself performed as part of the comedy character.

Indeed, what remains crucial in both Žižek (2012, 2015) and Zupančič's (2003, 2008) approaches is the ontological separation or the 'gap', which, rather than being subsumed in synthesis, is maintained by a minimal difference. Consequently, we can begin to see how examples of multiculturalism and calls for political correctness frequently stand opposed to such understanding. In view of Alan Badiou and Frederic Jameson, Žižek notes how 'today's multiculturalist celebration of the diversity of lifestyles and thriving of differences relies on an underlying One – that is, a radical obliteration of Difference, of the antagonistic gap' (2006c: 35). As a consequence, 'the moment we introduce the "thriving multitude" what we effectively assert is its exact opposite, an underlying all-pervasive Sameness – a non-antagonistic society in which there is room for all manner of cultural communities, lifestyles, religions, sexual orientations' (Žižek, 2006c: 35) – in other words, a reductive multitude. If we consider that it is this 'thriving multitude' which finds itself expressed in the rise of identity politics, then it is a complete lack of radical politicisation which underscores this 'politics'; as Flisfeder asserts: 'the problems with identity politics is that there is nothing inherently radical about them. Identity, like culture, is perfectly commodifiable, and diffusible into the mainstream of capitalist society' (2017: 150).

Instead, it is through a 'tyranny of difference' (Žižek and Daly, 2004: 14) that Real difference is obliterated. What is achieved in such obliteration is the obscuration of the lack that characterises the material One. It is this lack, and its excessive differentiation, which constitutes subject-object relations and, as a consequence, the subject's acceptance of objective reality (Dolar, 1991). Yet, it is also that which, in a rather paradoxical way, submits both the subject and the other to an inverted form of in-visibility. That is, in ensuring that every difference is celebrated through forms of diversity, *that* which makes the other 'unique', becomes lost to the multitude of differences. In a certain way, an inverted form of racism occurs which continues to ignore *that* which makes the other, *other*. Accordingly, instead of succumbing to the postmodern multitude, true comedy can stand apart from any shallow acceptance of difference based upon tolerance and distance, and instead acknowledge how such difference is fundamentally marked by an antagonistic split that is brought to bear by the 'very thread' that inseparably performs this minimal difference – the irreducible difference in the same.

The big Other's lack

When tackling political correctness and multiculturalism, it is comedy which can help achieve a sustained critique of the 'empty' universality which both political correctness and multiculturalism achieve (Žižek, 1998). It is important to remember that Lacan's symbolic order is that which 'is ultimately comprised of chains of signifiers, provid[ing] a regulatory framework for intersubjective relations insofar as its various participants collectively invest in and are represented by its system of signs and values' (Kingsbury, 2017: 2). Indeed, what this effectively captures is the 'regulatory' nature of the symbolic order, not in any deterministic way, but in the collective investment which underscores intersubjective relationships constituting daily life. Such investments are brought to bear through the Lacanian big Other. This investment is reflected in the level of 'trust' that is afforded to 'the Symbolic Order (big Other)', a trust that is dependent on both 'the explicit symbolic rules that regulate our social interactions, but also the shadow side of unwritten "implicit" rules' (Jagodzinski, 2004: 148). Such rules provide a dependence that both explicitly and implicitly frames how the subject *should* behave in certain situations.

It is in this vein that we can consider how the big Other works from 'a non-existent locus or point of reference that tacitly anchors, mediates, and gives consistency to symbolic rules, conventions, and mandates' (Kingsbury, 2017: 2). Indeed, the big Other is always the third that permeates the interactions between human beings (Žižek, 2006e), which, much like the subject, are constituted through a shared sense of lack that binds the subject to the big Other and which manages our inclusion in a shared social order:

> The individual's entrance into the social order and into language coincides with a lack that produces the desiring subject. … If the subject didn't lack a lost object, the subject would not desire and hence would not invest itself in the demands of the social order, which graft themselves onto this desire. … The social order redoubles the subject's lack and forces the subject to see itself as a being of lack, which prompts the subject to invest itself in this order. Lack in the subject ensures its adherence to the social order, which presents itself as harboring the solution to that lack in the form of belonging or possibilities for self-realization.
>
> *(McGowan, 2017: 19)*

However, one way of approaching this 'lack', shared by all, is through comedy. In commenting upon Žižek's use of jokes, especially in academic texts, Sigurdson highlights how 'The strategic aim of Žižek's theory is to get the reader/analysand to the point of realizing that "the big Other does not exist"' (2013: 246). This certainly seems like a paradoxical assumption, especially when one considers the importance of the big Other in maintaining intersubjective relations. Yet, what both Lacan and Žižek draw attention to is the socially constructed and significantly fragile form in which such eligibility is founded. It is this 'fragility' which is reflected in Žižek's (2006a) attempts to provide a parallax view that allows us to conceive of reality's 'indeterminate and never fully constituted' quality (Wood, 2012: 239). For Wood, this 'is another way of saying that the big Other does not exist' (2012: 239).

Certainly, this is not to suggest 'that the big Other is just a retroactive illusion masking the radical contingency of the real, [and] that we can simply suspend this "illusion" and "see things as they really are"'; instead, 'The crucial point is that this "illusion" structures our (social) reality itself: its disintegration leads to a "loss of reality"' (Žižek, 1991: 71). Accordingly, while the above process highlights how the big Other can collapse into the small other/fantasy object (the *objet a*) (Žižek, 2005), at the same time, this process can, in the form of comedy, prescribe an over-realisation of reality that works to short circuit the symbolic order.

Establishing this realisation, however, is clearly paradoxical and, as a result, bears an approach to the Real which is grounded in the big Other's lack, or, in the case of the other, as that unknowable 'X' which forever marks our proximity with the other (Žižek, 2002). Accordingly, when we share an obscene joke, we reflexively acknowledge the implicit difference that frames our proximity to the other; a proximity which is guaranteed in the big Other. By openly acknowledging the racist performance, we can achieve a shared sense of the big Other's obscene (or 'vulgar') underside, allowing us to bear witness to the object of racism via a comic space that reflexively alerts us to our shared strangeness and to the strangeness of racism itself. Such an approach diverts us from the 'safe spaces' and easy 'compassion' of political correctness towards a form of subversion that draws attention to the fantasies which underscore our relations with the other/big Other.

Furthermore, what the above discussion steers towards is a form of critical thinking that bears a notable resemblance to the type of critical analysis which postmodernism has sought to achieve, but which, as noted in Chapter One, remains grounded in forms of cynical distance and ironic expression. Significantly, it is through employing irony and self-parody that postmodernism can self-reflexively acknowledge that no representation is free of its political context and, as a result, no representation is ever neutral (Flisfeder, 2017; Hutcheon, 2002). Flisfeder draws upon this assertion to highlight how, in postmodern consumer culture, any commodity can be both art and commodity, so that when comparing Andy Warhol's *Campbell's Soup Cans* (1962) or in exploring the significance of the film *Blade Runner* (1982), in both instances, the painting and the film are 'doubly coded' (Flisfeder, 2017: 155). It is this 'double coding' that allows postmodernism to subvert both high and mass culture:

> Recognizing this, becoming self-aware, and being self-reflexive of the fact that our knowledge about the world comes pregnant with social and ideological meanings – that it never comes pure, from some neutral/objective place of understanding – is how postmodernism aims to dedoxify cultural representations.
>
> *(Flisfeder, 2017: 73)*

To this end, while such forms of analysis have, in most instances of popular culture (including comedy), become subversively un-subversive, in part, it is through acknowledging this 'redoubling' ('doubly coded') – as that which works to mask reality's inherent 'gap' – that the necessary redoubling of the social system, and the inherent transgressions which work to maintain the social symbolic order, can be identified and dedoxified (Flisfeder, 2017; Vogt, 2007).

When considered in relation to the parallax view, it is this 'redoubling' which underscores the 'self-division of the One' (Žižek, 2006a: 184) as well as the possibility of a self-reflexive subject.[4] To repeat McGowan's previously cited claim:

> The social order *redoubles* the subject's lack and forces the subject to see itself as a being of lack, which prompts the subject to invest itself in this order. Lack in the subject ensures its adherence to the social order, which presents itself as

> harboring the solution to that lack in the form of belonging or possibilities for self-realization.
>
> *(2017: 19 [italics added])*

Recognising this redoubling, or the lack in the subject, can, in the case of true comedy, help us to reflexively acknowledge our own capacity to critically identify with the big Other.[5] In this sense, it is not simply the case that one acts in defiance of the big Other – that one merely acknowledges and proclaims the lack at the heart of both the subject and the big Other – but that a more radical subversion can be achieved when the big Other is made to acknowledge and even perform its own prohibitions. Following the above assertions from McGowan this can be achieved when one comically overperforms (excessively performs) those 'solutions to the lack' that reside in the big Other or when one openly identifies with the illicit pleasures that remain curtailed and/or prevented by the symbolic authorities that are enacted in the aegis of the big Other. In a way, this requires forcing the authority to enact what it usually prohibits, so that a shift in the big Other – a parallax shift – can be achieved via a redoubling of that obscene underside that remains disavowed. In other words, the obscene injunctions of the big Other, its vulgar underside, are exposed through its own ambiguity and via the capacity for the big Other to perform and display its own obscenities.

This 'reflexive twist' is what posits a comic subversion that induces a parallax shift in the fundamental coordinates of the big Other and our relation to it. This can occur through the various ways in which jokes and comedy play a key role in reflexively drawing attention to the fragility of the big Other. Sigurdson explains that:

> Through the joke, the big Other is exposed as floating on air, not having any support except in the fantasy of our own identification with it. The joke … succeeds when it becomes clear to us, not only intellectually but most of all existentially, that, to speak figuratively, the king has no clothes.
>
> *(2013: 247)*

What this suggests, therefore, is that there is a space – a certain social efficacy – that can be approached if we are to subvert the symbolic/big Other through its own 'redoubling' ('when it becomes clear to us'). This subversion can be achieved, not by confronting the big Other, but by performing certain universal, abstract notions in a concrete form; that is to say, through performing comedy as concrete universal.

The universal is subverted: From Master-Signifier to concrete universal, from exception to included exclusion

It was argued in Chapter Two that the universal's contingency can be brought to bear in Hegel's notion of the 'concrete universal', which denotes 'the manifestation of the universal *in* the material' (Ladegaard, 2017: 182). While humanity often creates and recreates a search for universal meaning, such processes are always marked by failure, by exceptions, and by an inherent indeterminacy; indeed, it is such failure which underscores Hegel's, and later Zupančič's (2008) and Žižek's (2006b, 2012), interpretation of the concrete universal. This inherent failure, forged upon certain exclusions, is reflected in McGowan's reference to the Declaration of Independence:

> When Thomas Jefferson claims that 'all men are created equal' in the Declaration of Independence, everyone knows that this universality does not apply to women or slaves. But it is important to see that this exclusion is not merely historical or contingent. ... By seeing that they are not women or slaves, men of Jefferson's epoch can see equality among themselves where there is rampant inequality.
>
> *(2018: 202)*

McGowan's (2018) example can be allied with Hsiao's (2010) spectacle and spectre distinctions by considering how it is through the spectacle of declaring 'all men' equal that the spectre of exclusion is enacted – in this case, the exclusion of women and black slaves. In sum, it is through their exclusion that the universal relies upon an excluded group, from which the abstract universality of a particular Ideal is performed (Moolenaar, 2004). This performance highlights how it is through the universal that the legitimisation of encoded social divisions, which are subsequently separated from the abstract universal's 'real/impossible' demands, can be approached through their own excessive destabilisation (Moolenaar, 2004). Over the course of this study, this division has been evident in the politically correct 'desire' for an abstract cross-racial/ethnic 'harmony' and its 'on-the-ground' regulated enforcement of social divisions through coded forms of 'correct' behaviour. Approaching this division requires a dialectical perspective that performs – in a concrete form – this division within the universal.

Nevertheless, if 'the symbolic order is by definition antagonistic, thwarted, non-identical-with-itself, marked by a constitutive lack, virtual – or, as Lacan put it, "there is no big Other"' (Žižek, 2006b: vii) – then, to what extent is it possible to achieve this acknowledgment and, more importantly, subvert it? In addition, if we consider Žižek's (2008a) claims that, under postmodernism, the significance of the big Other has declined – evident in the postmodern declaration that there are no meta-narratives – then, to what extent can we even begin to acknowledge its non-existence? In answer to these questions, it is possible to assert that 'the absence of such a master might seem to produce a situation of complete openness and freedom' (Dean, 2014: 213). Yet, such openness is inherently not open, with 'the result [... being an] unbearable, suffocating closure' (Dean, 2014: 213). With no authority to prohibit enjoyment, we find that 'ideology, today, works by practices of willing back into existence forms of authority ..., or what Lacan called the "big Other"' (Flisfeder, 2017: 140). As Flisfeder notes, 'Even our activity on social media, the construction of self through the public profile, is a form of willing into existence the form of the big Other as those social networks that confer existence upon our constructed identities' (2017: 140).

To this extent, we can assert that 'willing' into existence some form of big Other finds itself enacted in examples of political correctness which seek to manage and regulate our contact with the other. Furthermore, by following the decline in symbolic efficiency (Dean, 2014; Flisfeder, 2017; Žižek, 2008a), we can observe how such management is inherently inconsistent. That is, political correctness obtains the position of a hegemonic universal by offering opportunities for *both* its advocation and criticism. Accordingly, though on the one hand, traditional forms of authority start to wane, on the other, new forms of 'politically correct' authority are established, which, despite their criticisms, continue to maintain an authoritative status.

Moreover, it is the failure of political correctness to effectively curtail racism which points to the spectral presence of race and the inherent inconsistencies of the symbolic order, big Other and the universal. While openly deriding forms of racial discrimination, examples of political correctness, and its calls for racial 'openness', are excessively bounded by coded forms of how one should and should not behave, resulting in examples of ambivalence, confusion and frustration. It is this sense of uncertainty that underscores discussions on multiculturalism and political correctness which have subsequently obtained a hegemonic universality, grounded in an implicit form of 'cultural' superiority and liberal autonomy. This sense of individualism is supported by the affirmation that one can maintain an abstract neutrality when engaging in cultural diversity. As argued in Chapter One, it is the multicultural, politically correct subject who 'retains this position as the privileged empty point of universality … the multiculturalist respect for the Other's specificity is the very form of asserting one's own superiority' (Žižek, 1997: 44). While acting as a hegemonic universal form, multiculturalism, and its politically correct codes of forbidden practices, are never neutral, but dialectically rendered in the antagonisms between the universal and the particular.

Consequently, if we accept the hegemony of political correctness, then to what extent can this hegemony be challenged through its own universal dimension? In approaching this dynamic, McGowan (2018) draws a connection between the universal and Lacan's Master-Signifier. As previously noted, the Master-Signifier is what stalls the endless deferment of signifiers, allowing signification to occur. For McGowan (2018), it is this interpretation which bears a resemblance to the universal: as that which behaves like a Master-Signifier via its ability to organise particular signifiers and to assert a certain orientation and direction to their meaning. Central to such orientation, however, is the universal's ability to contain opposing particularities. For example, with regards to the universal notion 'freedom' we can see how 'in 2003 the United States invade[d] Iraq in the name of this universal – going so far as to title its invasion "Operation Iraqi Freedom" – while the same term at the same time also inform[ed] the worldwide opposition to the American war' (McGowan, 2018: 196). Here, McGowan highlights that:

> The contradictory nature of these examples reveals that freedom operates as a master signifier. Rather than having a clear signification like other signifiers (*birch tree*, for example, which allows us to classify birch trees as distinct from oaks), *freedom* has no signified at all … Freedom seems to place the complete coincidence of the universal with the master signifier beyond any dispute.
>
> (*McGowan, 2018: 197*)

If we consider that the critique of political correctness, as outlined above, relies primarily on drawing upon those areas where political correctness is paradoxically performed, then we can begin to see how, much like McGowan's freedom example, political correctness provides a similar function. That is, political correctness serves as an abstract universal, which behaves like a Master-Signifier. Just like 'freedom', debates on political correctness remain antagonistic, confused and problematic, suggesting that it bears no clear, or definite, signification.

As noted by McGowan (2018), it is this lack of clarity that underscores Laclau's 'radical democracy' (Laclau and Mouffe, 1985), an argument that 'entails accepting the evanescent particularity of every universal master signifier' (McGowan, 2018: 198). As a result, 'Once one adopts this position, one retains the mastery of the universal, but one exposes this mastery as mortally wounded' (McGowan, 2018: 198). For McGowan (2018), Laclau's approach remains decidedly conservative in that while accepting the particularity of the universal (and, thus, its inherent inconsistencies), one is left *accepting* this particularity: a conservative gesture that serves to protect particular identities. Consequently:

> Though Laclau is not some type of closet conservative, his attempt to undermine universality by exposing its underlying particularity runs counter to the emancipatory political project that he attempts to advance. Laclau's solution to the problem generated by the identity of the universal and the master signifier is to accept this identity as given and subsequently denigrate the universal in order to undermine its mastery.
>
> (*McGowan, 2018: 199*)

Thus, it would seem that, from the aforementioned critique, the position advocated in this study shares Laclau's (2000) approach. As noted in Chapter Two, it is in enacting a certain concrete situation (particularity) that the inherent inconsistencies of the universal are performed. For McGowan (2018), such an approach presents a conservative error in that it permits the universal/Master-Signifier a significance which echoes Žižek's (2008a) contention that hegemonic ideologies work by containing their own disavowal. It is in this way that the Master-Signifier, referred to by Laclau as an 'empty signifier' – a signifier that joins together disparate elements through its 'emptyness' – is subsequently able to achieve a unifying (i.e. universal) significance.

Instead, according to McGowan, 'One of the key political struggles today – perhaps the key political struggle – consists in thoroughly divorcing the universal from the master signifier' (2018: 199). Indeed:

> Universals are not only not master signifiers. They are not present within the field of signification at all. Universals exist on the basis of what is missing in signification. We discover the universal through what cannot be said, even as we name this absence. Every authentic universal refers to a signifying absence.
>
> *(McGowan, 2018: 200)*

Accordingly, what remains key to McGowan's (2018) argument is the extent to which the universal remains an absent objective, something that is not present, but, in the desire for its actualisation, can help achieve emancipatory effects. Here, '*The absence of a fully realized universal is the essence of universality* … we access it only through articulating the struggle to realize it, not through proclamations about its reality' (McGowan, 2018: 212 [italics added]). Indeed, if we were to 'realise' the universal, it would begin to share the characteristics of the Master-Signifier, through achieving a sense of wholeness, undergirded by some form of inherent exclusion. Instead, 'The point is rather that we access the universal through the exception that appears to be excluded from it, through the moment where the universal appears not to hold' (McGowan, 2018: 207).

Yet, perhaps such an approach is just as easily subject to a certain impasse that fails to achieve its intended 'subversive' aims. That is, if following McGowan (2018), we attempt to realise (not achieve) the universal by acknowledging that which appears excluded from it, then, equally, such struggles can just as easily result in a form of generic inertia – indeed, a constant, frenzied turn to that which is always excluded; or, worse, a constant, frenzied attempt to *find* that which is always excluded. More to the point, is there *one* form of exclusion which stands separate to the universal? How do we decide which exclusions to argue for? Ultimately, these questions can result in frenetic attempts to continually change a system which very easily manages to catch up with the protested intentions. Though 'we' may be able to look for that which appears excluded, in the end we simply remain tied to the same horizons that determine this exclusion in the first place, thus immunising any attempt to subvert the universal. In short, while looking for the exception/exclusion, we miss the very obscenities that underscore hegemonic power structures; the Achilles heel which maintains and relies upon a certain (un)acknowledged exclusion in order to function.

Rather, in view of these questions and in view of the concrete universal, we can offer an extension to McGowan's (2018) approach. As is evident in his desire to 'access the universal through the exception', it is, nonetheless, an *exception* that remains *excluded* and, thus, separate, from the social order. It is in this way that such exclusion serves to combine the Master-Signifier's inherent exclusion with a universal significance. By implementing a slight revision to McGowan's (2018) account, we can instead view this 'exception' in accordance with his 'included exclusion' example, drawn from his analysis of Buster Keaton (McGowan, 2016). In fact, whereas Keaton's comedy exposed the exclusion at the heart of the social order, his comic subversion emanated from his ability to highlight the inconsistencies of this system through its own 'excess' – that is, through his own 'inclusion' in a system of 'exclusion'. Again, this points to the importance of the divided One and how, even when excluded, certain exceptions are nevertheless constitutive of the One's division; indeed, their exclusion posits this division.

This presents a dialectical approach to our understanding of inclusion and exclusion (Black, 2019). What is significant here is that while particular individuals/groups may be excluded from a certain universal claim, it is their *exclusion* which has to be *included* in order for the parameters of this universal claim to be established. In other words, one cannot posit the limits of a universal without *including* what is inherently *excluded* beyond these limits. In fact, even when certain excluded individuals/groups are included, they can often find that their inclusion rests upon certain contingencies that work to maintain the hegemonic group (Black, 2016; Black and Fielding-Lloyd, 2019). Moreover, such an inclusion-exclusion dialectic proves amiable to our understandings of the concrete universal.

For example, in accordance with McGowan's 'freedom' example, we can see this inclusion-exclusion dialectic reflected in McMillan's (2013) comments on 'freedom'. He notes that:

> If liberal capitalism is based around an empty signifier of freedom, which becomes universalized through an abstract hegemonic horizon, then this notion is subverted by the freedom to sell one's labour on the market. ... It is this freedom to sell labour power which is the universal exception to the abstract universality of bourgeois freedom.
>
> *(McMillan, 2013: 90)*

What McMillan's (2013) example points to is the *inherent exception* which underscores liberal capitalism's universality. Importantly, 'we can identify a formal necessity *within* the wage-labour system to have an element incommensurable with its ideological narrative that cannot be acknowledged *within* this narrative' (McMillan, 2013: 92 [italics added]). Key here is that while this element 'cannot be acknowledged', it nonetheless helps to constitute the 'formal necessity' of the system itself. That is, in other words, it is paradoxically both included and excluded *within* the universal. This approach draws attention to the ways in which universal forms can be used to identify the exceptions that remain inherent to the Master-Signifier's 'empty presence': a form of extimacy that stands apart from the Master-Signifier, but which helps to establish its constitution.

By returning to McGowan's (2018) marriage example (see Chapter Two), we can begin to see how it is in the claims of marriage equality proponents that the universal is performed, so that 'By pointing out what is missing for the symbolic field – gay marriage – they articulate universal equality' (McGowan, 2018: 207 [italics added]). While gay marriage is excluded from heterosexual claims of marriage equality, they nonetheless remain that point of *exception* from which their own exclusion is dialectically *included as that point of exception*. As a result, it is by excessively performing, highlighting and arguing for the point of exception that they can serve to challenge and subvert the false universality of marriage equality. It is in 'saying what is missing' that the claims made by those campaigning for marriage equality embody the 'gap, antagonism or obstacle which holds this field together' (Žižek, 2016: 18), a process that serves to render the concrete universal by concretely performing the 'gap, antagonism or obstacle' *within* the universal.

Furthermore, if we consider McGowan's contention that 'the unsayable is never just absent. It is always present within the signifying structure as an absence. When we express it, we express universality' (2018: 207), it is possible to adapt these remarks with regards to the spectacle and spectre of race. That is, the spectre of race *is never just absent*, but rather its absent-presence is always located in the spectacle itself. What this requires is a process that draws attention to this absence (spectre) within the universal, via comic examples that excessively perform the universal and its inherent inconsistencies. Such comic examples are depicted in those moments when the universal appears not to hold (McGowan, 2018). More to the point, it is by returning to those cultural excesses, which are so often framed as the 'problem' in accounts of political correctness (Žižek, 1998, 2006c, 2006d), that we can begin to undermine the universal significance of such politically correct assertions by comically performing this cultural excess (including its 'racist' manifestations) in a manner which serves to undercut its significance. Again, it is here that comedy's subversive significance aligns with its capacity to draw attention to the inherent lack that constitutes such excess (McGowan, 2017).

Thus, if it is through the Master-Signifier that the subject gains purchase on social reality, serving as that which allows the subject to locate themselves within a signifying system, then, evidently, its informative role cannot be dismissed. To this end, what comedy achieves is a form of subversion which draws attention to the comic significance of the Master-Signifier and of the presupposition that one requires in order to situate oneself within a signifying system. Here, every subject is orientated towards a missing signifier, which seeks to suffice the subject's inherent lack. Accordingly:

> The missing signifier is unavoidable for all subjects. It forms how they relate to themselves and to the social structure. The role of the missing signifier allows us to distinguish the universal from something held in common, which is precisely the conception of the universal that always sets us on the wrong path. *The universal is not what subjects have in common but what they don't have in common, the cut that blocks the social structure's completion for the subject.* It is an absence that all subjects partake in. This insight cuts against the commonsense conception of universality that associates it with the master signifier.
>
> *(McGowan, 2018: 201 [italics added])*

Key to McGowan's remarks is the importance of recognising that this 'lack' is shared; a point that is echoed in Žižek's (1998, 2004, 2017b) comments on the other. Subsequently, while 'The universal struggle aims at drawing attention to the universal as a lack in signification' (McGowan, 2018: 213), it is through the concrete universal that comedy can lay bare this lack via the comic performance: 'What all subjects have in common is what they don't have' (McGowan, 2018: 200). It is in sharing this common lack that comedy's 'shared obscenities' can transpose the burden of lack through the risk that is involved in being with the other and in approaching their as well as our difference – the commonality of what we 'don't have in common' (McGowan, 2018: 201). To this end:

> Because the universal is a shared lack, one cannot articulate it directly. It is not as simple as saying, for example, that all people are free or everyone is equal. This attempt to transform the universal, which is an absence in signification, into a positivity necessarily misses it. Rather than expressing universality, one erects a master signifier that functions through exclusion.
>
> *(McGowan, 2018: 202)*

Importantly, this exclusion does not rest upon the other, but instead provides a reflexive short circuit which draws attention to the shared lack (the shared strangeness in difference) between the subject and the other. Moreover, it is this absence (universal) through exclusion (Master-Signifier) which alludes to the spectre of race as it is performed in the comic spectacle. As an absent-presence, it is the spectre which is approached through shared obscenities which deliberately lay bare the subject's vulnerability *to/with* the other. This prescribes a space in which what cannot be said (spectre) can at least be approached via a form of interaction grounded in an acknowledgment of absence and (possible) exclusion (Žižek, 2004, 2017b). Indeed, 'Since the universal is an absence within signification' and 'one must look for it in what is not said' (McGowan, 2018: 204), under such circumstances, a joke can say more than the 'safe spaces' and fake compassion that is inscribed within the regulated nature of political correctness and which ultimately obscures any Real engagement with the other.

Coupled with the work of Zupančič, we can begin to see how it is in the relation between the 'empty' Master-Signifier and the universal that comedy's subversive potential can be performed. That is, it is in the performance of comedy that 'humour can generate a process of contamination of the empty signifier by infusing it with diverse, incongruent content, [and] thereby "overburdening" its universalizing function' (Karlsen and Villadsen, 2015: 527). This, it is argued, can only be achieved by drawing attention to the 'fragility and fictive universality' which is brought to light via the concrete universal (Karlsen and Villadsen, 2015: 527).

This professes a new approach to political correctness, one that does not ignore political correctness by simply dissolving into open racism, but rather re-approaches it as a universal that, through a comic process, can be subversively performed. To return to the discussion of the concrete universal in Chapter Two, it is in particular examples of political correctness that a certain racist exception can be universally performed. Key here is that rather than presenting racism as *the* concrete universal, such performances can instead expose the coinciding inconsistencies in both racism *and* political correctness. If we remember that the 'gap' between the particular and universal is transposed into the particular itself, then it is in this sense that particular examples of political correctness can follow a process of transposition which reveals its own universal inconsistency, performed through its own inherent exceptions. It is in this way that:

> comedy has the ability to reveal division or splitting where we perceive wholeness, and when it sustains this revelation, it functions successfully as a critical comedy or a comedy of critique. The comedy of critique exposes the incompleteness of the social order and of the subject who exists within this order. In the comedy of critique, both the source of the comedy and its target appear divided internally, and it is the emergence of this internal division that enables us to laugh while also facilitating critique.
>
> *(McGowan, 2015: 205)*

Over the course of this discussion, such internal division has been approached via Zupančič's (2008) Hegelian adoption of the concrete universal, Žižek's (2006a) parallax view and McGowan's (2017) lack and excess. Central to each of these concepts is the desire for comedy to reveal the internal divisions (the division of the One) of a symbolic order that has increasingly been subjected to forms of 'politically correct' regulation. It is through this regulation that we see the spectacle of race work to obfuscate or even ignore the spectre of race (Hsiao, 2010). Such obfuscation accentuates racism's Real effects, by foreclosing the capacity to engage with the Real other.

Comedy's Real subversion: Subverting political correctness through comedy

As a hegemonic universal notion, political correctness fails to elicit a short circuit between its celebration of diversity and the concrete materiality of this diversity in action. This separation between multiculturalism's ideals and it's 'on-the-ground' reality ignore the Real antagonisms that constitute its universality via a proliferation of differences that merely propose a detrimental sameness. Certainly, this is not to suggest that we ignore these differences, but rather consider how such differences can serve as an exception to the universal.

Both this chapter and the preceding chapter have argued that in order 'to contest the concrete existing universal order on behalf of its "symptom", that is to say, on behalf of the part which, although inherent to the existing universal order, has no proper place within it' (Moolenaar, 2004: 289), this requires drawing upon those 'excessive' elements that effectively distort the universal symbolic order. It has been claimed that this 'excess' can occur in those moments when an obscene or racist joke is shared with the other. Instead of simply acknowledging and critiquing the symbolic's excess (bearing in mind that the symbolic maintains its ideological function through excessive forms that preserve the big Other), we can, via our understanding of the concrete universal, provide a comical rendering of such excess so as to potentially subvert the inconsistencies of the symbolic order. In other words, it is through approaching this excessive element that comedy performs, in often-exaggerated ways, the inherent contradictions within a particular (politically correct) position. Rather than subsuming or denouncing one position over another, these contradictions can be viewed in a parallax form that maintains the tension.

To this end, we can now draw a connection between political correctness – in all its abstract universality – and the significance of true comedy in performing this abstract universality through the concrete universal. This becomes apparent when we recount Zupančič's assertion that 'Comedy … is not an objection to the universal, but the concrete labor or work of the universal itself' (2008: 27). In other words, comedy takes place when we consider 'the relation of the universal *to itself* in and through the concrete individual' (Ladegaard, 2014: 116 [italics added]). Importantly, it is in this 'relation … to itself' that the concrete universality of comedy can be used to subversively expose abstract universal notions. Notably, this argument has integrated the concrete universal with a wider discussion on parallax, the spectre and spectacle of race, the other and the Real – all of which have been used to expose comedy's Real subversion. Following this path, it is argued that such subversion can be achieved through comedy inducing a parallax shift that draws attention to the inherent fissures within the social order. It is this shift which works alongside the concrete universal and which helps to expose that constitutive exception which remains excluded from the universality of political correctness.

If we consider that, while political correctness seeks to promote an abstract form of equality which ignores latent forms of systematic inequality, then it is the 'gap' between the universal's abstract claims and its point of exception which avers the Real. What is significant here is that 'the Real can have an existence, or at least a non-existence in Lacanian parlance, outside the discursive construction of a certain narrative' (McMillan, 2013: 91) and it is this 'non-existence' which underscores the spectacle of race and which points to its spectral dimensions (Hsiao, 2010). It is through comedy, therefore, that examples of political correctness can be subverted by identifying and performing that point of distortion – that point of lack/excess – which proffers 'the anxiety of the Real' (McMillan, 2013: 163).[6] In fact, comedy can prove adept at performing and approaching this anxiety by framing our aversion to the Real as well as revealing that which underscores our relations with the other. What remains subversive in this approach is not the direct critique of political correctness, but rather the ability to comically perform those inherent exceptions that underscore the universality of political correctness. It is in this sense that the risk and anxiety that occurs when one shares an obscene joke – a sense of risk and anxiety which underscores our relations with the other – can be used to perform this exception.

Finally, it is important to note that the above discussion has not sought to reify racial differences as in some way innate to the individual and/or fixed across different historical and social contexts. On the contrary, the above argument has emphasised that, when race is conceived as a symbolic (discursive/socially constructed stereotype) and imaginary (fantasy) phenomenon, there arises the opportunity to traverse racial distinctions by approaching those inherent incongruities that frame examples of racial stereotyping. This can be achieved in examples of comedy that draw attention to this incongruity. As will be discussed in further detail, this is undoubtedly a risky and alternative path. What Žižek's (2006a) conception of parallax affords, however, is not the resolution of these difficulties, but an acceptance of their constitutive role in providing forms of 'fantasmatic dexterity' (McGowan, 2015: 80). Such dexterity will be sought in the following analysis.

Notes

1 When K. examines the Law books, he sees a picture of a man and a woman sitting naked on a sofa.

2 In the UK, the often-cited 'I beg your pardon' when you mishear someone – does anyone really *beg the pardon* of their companion?

3 It is a 'void', as noted by McGowan's (2007) account of the 'sled' (Kane's 'Rosebud') in Orson Welles's *Citizen Kane* (1941).

4 Equally, this redoubling is akin to the topological structure of the Mobius Strip: a surface where, while remaining on one side, we eventually end up on the other.

5 It is this identification which is echoed in Žižek's (2006a) dialectical materialism. He notes that 'Materialism is not the direct assertion of my inclusion in objective reality (such an assertion presupposes that my position of enunciation is that of an external observer who can grasp the whole of reality); rather, it resides in the reflexive twist by means of which I myself am included in the picture constituted by me – it is this reflexive short circuit, this necessary redoubling of myself as standing both outside and inside my picture, that bears witness to my "material existence." Materialism means that the reality I see is never "whole" – not because a large part of it eludes me, but because it contains a stain, a blind spot, which indicates my inclusion in it' (Žižek, 2006a: 17).

6 See also McGowan (2017).

References

Alonso, P. 2016. Sacha Baron Cohen and *Da Ali G Show*: A critique on identity in times of satiric infotainment. *The Journal of Popular Culture*, 49 (3), 582–603.

Apocalypse Now. 1979. Film. United Artists.

Bakhtin, M. 1984. *Rabelais and His World*. Bloomington, NI: Indiana University Press.

Baudrillard, J. 1994. *Simulacra and Simulation*. Ann Arbor, MI: The University of Michigan Press.

BBC. 2018. Comedian refused to sign 'behavioural agreement' before gig [online]. *BBC News*. Available from: www.bbc.co.uk/news/newsbeat-46541002 [Accessed 1 March 2019].

Beck, U. 2005. *Risk Society: Towards a New Modernity*. London: Sage.

Berlant, L. and Ngai, S. 2017. Comedy has issues. *Critical Inquiry*, 43, 233–249.

Billig, M. 2005. Comic racism and violence. In: S. Lockyer and M. Pickering, eds. *Beyond a Joke: The Limits of Humour*. Basingstoke: Palgrave Macmillan, 25–44.

Black, J. 2016. 'As British as fish and chips': British newspaper representations of Mo Farah during the 2012 London Olympic Games. *Media, Culture & Society*, 38 (7), 979–996.

Black, J. 2019. Conviviality and parallax in David Olusoga's *Black and British: A Forgotten History*. *European Journal of Cultural Studies*, 22 (5–6), 979–995.

Black, J. and Fielding-Lloyd, B. 2019. Re-establishing the 'outsiders': English press coverage of the 2015 FIFA Women's World Cup. *International Review for the Sociology of Sport*, 54 (3), 282–301.

Blade Runner. 1982. Film. Warner Bros.
Blanchot, M. 1997. *Friendship*. Stanford, CA: Stanford University Press.
Bonic, N. 2011. Psychoanalysis and comedy: The (im)possibility of changing the socio-symbolic order. *S: Journal of the Jan Van Eyck Circle For Lacanian Ideology Critique*, 4, 91–108.
Buk-Swienty, A. 2016. The law ex-ists: Reading Kafka with Lacan [online]. *Ark Books*. Available from: http://arkbooks.dk/the-law-ex-ists-reading-kafka-with-lacan/ [Accessed 2 April 2018].
Casablanca. 1942. Film. Warner Bros. Pictures.
Chow, B. 2014. The tickling object: On Žižek and comedy. In: B. Chow and A. Mangold, eds. *Žižek and Performance*. Basingstoke: Palgrave Macmillan, 224–252.
Citizen Kane. 1941. Film. RKO Pictures.
Conrad, J. 2008. *Heart of Darkness and Other Tales*. Oxford: Oxford University Press.
Contu, A. 2008. Decaf resistance: On misbehavior, cynicism, and desire in liberal work-places. *Management Communication Quarterly*, 21 (3), 364–379.
Critchley, S. 2002. *On Humour*. London: Routledge.
Das, R. and Graefer, A. 2017. *Provocative Screens: Offended Audiences in Britain and Germany*. Gewerbestrasse, Switzerland: Palgrave Macmillan.
Dead to Me. 2019–present. TV Series. Netflix.
Dean, J. 2006. *Žižek's Politics*. New York, NY: Routledge.
Dean, J. 2014. The real internet. In: M. Flisfeder and L.-P. Willis, eds. *Žižek and Media Studies: A Reader*. Houndsville: Palgrave Macmillan, 211–228.
Dolar, M. 1991. 'I shall be with you on your wedding-night': Lacan and the uncanny. *October*, 58, 5–23.
Flisfeder, M. 2012. *The Symbolic, The Sublime, and Slavoj Žižek's Theory of Film*. New York, NY: Palgrave Macmillan.
Flisfeder, M. 2017. *Postmodern Theory and Blade Runner*. New York, NY: Bloomsbury.
Freud, S. 2003. *The Joke and its Relation to the Unconscious*, trans. J. Crick. London: Penguin.
Friedman, S. 2014. *Comedy and Distinction: The Cultural Currency of a 'Good' Sense of Humour*. Abingdon: Routledge.
Gilroy, P. 2004. *After Empire: Melancholia or Convivial Culture?* Abingdon: Routledge.
Grant, L. 1994. Sex and the single student: The story of date rape. In: S. Dunant, ed. *The War of the Words: The Political Correctness Debate*. London: Virago Press, 76–96.
Hegel, G. W. F. 1998. *Phenomenology of the Spirit*, trans. by A. V. Miller. Delhi, India: Motilal Banarsidass Publishers.
Heller, A. 2005. *Immortal Comedy: The Comic Phenomenon in Art, Literature, and Life*. Lanham, MD: Lexington Books.
Hsiao, L.-C. 2010. Color (un)conscious: Psychoanalysis, resistance, and the specter/spectacle of race. *Concentric: Literary and Cultural Studies*, 36 (1), 159–187.
Hutcheon, L. 2002. *The Politics of Postmodernism*. New York, NY: Routledge.
Jagodzinski, J. 2004. *Youth Fantasies: The Perverse Landscape of the Media*. New York, NY: Palgrave Macmillan.
Jeffries, S. 2014. The science of comedy: Can humour make the world a better place? [online]. *The Guardian*. Available from: www.theguardian.com/stage/2014/feb/11/science-comedy-academics-social [Accessed 1 March 2019].
Kamm, J. and Neumann, B. 2016. Introduction: The aesthetics and politics of British TV comedy. In: J. Kamm and B. Neumann, eds. *British TV Comedies: Cultural Concepts, Contexts and Controversies*. Basingstoke: Palgrave Macmillan, 1–22.
Karlsen, M. P. and Villadsen, K. 2015. Laughing for real? Humour, management power and subversion. *Ephemera: Theory & Politics in Organization*, 15 (3), 513–535.

Kingsbury, P. 2017. Uneasiness in culture, or negotiating the sublime distances towards the big Other. *Geography Compass*, 11 (6), 1–11.

Kisin, K. 2018. What a joke! His dissident grandfather fled Russia for the freedoms of Britain. Now comedian Konstantin Kisin has faced ludicrous censorship by snowflake students here. His withering response? [online]. *Daily Mail*. Available from: www.dailymail.co.uk/news/article-6493921/Comedian-signed-behaviour-agreement-reveals-family-fled-censorship-Soviet-Russia.html [Accessed 21 December 2018].

Kottman, P. A. 2008. Slipping on banana peels, tumbling into wells: Philosophy and comedy. *Diacritics*, 38 (4), 3–14.

Kottman, P. A. 2009. *Tragic Conditions in Shakespeare: Disinheriting the Globe*. Baltimore, MD: The John Hopkins University Press.

Kunkle, S. 2008. Embracing the paradox: Žižek's illogical logic. *International Journal of Žižek Studies*, 2 (4). Available from: http://zizekstudies.org/index.php/IJZS/issue/view/10 [Accessed 30 November 2020].

Laclau, E. 2000. Identity and hegemony: The role of universality in the constitution of political logics. In: J. Butler, E. Laclau and S. Žižek, eds. *Contingency, Hegemony, Universality: Contemporary Dialogues on the Left*. London: Verso, 44–89.

Laclau, E. and Mouffe, C. 1985. *Hegemony and Socialist Strategy: Towards a Radical Democratic Politics*. London: Verso.

Ladegaard, J. 2014. Laughing matters: Four Marxist takes on film comedy. In: E. Mazierska and L. Kristensen, eds. *Marx at the Movies: Revisiting History, Theory and Practice*. Basingstoke: Palgrave Macmillan, 102–122.

Ladegaard, J. 2017. The comedy of terrors: Ideology and comedy in Marlowe's *Doctor Faustus*. *Textual Practice*, 31 (1), 179–195.

Lentin, A. 2018. Beyond denial: 'Not racism' as racist violence. *Continuum*, 32 (4), 400–414.

Loughrey, C. 2018. Comedians asked to sign 'behavioural agreement' for London University gig [online]. *Independent*. Available from: www.independent.co.uk/arts-entertainment/comedy/news/soas-comedians-behavioural-agreement-london-university-a8679026.html [Accessed 1 March 2019].

Mangold, A. 2014. Introduction: Performing Žižek: Hegel, Lacan, Marx, and the parallax view. In: B. Chow and A. Mangold, eds. *Žižek and Performance*. Basingstoke: Palgrave Macmillan, 1–12.

Martín-Lucas, B. and Ruthven, A. 2017. Introduction: Interrogating the production, circulation and reception of 'difference' in globalized cultures. In: B. Martin-Lucas and A. Ruthven, eds. *Narratives of Difference in Globalized Cultures*. Gewerbestrasse, Switzerland: Palgrave Macmillan, 1–12.

McGowan, T. 2007. *The Real Gaze: Film Theory after Lacan*. Albany, NY: State University of New York Press.

McGowan, T. 2015. *Psychoanalytic Film Theory and the Rules of the Game*. New York, NY: Bloomsbury.

McGowan, T. 2016. The location of silent comedy: Charlie Chaplin's outsider and Buster Keaton's insider. *Quarterly Review of Film and Video*, 33 (7), 602–619.

McGowan, T. 2017. *Only a Joke Can Save Us: A Theory of Comedy*. Evanston, IL: Northwestern University Press.

McGowan, T. 2018. The absent universal: From the Master Signifier to the missing signifier. *Problemi International*, 2 (2), 195–214.

McMillan, C. 2013. *Žižek and Communist Strategy: On the Disavowed Foundations of Global Capitalism*. Edinburgh: Edinburgh University Press.

Moolenaar, R. 2004. Slavoj Žižek and the real subject of politics. *Studies in Eastern European Thought*, 56, 259–297.

O'Hara, M. 2016. How comedy makes us better people [online]. *BBC*. Available from: www.bbc.com/future/story/20160829-how-laughter-makes-us-better-people [Accessed 1 March 2019].

Pérez, R. 2013. Learning to make racism funny in the 'color-blind' era: Stand-up comedy students, performance strategies, and the (re)production of racist jokes in public. *Discourse & Society*, 24 (4), 478–503.

Peters, L. and Becker, S. 2010. Racism in comedy reappraised: Back to Little England? *Comedy Studies*, 1 (2), 191–200.

Raisborough, J., Frith, H. and Klein, O. 2012. Media and class-making: What lessons are learnt when a celebrity chav dies? *Sociology*, 47 (2), 251–266.

Rudge, T., Mapedzahama, V., West, S. and Perron, A. 2012. The violence of tolerance in a multicultural workplace: Examples from nursing. In: D. Holmes, T. Rudge and A. Perron, eds. *(Re)Thinking Violence in Health Care Settings: A Critical Approach*. London: Routledge, 31–46.

Sayeau, M. 2013. Enjoy his symptoms? [online]. *The White Review*. Available from: www.thewhitereview.org/feature/enjoy-his-symptoms/ [Accessed 3 March 2019].

Sharpe, M. and Boucher, G. 2010. *Žižek and Politics: A Critical Introduction*. Edinburgh: Edinburgh University Press.

Sharpe, M. and Turner, K. 2018. Fantasy. In: Y. Stavrakakis, ed. *Routledge Handbook of Psychoanalytic Political Theory*. London: Routledge.

Sigurdson, O. 2013. Emancipation as a matter of style. *Political Theology*, 14 (2), 235–251.

Stavrakakis, Y. 2016. Ambiguous ideology and the Lacanian twist [online]. *Journal of the Centre for Freudian Analysis and Research*. Available from: https://jcfar.org.uk/wp-content/uploads/2016/03/Ambiguous-Ideology-and-the-Lacanian-Twist-Yannis-Stavrakakis.pdf [Accessed 9 December 2020].

Verhaeghe, P. 2018. Lacan's answer to alienation: Separation. *Crisis and Critique*, 6 (1), 365–388.

Vogt, E. 2007. Exception in Žižek's thought. *Diacritics*, 37 (2–3), 61–77.

Vonnegut, K. 2009. *Slaughterhouse Five*. New York, NY: Dial Press.

Weaver, S. 2010. The 'Other' laughs back: Humour and resistance in anti-racist comedy. *Sociology*, 44 (1), 31–48.

Weaver, S. 2011. Liquid racism and the ambiguity of Ali G. *European Journal of Cultural Studies*, 14 (3), 249–264.

Wood, K. 2012. *Žižek: A Reader's Guide*. Chichester: Wiley-Blackwell.

Yao, D. 2012. Learning to tickle: How to transmit knowledge as if re-telling a joke. *The International Journal of Žižek Studies*, 6 (2), 1–12.

Žižek, S. 1991. *Looking Awry: An Introduction to Jacques Lacan through Popular Culture*. Cambridge, MA: MIT Press.

Žižek, S. 1997. Multiculturalism, or, the cultural logic of multinational capitalism. *New Left Review*, 1 (225), 28–51.

Žižek, S. 1998. *Tarrying with the Negative: Kant, Hegel, and the Critique of Ideology*. Durham, NC: Duke University Press.

Žižek, S. 1999. You may! [online]. *London Review of Books*. Available from: www.lrb.co.uk/v21/n06/slavoj-Žižek/you-may [Accessed 10 January 2019].

Žižek, S. 2002. The only good neighbor is a dead neighbor. *Identities: Journal for Politics, Gender and Culture*, 2 (2), 9–31.

Žižek, S. 2004. The structure of domination today: A Lacanian view. *Studies in Eastern European Thought*, 56, 383–403.

Žižek, S. 2005. *The Metastases of Enjoyment: Six Essays on Women and Causality*. London: Verso.

Žižek, S. 2006a. *The Parallax View*. Cambridge, MA: MIT Press.

Žižek, S. 2006b. Preface to the paperback edition: The big other between violence and civility. In: R. Butler and S. Stephens, eds. *Slavoj Žižek: The Universal Exception*. London: Continuum, vii–xxxii.

Žižek, S. 2006c. Why we all love to hate Haider. In: R. Butler and S. Stephens, eds. *Slavoj Žižek: The Universal Exception*. London: Continuum, 33–41.

Žižek, S. 2006d. A leftist plea for Eurocentricism. In: R. Butler and S. Stephens, eds. *Slavoj Žižek: The Universal Exception*. London: Continuum, 183–208.

Žižek, S. 2006e. *How to Read Lacan*. London: Granta Books.

Žižek, S. 2008a. *The Sublime Object of Ideology*. London: Verso.

Žižek, S. 2008b. *The Plague of Fantasies*. London: Verso.

Žižek, S. 2010. *Living in the End Times*. London: Verso.

Žižek, S. 2012. *Less Than Nothing: Hegel and the Shadow of Dialectical Materialism*. London: Verso.

Žižek, S. 2015. *Absolute Recoil: Towards a New Foundation of Dialectical Materialism*. London: Verso.

Žižek, S. 2016. *Disparities*. London: Bloomsbury.

Žižek, S. 2017a. *In Defense of Lost Causes*. London: Verso.

Žižek, S. 2017b. *Against the Double Blackmail: Refugees, Terror and Other Troubles with the Neighbour*. London: Penguin.

Žižek, S. 2018a. *Like a Thief in Broad Daylight: Power in the Era of Post-Humanity*. London: Allen Lane.

Žižek, S. 2018b. Ernst Lubitsch, censorship, and political correctness. *American Affairs*, 2 (3). Available from: https://americanaffairsjournal.org/2018/08/ernst-lubitsch-censorship-and-political-correctness/ [Accessed 30 November 2020].

Žižek, S. and Daly, G. 2004. *Conversations with Žižek*. Cambridge: Polity Press.

Zupančič, A. 2003. *The Shortest Shadow: Nietzsche's Philosophy of the Two*. Cambridge, MA: MIT Press.

Zupančič, A. 2008. *The Odd One In: On Comedy*. Cambridge, MA: MIT Press.

Zupančič, A. 2017/18. The apocalypse is (still) disappointing. *S: Journal of the Circle for Lacanian Ideology Critique*, 10/11, 16–30.

5

THE OFFICE

The Office: 'a small show, set in a bland, insignificant and grey place'

The Office was a British sitcom which aired on the BBC from 2001 to 2003. The series was created, written and directed by Ricky Gervais and Stephen Merchant, with Gervais playing the show's protagonist, David Brent. After first airing in July 2001, the show continued for two series and two Christmas specials as well as spawning international adaptations, the most successful being *The Office* (US), which aired from 2005 to 2013.

Widely successful, both abroad and in the UK, the series garnered critical and popular acclaim, helping to form part of a lineage of TV comedies which have sought to address and perform underlying contradictions and inherent inconsistencies in British cultural values. In the case of *The Office*, these values would centre around a group of staff working for a fictional paper merchants, Wernham Hogg, in offices that were located in Slough, Berkshire (UK). For Brabazon, the location proved crucial to the show's significance:

> It is a small show, set in a bland, insignificant and grey place, with minor and irrelevant cities encircling it. … The global, cosmopolitan citizen, unrestrained by location, is not part of *The Office's* world. The programme is strained and conflictual in the presentation of race, gender, sexuality and age, probing how these differences operate through labour.
>
> *(2005: 105)*

Indeed, as will be discussed, it was *The Office's* ability to perform these conflictual representations that afforded it a significant and important position in UK popular culture, emerging during a period where an apparent media bias towards ethnic minority groups and the questioning of hegemonic discourses pertaining to race, gender, homosexuality and disability were being acknowledged and debated. In fact, amidst wider derisions of political correctness, the series would also critique the mundanity of popular commercial culture and celebrity discourse. In his appraisal of the series, Gilroy notes how:

> *The Office* offered a distorted-mirror microcosm of Tony Blair's Britain in a peculiar collection of working people whose very ordinariness supplied the magic element that drew us into their narrow, suburban orbit and celebrated the country's slow but profound adaptation to the new tempo of its multi-cultural life. All of old Britain's obsessions with class, race, gender, tradition, national identity, and even with the propriety of laughter itself were present here. *The Office* acknowledged them and then dramatized and celebrated their still-incomplete overcoming.
>
> *(2004: 149)*

Central to this presentation was the Slough branch manager, David Brent, who spends the majority of each series stumbling through a number of comic gaffes in his attempts to impress his colleagues and managers. Tyler and Cohen note that much of the comedy stems from 'Brent's desperation to be both popular, "one of the lads", and at the same time revered for his (self-professed) managerial acumen and charismatic style of leadership' (2008: 115). In many ways, David reflects Žižek's account of the 'postmodern boss', where, in contrast to a strict authoritarianism, David seeks to be both boss and friend to his subordinates:

> A 'postmodern' boss insists that he is not a master but just a coordinator of our joint creative efforts, the first among equals; there should be no formalities among us, we should address him by his nickname, he shares a dirty joke with us … but during all this, he remains our master. In such a social link, relations of domination function through their denial: in order to [be] operative, they have to be ignored.
>
> *(2015: 115)*

In fact, such denial was cleverly presented in Gervais's performance, with David's awareness of the watching camera offering him the opportunity to present his pseudo-philosophical wisdom to staff as well as 'us' the audience. In this regard:

> *The Office* brilliantly portrays the life of David Brent, a man of many moral shortcomings, whose main moral flaw is that he is too busy with *looking* good, instead of *being* good. When the cameras are rolling, Brent is very much aware of the demands of PC, because he does not want to seem intolerant, or judgmental, narrow-minded, or illiberal. Instead, he wants to be remembered for his humanity, his charity, and his humour. Brent therefore tries to present himself as a person of moral excellence. Yet, as we all know, this attempt fails

> miserably because his commitment to the values he wants to uphold is only skin-deep. Even his charity work is just a means for personal glorification.
>
> *(Nys, 2008)*

Often in full view and acknowledgment of the camera, it was evident that David sought to use his humour as an attempt to promote his own celebrity. To this extent, the series was able to perform and play with a number of instances where the cast sought to present a politically correct persona, which, in most cases, was comically performed in a politically incorrect way. This was apparent in one 'talking head' scene where the writers were able to portray the complexities and cultural sensitivities regarding the correct terminology that one should and shouldn't use. In a scene involving the character Gareth (Mackenzie Crook), we watch Gareth provide the following explanation:

> That's it, see, a lot of people can't keep up with what words are acceptable these days and what words aren't. It's like my Dad, for example, he's not as cosmopolitan or as educated as me, and… it can be embarrassing. You know, he doesn't understand all the new trendy words. Like, he'll say… umm… 'poofs' instead of 'gays', 'birds' instead of 'women', 'darkies' instead of 'coloureds'.
>
> *(*The Office*, S2E01, 2002)*

In this scene, Gareth reflects upon as well as performs many of the contradictions and inconsistencies enveloped in political correctness, including: the patronising portrayal of his father, not as cosmopolitan or as educated as him; the personal embarrassment that this causes for Gareth; and, perhaps most importantly, his inability to stick to a politically correct terminology, as made clear in his reference to 'coloureds'. As a result, it is in 'their skirmishes with the politically correct directives of corporate multiculturalism' (McNeil, 2010: 108–109) that characters such as Gareth would serve to comically perform the inherent limitations within political correctness.

These performances were neatly captured in the show's use of the sitcom genre. Emerging in the 1960s, situated comedy would prove a useful format for television writers seeking to explore new political trends and 'new forms of political satire' (Bebber, 2014: 254). During this time the BBC Director-General, Hugh Greene, alongside Michael Mills (Head of Comedy) and Tom Sloan (Head of Light Entertainment), adopted the sitcom format in order to help create characters that were not only easy to identify with but who would also be situated in recognisable locations (Kamm and Neumann, 2016). Various sitcoms would often centre around the family, with 'characters who debated salient conflicts in Britain like the rise of social democracy, the loss of British gentility and national tradition, and the decline of the empire that marked the first few decades after the Second World War' (Bebber, 2014: 253). The success of the sitcom genre would consolidate its position in British television comedies, offering an opportunity to help air the UK's cultural, political and social tensions (Bebber, 2014).

However, in *The Office*, the sitcom genre underwent a certain revamp in its format, with the series drawing upon a 'mockumentary' style: a comic subgenre which creates fictional events but portrays these events as 'real' (Wallace, 2018). This was achieved via a fictional camera crew who were making a 'documentary' on 'the office', filming and interviewing its staff as they went about their day-to-day roles. Consequently, in its attempts to maintain a realistic documentary style, the show would refrain from using standard sitcom techniques, such as laugh tracks or live audiences, and would, for the majority of its script, refrain from one-liners or the use of catchphrases. This put the audience in a unique position, with no explicit reference as to what should be laughed at (De Jongste, 2017). Instead, as Soper highlights, 'we laugh or cringe as we observe people much like ourselves unwittingly revealing their foolishness through talking head interviews, banal every-day situations, and seemingly unscripted exchanges with office mates' (2009: 83). For the series as a whole, however, its 'downbeat style' allowed the show's characters to comically perform and reflect upon the real and lived experiences of a post-imperial, neoliberal UK – a UK that, for many, was struggling to come to terms with its cultural diversity in the new millennium (Gilroy, 2004). In doing so, the series presented a unique insight into the everyday banality of office-culture under New Labour, one marked by an increasing knowledge of politically correct behaviours and cultural sensitivities. Furthermore, through its use of the mockumentary format, the series was able to mimic the Reality TV genre popular at the time (Schwind, 2014: 23). Alongside the use of 'talking head' sequences, various characters would deliberately acknowledge the camera, revelling in their chance to be on TV (Kilborn, 2003). For David, it was this opportunity which underscored his, often misplaced, ambitions.

Though many sitcoms have centred on the family, with the family home being the prime location, *The Office* shifted its focus towards 'the office' workspace and a '9 to 5' neoliberal working environment. Consequently, whereas the setting would echo the humdrum mundanity of office culture, its 'semi-public' environment also ensured that a number of 'everyday' situations could be comically performed with embarrassing potential (Jacobi, 2016). These 'everyday' interactions were crucial to *The Office* narrative, with the 'camera crew observing the employees of Wernham Hogg's Slough branch in their everyday work routines and conversations' (Schwind, 2014: 23). Certainly, as Gilroy (2004) highlights, these workplace interactions were not reducible to race but included wider tensions and observations on sexism, disability, homophobia and masculinity, all portrayed within a 'postmodern' working environment shaped by company mergers, bureaucratisation and corporatism. As a result, the show afforded an insight into the ways in which these changes were managed by individuals from often diverse cultural backgrounds via scenes that sought to perform the 'taken-for-granted' ordinariness of professional work relations.

To this extent, the location of 'the office' helped to position the show within a corporate setting that has seen debates on political correctness and its effectiveness in managing workplace environments come under scrutiny (Goncalo et al., 2015). Such assessments clearly point to the hegemonic significance of political correctness and the concern that its use may either promote or curtail workplace relations. Indeed, these scenarios have been lampooned by comedians. In 2017, 'British actress Tracey Ullman released a satirical sketch involving a support group full of 20-somethings who were "too woke" to enjoy themselves or discuss anything' (Murray, 2018). Here, Murray notes:

> The sketch skewers politically correct culture in a social context, but it surfaces a concern that exists for many in the workplace; namely, how can people be authentic and productive if they're constantly worried about offending their colleagues through language that could be construed as offensive?
>
> *(2018)*

While Murray's (2018) questioning highlights the 'concern' surrounding political correctness, his brief assessments are geared towards evaluating whether political correctness is a productive instrument for business success. Of greater concern is the notable use of the term 'woke' alongside a – albeit comic – derision of political correctness. Emerging in the US, Cauley (2019) notes that the term 'woke' was originally used by black communities as a way of keeping them aware of examples of anti-blackness and social/racial injustice. Indeed, 'It acknowledged that being black meant navigating the gaps between the accepted narrative of normality in America and our own lives' (Cauley, 2019). Much like the use of the term 'politically correct', the term 'woke' has become desensitised to its original purpose, with Cauley highlighting that:

> after the deaths of Michael Brown and Eric Garner, 'Stay woke' became a rallying cry for the Black Lives Matter movement. But with its mass adoption, the word's black activist history has faded, and its urgency has dulled. Now it functions merely as a nod to the speaker's mainstream lefty positions, a smug confirmation that the speaker holds the expected progressive beliefs.
>
> *(2019)*

We can, in Cauley's references to the 'mainstream lefty positions' of those using the term, draw connections between the speaker's supposed 'progressive beliefs' and Žižek's criticisms of the ways in which politically correct assertions maintain the assumed 'neutrality' of the multicultural, cosmopolitan subject. If we compare this to Ullman's sketch then we can also observe how, in accordance with Zupančič's (2008) false comedy and true comedy distinctions, Ullman's example provides a source of resistance that, while making fun of political correctness, merely maintains its hegemonic role as some*thing* to be resisted. Whereas the Ullman sketch highlights how the term 'woke' has been appropriated beyond its original use as a signifier of Black disenfranchisement, of greater concern is the difficulty in determining whether Ullman's sketch is lampooning politically correct behaviour; deriding those who seek to blame political correctness for preventing them from telling racist, sexist and homophobic jokes (in the scene, the councillor is the one suggesting to the support group not to worry, they'll be 'right-wing' by the time they're thirty); or drawing attention to the fact that we should be 'woken' to examples of discrimination. What is clear is that though Ullman provides a concrete example of the frustrations regarding political correctness, we are instead encouraged to laugh at the irony of the fictional setting as well as the support group participants who find themselves unable to stop making politically correct assertions. Though the sketch is funny, unfortunately it simply maintains political correctness as an abstract universal, which, through a self-detached irony, works to direct its comedy on those individuals who remain offended at every form of social labelling.

While the analysis presented here will steer clear from assessing whether political correctness may improve or even hinder employee productivity – indeed, a clear reminder of the ideological manipulation that the term prescribes, as reflected in the apparent ease in which it can be administered to support capitalism – it will consider how examples of political (in)correctness can prove useful in examining the relation between comedy, race and racism, as performed in the fictional Slough office (Nys, 2008).

In what follows, consideration will be given to examining the performance of a racist joke from episode one, series two, 'Merger'. Specifically, this analysis will first provide a synopsis of the episode, before presenting a scripted account of each scene. Drawing upon the theoretical analysis that was built in Chapters One to Four, the remainder of the chapter will offer a considered and critical appraisal of each scene.

The Office: 'Merger'

'Merger' is the first episode of the second series of *The Office*, which aired on 30 September 2002. The episode follows the merger of the Swindon and Slough branches of Wernham Hogg, with the Swindon staff joining the Slough team (this plotline was followed during the first series). As part of the merger, Neil, previously the Swindon manager and David's former equivalent, is now David's boss, with David managing the expanded branch at Slough. Neil is popular with staff and, to the frustration of David, is able to effortlessly maintain a certain professional sensitivity and sense of humour with his colleagues. Over the course of the second series, David's many attempts to be perceived as the 'cooler' boss result in a number of gaffes, faux pas and errors. Moreover, while David remains socially aware of the judgements surrounding political correctness, he is a character who, in his attempts to be politically correct, often fails and, as a result, finds himself failing to meet both his employer's and, perhaps, our own, expectations. This is echoed in the episode where, during an introduction between David and the 'new' (Swindon/Slough) team, David introduces himself by typically misjudging the appropriateness of the situation, performing what can only be described as a well-prepared, yet badly performed, 'stand-up routine'. Unsurprisingly, David's attempt to impress the staff fails, with David making a number of awkward statements throughout the scene, one of which involves doing an impression of a disabled member of staff.

However, as will become clear in the following analysis of notable scenes drawn from the episode, much of this episode centres around the performance of a 'black man's cock' joke. While the joke's content draws upon the popular stereotype that all black men have large genitalia, the prevalence of this imagery is one that is vividly recalled by Boakye, who, as a child, recounts the media's 'feverish excitement' regarding the Jamaican-born British Athlete Linford Christie and his 'lunchbox'. Boakye notes, 'I remember because growing up, it was patently obvious to me that one of the big black stereotypes was that black men have big black penises' (2019). Never funny and always uncomfortable, 'the objectification, the belittling, [and] the basic disrespect of reducing an entire person to the sum total of their genitals' remains, for Boakye (2019), attributable to those 'many indirect comments about having a big penis' which have been directed at him. Indeed, though the reference would often be made by people he knew, and while never meant 'in malice', it stands as 'Further evidence of the nervous affinity between dominant whiteness and a blackness it doesn't quite understand' (Boakye, 2019).

Boakye's comments draw attention to the subtlety of certain racist associations and how, much like Brent, though never made in enmity, they remain attributable to a misguided form of 'banter' (Boakye, 2019). This 'nervous affinity' is clearly exposed in the scenes' performances, with David's initial hesitancies giving way to the assumption that he has, on a certain level, achieved a banterous exchange with a black colleague, Oliver (Howard Saddler). While it is acknowledged that the reference to a 'black man's cock' is a racial stereotype, what the following analysis will consider is the way in which David's attempts to build morale amongst his colleagues clashes with his politically (in)correct intentions. Evidently, the purpose here is not to expose the joke as racist – the remainder of this analysis will work off the assumption that the reader is clearly aware of this – rather, what will be considered is how this racial exchange can subversively be used to challenge examples of political correctness. This is most notable in the performance of David, who, despite his various faux pas, continues to maintain the presumption that he is being politically correct.

In the following analysis, specific attention will be paid to examining four related scenes from the episode, each of which will be considered in chronological order. In reflecting upon the episode and the joke, Gilroy notes:

> The country's time-worn habit of dealing with racism through the ritual activity of having a laugh was dealt with directly in one extra-ordinary episode of *The Office* in which David Brent, the principal character, who is both office manager and a would-be comedian, gets rebuked for telling a racist joke in the presence of a black colleague and is then exposed to the lucid objections of his fellow workers who found it offensive. The joke in question will have

offended monarchists as well as anti-racists by suggesting that the members of the royal family were intimately familiar with a 'black man's cock'.

(2004: 150)

Accordingly, consideration will be given to examining how such an 'extra-ordinary' performance can expose a number of important contentions in the performance of comedy and, more specifically, in examples of political correctness. Implicit within this analysis will be the underlying concern that the performance of the 'black man's cock' joke represents a parallax shift that reveals the joke's, and the scene's, subversive significance.

'I've got a joke you can use': The spectacle and spectre of race

In the first scene, before David's introduction with the new members of staff, David approaches his colleagues, Gareth and Tim (Martin Freeman), in order to explain that he has prepared a short comic routine for the introductory meeting. Gareth explains that he has a joke David can use:

GARETH: I've got a joke you can use.

DAVID: Well, you don't usually do jokes, but go on…

GARETH: Alright, it's Christmas dinner… Royal Family having their Christmas dinner… Camilla Parker Bowles goes: 'OK, we'll play twenty-questions, I'll think of something, you'll have to ask me questions and guess what it is…' and what she's thinking is a black man's cock.

DAVID: (*giggles*) Trust Camilla.

David looks at the camera.

DAVID: It's not racist, is it? Because…

GARETH: (*quickly*) No…

Tim, bemused, looks at the camera.

GARETH: Um… so, Prince Phillip goes… 'Is it bigger than the bread bin', she (Camilla) goes… 'Yeah'. Prince Charles goes… 'Is it something that I can put in my mouth', she goes… 'Yeah'. Queen goes… 'Is it a black man's cock?'

David bursts-out laughing.

There are a number of important significances that can be drawn from the first scene. Notably, it is here that we witness the initial performance of the racist joke, as told by Gareth to David. The laughter of both men, while Tim sits quietly, provides the scene an undeniable awkwardness. This is reflected in Tim's facial expressions, which serve to highlight his disbelief in the joke being told. Consequently, in contrast to Tim, it is clear that David and Gareth obtain a certain level of enjoyment from the joke. Both men laugh and snigger at the joke's punchline and, towards the end of the scene, David congratulates Gareth for telling the joke. In comparison to Tim, both David and Gareth reflect a clear lack of reflexivity. This is evident in their open enjoyment of the joke (both men laugh) and their subsequent failure to perceive its racist significance, despite David's initial questioning ('it's not racist, is it?'). To this extent, the scene serves as a demonstration of how the other (the 'black man') is used 'as a means of relating to our own enjoyment, [and] as a screen for our fantasy' (Zupančič, 2003: 180). This is brought to light in the joke's punchline, which serves to reproduce the racist fantasy that all black men have large genitalia.

Yet, it is in the context of the joke's performance that we can begin to draw further connections between the formal structure of the joke and the previously discussed spectacle and spectre of race. As noted, Hsiao's analysis of black minstrelsy revealed how 'the spectral existence of racial trauma is occluded or concealed precisely by means of exposing racial difference in full view' (2010: 182). These differences were often performed through the spectacularisation of racial fantasies that ensured that the audience never had to encounter the Real presence of race, reducing it instead to a spectral presence. In similar fashion, while, in the above scene, the joke is not performed by a black colleague, we nevertheless see a similar relation being presented. That is, although the spectacle of race is performed – via the racist fantasy that all black men have large genitalia – the spectre of race is kept hidden through its obfuscation. This occurs in a very particular way.

For example, if we consider that the symbolic order is not undermined, but rather formed through 'transgressive fantasies' that 'are constitutive and supportive of this order since they rely on what they desire to be transgressed' (Bergmann and Højlund, 2019: 266), then it is apparent that examples of self-censorship can help to promote racism through forms of inherent transgression (Žižek, 2008a). Equally, David is a master at using the camera as a form of self-promotion, with many of his talking-head sequences and filmed scenes involving him looking directly at the camera from which he seeks approval. Westwood and Johnston note how:

> The notion of 'performance' is apposite since Brent often expressly plays to camera when wanting to signal that he is being PC – note … when Gareth begins his joke and Brent looks nervously at the camera and asks 'It's not racist is it?'. He invites the audience to monitor his performance and validate his appropriateness and political correctness.
>
> *(2011: 796)*

Accordingly, it is when David is aware of the camera that we witness his 'politically correct' performance. Indeed, this acknowledgment of the camera will prove important to the analysis below. When we consider the scene in question, it is clear that David knows the joke is racist. In doing so, David adequately executes the politically correct rhetoric, by knowingly performing the 'correct' behaviour to 'us' the audience (Westwood and Johnston, 2011).

However, what we see here is how such acknowledgment provides an inherent transgression that serves as 'a form of ideological inscription that is central to the maintenance of numerous social bonds, especially those that comprise institutions, bureaucracies, and communities' (Kingsbury, 2017: 5). That is, although

David questions whether the joke is racist, his clarification and later actions (laughing) tell a different story. In fact, whereas political correctness emerges in David's questioning of the joke, his remarks neither prevent the joke being told nor are they followed. Instead, such political correctness, while duly noted, is 'sustained by an obscene supplementary element that transgresses the conscious element' (Delay, 2014: 1). It is under these circumstances that political correctness maintains a symbolic efficiency, even in the face of open racism. As a result, David's politically correct acknowledgment admits him to transgress the joke's racism, and thus allows him to enjoy its racist significance. Though the spectacle of race is acknowledged and performed, the racial significance of the joke – the spectre of race – remains disavowed.

Furthermore, it is in this first scene that the joke echoes Zupančič's (2008) false comedy by maintaining a certain level of distance between the concrete (the performance of the joke) and the universal (political correctness can be maintained and followed via David's initial response: 'it isn't racist, is it?'). In doing so, both the universal and the concrete remain separate. As a result, what we witness in this performance is a racist joke that is sustained by a level of political correctness that ensures the joke's continuation.

'Here's what I should have told you...': Comedy, parallax and the other – identifying the comic shift

In a second scene, following David's disastrous introductory meeting, we cut to David and a small group of Wernham Hogg staff. Clearly annoyed that the new staff members did not find his prepared jokes funny, and with the camera positioned from across the room, David leans into the huddled group and begins to tell Gareth's joke:

DAVID: ... Here's what I should have told you. Right, Royal Family, yeah, Christmas Day, they've had lunch, sitting down, Camilla goes, 'Let's play a game. Let's play twenty-questions. I'll think of something and you've got to guess what I'm thinking of.' And what she's thinking of is a black man's cock. So, Charles goes... 'Is it bigger than the bread bin?'. She says, 'Yes'. Phillip goes... 'Can I put it in my mouth?' She goes... 'Yes'. So, the Queen goes... 'Is it a black ma...'

Just before David reaches the punchline, Oliver, a black colleague, enters the group.

OLIVER: Hiya!

David gives a quick thumbs-up, acknowledging Oliver's presence. He stands straight, looks at the group and straightens his tie. Evidently, he doesn't intend to finish the joke.

OLIVER: Sorry... were you telling a joke?

It's clear that Oliver is aware that his entrance has interrupted David speaking.

DAVID: No. That was it.

David smiles, awkwardly nodding to the rest of the group.

COLLEAGUE: What did the Queen say?

David shrugs his shoulders and shakes his head.

DAVID: Didn't...

(clearly embarrassed, David looks nervously at the group's members)

OLIVER: Come on, what was the joke?

COLLEAGUE: It's about the Royal Family playing twenty-questions.

OLIVER: Aww... (*Oliver stops to think*) it's not the black man's cock one, is it?

DAVID: (*nervously playing with his tie*) It might be, but... (*stumbling*) it's bad ain't it?

OLIVER: No, no, it's alright... funny.

David turns to the group, still nervously smiling.

DAVID: Harmless... (*David turns to Oliver*) Well done!

Oliver, looking at David, slowly sips his drink. He stops sipping and, uneasily, stands straight as he hears David's 'well done'.

The camera zooms out to reveal the group to be much larger. One of the members of the group is in a wheelchair.

DAVID: (*stumbling for words*) Have you all met the... this little lady... this lady?

(he gives her a thumbs-up).

If we return to the Real, then, in accordance with the analysis of the first scene, it is apparent that any symbolisation is always marked by a 'remainder' or an 'excess' that is omitted from the process of symbolisation (Swyngedouw, 2015). This excess is brought to bear in this scene, where, in contrast to the first, the spectre of race is made 'present' in the sudden and surprising appearance of Oliver (a black colleague). Deliberately refraining from the punchline, David acknowledges the spectre of race, via the remark: 'bad ain't it?' From this point onwards, it is not the spectacle of race which garners attention, but instead its political significance as the spectre of race is recurrently acknowledged in the ensuing events.

It is this spectre and spectacle distinction which bears witness to the parallax within content and form. Indeed, for Žižek 'if we want to reconstruct "all" of the narrative content', evident in the scene's repeated performance of the racist joke, 'we must reach beyond the explicit narrative content as such, and include some formal features which act as the stand-in for the "repressed" aspect of the content' (2001: 58 [italics removed]). In the case of the above scene, the character, Oliver, reflects a formal feature who 'stands-in' for what was repressed within the narrative content of the first scene (the absence of the 'black man'). This highlights that we are not just dealing with an excessive racist joke (content), but with a performance that seeks to deliberately draw attention to the spectre of race *within* the formal (re)structuring of the joke's performance (Oliver's 'included' presence). In other words, our focus moves from the content of the joke to the scene's formal structure; in this case, Oliver's unexpected presence.

In view of Oliver's inclusion in the scene, and in accordance with Žižek's (2006c) extension of Lacan's Real, we can conceive of Oliver's presence as mirroring Žižek's (2006c) Imaginary Real: a form of the Real which is brought to bear when one's imaginary fantasies have a very Real impact on the subject. Indeed, as Žižek highlights, 'it is this real, foreclosed from the symbolic fiction, that returns in the guise of spectral apparitions' (2012: 26). This spectral appearance of the Real occurs when David is confronted with the obscene enjoyment which sits at the heart of the joke's racist fantasy and which is subsequently brought to bear via the emergence of the 'black man', Oliver. In this singular moment, the symbolic consistency of the scene is fractured and 'in a contingent moment of encountering an excess' (Kunkle, 2012: 11), David is confronted with the Real of the other in all their traumatic dimensions – their Real presence. Here, Oliver's Real presence leaves David confronting the imaginary 'butt' of the joke.

To further elucidate this confrontation, consider the following example from McGowan:

> The trauma of the real becomes readily apparent when we consider social instances where the real manifests itself. It emerges whenever there is a hitch in the usual order of things. It occurs when a teacher is giving an account of something and a student asks a question that disturbs that account in a way that the teacher can't answer. The teacher's failure of mastery and evident discomfort is a trauma of the real. The symbolic authority reveals at this moment its lack of authority and the inability of the symbolic to cover everything. Or this trauma occurs when a child continues to ask why. At some point, the parent just says, 'Because I said so.' This is the real that interrupts the flow of the symbolic order.
>
> *(2015: 37)*

Accordingly, the scene's comic suspense is effectively rendered as we wait to see how David will respond to Oliver's presence. In much the same way that the socio-symbolic status of 'the teacher' and 'the parent' is challenged in McGowan's (2015) example, in this scene the Real 'interrupts' when we witness David's socio-symbolic status as 'manager' undermined, with Oliver's interruption and finishing of the joke subverting David's symbolic authority. In the case of David, this authority is conferred on his role as office manager, but also in his position as the joke-teller. Here, Oliver's attempts to hear the joke's punchline deliberately draw upon 'the embarrassing idiosyncrasy of the obscene enjoyment' (Žižek, 2002: 12), with Oliver's delivering of the punchline locating *him* in the position of enunciation. This interruption fundamentally re-orientates the passage of the joke, dislodging the 'wholeness' granted to David's authority and relinquishing the 'false solidarity' that works to disguise the power of those who hold authority (Žižek, 2002). Instead, in his moment of authoritative abandonment, David's failure to finish the joke, and his subsequent attempts to defend it, reveal a form of self-estrangement, or, as McGowan notes, 'One … divided against oneself' (2014: 213). The effect of this subversion is that David's authoritative status is divided against him*self*; a self-division which leaves David in the awkward position of beginning, but not finishing, the joke's punchline. What is significant, however, is that it is in the joke's formal performance that this division in David's authority and his 'politically correct' persona is enacted and repeated. As will be discussed below, it is

David's (the comic persona) ability to perform this self-division which underscores his role as a subversive comic character.

For now, if we consider the importance of Oliver in this scene, then it is evident that his presence is not viewed as in some way legitimising the joke's racism; nor should it be suggested that his actions simply relieve David from telling the joke. Certainly, we could interpret Oliver's response as 'a tactical mimicry of the other's mimicry of the mimicked subject's misrecognized and fantasized image' (Hsiao, 2010: 178), reflected in the contention that Oliver is merely performing how he believes he should behave in the presence of his (white) boss (keep your head down and laugh at your boss's jokes). Here, McGowan notes:

> Oftentimes, the type of subject and the type of object coincide: either the figure of authority finds comedy in mockery of the excluded, or one of the excluded tells a joke undermining symbolic authority. One can easily imagine a business leader recounting a racist or a sexist joke or laughing at satirical depictions of the excluded, just as one can also imagine a group of servants laughing at the foibles of the upper class families that they serve. In both cases, the political bearing of the subject and object of comedy line up exactly.
>
> *(2014: 204)*

Nevertheless, while aware of McGowan's concerns, it is argued that Oliver's performance requires a more nuanced approach. That is, though the joke deliberately objectifies 'black men', we see, in the case of Oliver, how such objectivisation is liberated by Oliver's active role in the scene: *he* states that he's heard it before; *he* chooses to finish the joke; and *he* suggests that it is funny. In addition, Oliver's role within the joke prevents any awkwardness or humiliation on his behalf. This is made apparent when we imagine an alternative scene, where, upon Oliver's arrival, David immediately stops telling the joke and, as they stand quietly, the group wait for someone to talk about something else. In this latter scenario, Oliver would be well aware that his presence has disturbed what was previously being said (we've all walked in on a conversation that we should not be privy too) and, in this instance, what is not said, thus, what is ignored, could have a more upsetting effect. Instead, we can view Oliver's response as an honest engagement, or perhaps a more deliberate engagement, to emphasise 'the embarrassing idiosyncrasy' (Žižek, 2002: 12) which structures the joke's racist fantasy. In doing so, Oliver's actions are presented as a performance that *subjects* David to the 'real Thing' – that is, the 'real black man'. In effect, Oliver's role in finishing the joke bears a more intrusive incursion that serves to reveal race's in-visibility (his real appearance), as opposed to merely presenting the spectacle of racial difference through examples of polite, and easily forgotten, apologies.

Furthermore, though the scene can be interpreted as a racist depiction that unnecessarily uses a racist joke in order to provide a politically incorrect gesture, at the same time, the scene re-uses the racist joke to make fun of Brent's naivety and his own racist fantasies. Central to each of these interpretations is the ambiguity of

Oliver's performance. Indeed, it is Oliver's acceptance of the joke and his finishing of the punchline which not only dislodges the joke and the scene's narrative, but which also allows the joke to be told, much to Brent's relief. Yes, Oliver is a fictional character, constructed by the two white writers, but his role within this scene provides a certain level of subversive agency – it is his presence and gesture which frames the awkward encounter. Moreover, rather than Oliver *being* the humour (McGowan, 2014), it is his response (his commendation of the joke) which proves integral to the narrative in scenes three and four.

To this extent, the presence of Oliver can be related to what Lacan believed to be a key structural feature in comedy – 'the appearance of the phallus' (Zupančič, 2016: 220). For Lacan, the phallus occupies a vital position in the signifying order and its associated power relations: it is the appearance of the phallus which brings this power to bear. Certainly, as Zupančič notes, 'The connection between comedy and the phallus is not Lacan's invention; it is pointed out by virtually all theoreticians and historians of comedy, especially with regard to the origins of comedy and its beginnings' (2016: 220). In Ancient comedy, the phallus would play a literal role, often being unveiled as a prop at certain comical moments (Gherovici and Steinkoler, 2016). However, for Zupančič:

> Lacan's contribution is to relate this comic usage of the phallic reference to his theory of the phallic signifier or, more precisely, to his theory of the place and the office that this signifier holds in the symbolic structure. To put it simply: the phallic signifier is a tautological signifier that signifies nothing but that it signifies; it functions as a hidden presupposition (and reference) of the signifying order, guaranteeing its meaning. Comedy plays with this hidden presupposition in different ways, exploring the fundamental function of this presupposition: the linking together of the field of signification and of the field of desire.
>
> *(2016: 220)*

Drawing from Zupančič's account, it is the phallus's 'hidden presupposition' which maintains the signifying order, and, in an analogous mode, we can see this 'hidden' importance echoed in the spectre of race which remains obfuscated in its spectacle. As noted in the analysis of scene one, it is this obfuscation which the current scene comically performs. Indeed, it is Oliver's sudden presence (and, to a certain extent, his literal black cock) which symbolically provides 'the comic "coming out" of the hidden signifier pertaining to the fundamental structure of the symbolic order and to its power relations' (Zupančič, 2016: 220). It is this sudden 'appearance' which provides Oliver's unexpected presence with a comic effect that subverts the scene's symbolic order and exposes David's diminished authority.

More importantly, it is in this scene that we can begin to examine Oliver's Real presence as inducive of Žižek's parallax shift and Zupančič's concrete universal. As previously noted, with Oliver finishing the racist joke, it is clear that he occupies the place of enunciation *and* the subject of the enunciated. Here, 'the place of enunciation does not undermine the universality of the statement but becomes its very internal gap, that which alone generates the only (possible) universality of the statement' – the concrete universal (Zupančič, 2008: 60). To this extent, it is not just that Oliver resides within the joke's content – he is a black man – but that rather than being excluded from the joke's performance, it is through Oliver's recounting of the punchline that a parallax shift – an exposition of the inherent 'gap' at the heart of the One – is achieved. In a paradoxical way, Oliver's place of enunciation reveals the 'gap' within the enunciated content, with his own intentions and the joke's political incorrectness being called into question. Oliver's finishing of the joke leaves one asking: is any individual free to partake in the performance of a racist joke? Is this not a form of *political correctness*?

In accordance with David's subverted authority, we can see how the position of the joke teller and their relation with the listening group, as considered by Heller, can further reveal the scene's parallax effect:

> The public and oral character of joke-telling creates a kind of silent conspiracy among the listeners. The readiness to laugh, like laughter itself, creates a bond of quasi-companionship among a group. This is why the narrator of a joke has to presuppose the relative homogeneity of the company attuned to mirth. One tells certain jokes to certain people from whom one expects the ability to grasp certain hints, background information, and the hidden message of the joke. One cannot tell jokes with footnotes. They would no longer be jokes. It may even be sufficient in a homogenous group of a certain joke-culture for someone to utter only the first sentence, or perhaps the punch line, or – according to a well known anecdote – the number of a joke, and everyone will burst out laughing, because they have heard the joke several times already, and one single word or even a number may work as a trigger to bring the joke back into the conscious mind and to simultaneously provoke the expression of laughter.
>
> *(2005: 126–127)*

It is important to highlight how Heller's notion of 'homogeneity', a homogeneity that stems from the shared cultural and social space of the joke-teller and its listeners, undergoes a parallax shift which bears witness to the inherent inconsistences of any 'homogenous' account. If we continue along the lines of Zupančič's materialist approach to comedy, and if we remember that, in Chapter Two, it was argued that through a parallax shift we can observe the self-division of the One – reflected in the acknowledgment of what was there, but ignored; what was invisible, but now visible – then, it is evident that in light of Heller's comments, the performance of the Royal Family joke presents a particularly subversive significance.

That is, as evident in the above analysis, it is Oliver's appearance which fundamentally ruptures the performance of the joke and which, through a parallax shift, undermines 'the relative homogeneity of the company attuned to mirth'

(Heller, 2005: 126–127). This prescribes a transference – a short circuit – from which the presence of Oliver (the content's absent-presence) reveals the inherent inconsistency of what was previously a homogenous performance (we've already heard the joke, we know its narrative and the joke's punchline). To this extent, Oliver's presence does not reflect the intrusion of an 'outside' element – this would only serve to ensure Oliver's 'outsider exclusion' – but, instead, Oliver's presence reveals the 'included exclusion' (the exception) within the homogenous group (McGowan, 2016). In fact, rather than remaining absent – indeed, rather than silently listening to the joke, with the spectre of race remaining invisible – Oliver's appearance induces a parallax shift and, thus, serves to reveal *that* which remains invisible in what is usually considered homogenous. What is significant here is that Oliver does not stand apart from this 'company', but, clearly, forms a constitutive member of the staff. Further compounding this 'shift', is the fact that Oliver has heard the joke before and, more importantly, can state the punchline. This locates the joke within a wider social context of racism, with Oliver's open acknowledgment positioning him as the universal exception in the 'homogenous' order.

Therefore, when considered in relation to Zupančič's account of the temporal differences between the joke and the comic sequence, we can assert how the Royal Family joke denotes 'the specific temporal modality of jokes' (2008: 133), reflected in the 'retroactive' surprise – the parallax shift – that occurs as part of the joke's narrative. This is performed when the Queen unexpectedly finishes the game. At the level of the joke's performance, however, David's awkward indecision on whether he should finish the joke's punchline, as well as Oliver's unexpected response to the joke, effectively renders the scene with a certain comic suspense that is, on the hand, orientated around Oliver's Real presence, but which, on the other, produces a parallax shift that brings to bear comedy's subversive capacity. What is important here is that, following the argument outlined in Chapter Four, such subversion requires a certain 'redoubling' which reveals the negativity at the heart of any socio-symbolic order. Consequently, in a formal process that resembles 'the experience of social fantasy as a screen masking the ultimate structural impossibility of society as nonantagonistic whole', we witness this same impossibility – this 'materialist moment' (Vogt, 2007: 63) – in the scene's self-relating negativity. It is this negativity which comically performs the (potential) failure of social interaction and which emphasises the scene's comic materiality: the ability to portray that particular idiosyncrasy, symbolic attachment or failure to communicate, through a self-negating gesture that bears witness to reality's conflicting heterogeneity (as opposed to some harmonious homogeneity). It is this process of self-negation that effectively posits the scene's subversion.

This can be given further elucidation via Chow's assertion that jokes offer the opportunity to '"look awry" at reality' (2014: 232). Drawing upon Žižek's notion of the 'tickling object', Chow details how:

> The 'tickling object' of the joke reveals the central concept of the parallax gap, and, when circulating in interpersonal discourse, its potential misfiring

> (its potential to provoke silence or bemusement rather than laughter) reveals the limits of the symbolic order to represent the Real, and the incommensurability between our symbolic universes.
>
> *(2014: 232)*

Here, the limits of the scene's symbolic order, and its (in)ability to account for Oliver's Real presence, point to 'the inconsistencies and contradictions of matter itself' (Zupančič, 2008: 47). This inconsistency is brought to bear in the scene's performed contradictions. Indeed, as noted in the previous discussion on Oliver, when we compare the first and second scenes, what surprises us is not the joke's punchline, but that a racist joke, told amongst a group of white colleagues, is subsequently followed by the unexpected entrance of a black colleague who continues to finish the joke. As a result, it is 'precisely the impossible sustained encounter between two excluding realities' – between a group of colleagues sharing a joke about a 'black man's cock' *and* a black man performing the punchline to a joke about a 'black man's cock' – that the second scene elicits an 'impossible sustained encounter' (Zupančič, 2008: 57). It is in this sense that:

> the two levels involved in a parallax shift are radically asymmetric: one of the two levels appears to be able to stand on its own, while the other stands for the shift as such, for the gap between the two.
>
> *(Žižek, 2006a: 42)*

Following this, it is the joke's performance in the second scene which stands for the shift in the joke's narrative, revealing the 'gap' that was inherent in the first scene. That is, while the second scene sees the same joke retold, rather than having the joke faithfully retold, we are introduced to a 'gap' in its retelling. As a result, there is a certain absurdity to the second scene that is forged from the unexpected response that Oliver provides. Indeed, we would not be wrong in expecting Oliver to find the joke offensive or for David to offer his sincere apologies for telling the joke in the first place. Instead, Oliver's finishing of the joke echoes Yao's assertion that:

> Though a joke's punchline is often based on a disgusting premise, there are certain moments in which this premise itself is subverted in the telling of a joke, say, by a member of the race or class which the joke is targeting.
>
> *(2012: 2)*

However, it is not simply the case that such subversion emerges from Oliver finishing the joke, but that in accordance with David and Oliver's maintained relationship, the initial absurdity of the scene *works*. In other words, it is 'illogical, yet logical' (Zupančič, 2008: 58). Rather than ignoring the joke or admonishing its racist significance, then, we get both realities performed in the scene: Oliver finishing the joke *and* David's retained self-esteem (moreover, from Oliver's performance we are led to believe that he 'genuinely' finds the joke funny). Importantly, it is in bringing these two realities together that we witness the joke's ability to draw attention to the inherent inconsistencies that constitute our 'coherent' reality and, more specifically, to the (possible) failure that underscores Real human interaction.

To help provide further clarification on this comic shift and its formal significance, we can turn to Dolar, who, while drawing upon a line from Pascal Blaise, cites the following: 'Two faces are alike; neither is funny by itself, but side by side their likeness makes us laugh' (1995: 58 cited in Dolar, 2017: 582). In explaining this line, Dolar notes:

> The beauty and the austere elegance of this line is that it tries to pin the comical by the very minimal, just by the mechanism of doubling. It brings it to this core: one is not funny, two is funny, but provided that two is the replication of one, its imitation, its likeness, its mimetic double, its similar twin. What happens between one and two to produce the comical effect? Not between one and two, but between two ones that don't quite add up to two; they are just clones of each other, same and different at the same time. Where there should be difference there is replication, a crack in the midst of the same. Two different faces are not funny, two similar ones are. So ultimately this is neither a two nor two ones, but a split one, where both parts can neither be counted as two nor made one. The comical object emerges in their very split.
>
> *(2017: 582)*

It is in scenes one and two (two *similar* scenes), then, that we observe 'a crack in the midst of the same'. That is, while we expect difference, we instead get the same joke performed but in two different forms. In fact, for Dolar, 'both parts can neither be counted as two nor made one' (2017: 583), and it is this same formal structure which is reflected in scenes one and two. Considered separately, neither scene would be funny (we wouldn't know the punchline if we only saw the second scene and, after the first scene, we are simply left with the performance of a racist joke); if merged together, then one would be left with the decision of choosing between *who* finishes the joke's punchline (Oliver or David?). This latter decision would subsequently lose the comedy that emerges from David's unashamed laughter in scene one *and* his embarrassment in scene two. Consequently, it is in the asymmetry between each scene (their minimal difference) that David's embarrassment and Oliver's acknowledgment provides a comic effect.

This 'minimal difference that cuts across and divides the same object among the various different perspectives' (Flisfeder, 2012) is given further consideration in what Žižek (2006a) refers to as a 'parallax Real'. For Zupančič, 'The Real is identified here with the gap that divides the appearance itself' (2003: 174). As a result, the Real occurs not when one side subsumes the other, but when two opposing sides meet in an impossible shared space (Zupančič, 2008). It is in this way that Oliver's presence in the scene is not one of a detoxified other, whose presence is kept at a tolerable distance, but, on the contrary, when confronted with the Real other – the object of the racist joke – David's political correctness is awkwardly performed via the comedy that ensues from him trying to maintain his politically correct status. He even states to Oliver that the joke 'is bad, ain't it?' When Oliver responds by stating that the joke is funny, he deliberately performs a certain 'excessive engagement' with the joke (Žižek, 2010). This proves to be a rather traumatic encounter for David, as is clear in his nervous responses and his over-emphasised relief. In fact, David's 'harmless' and 'well done' responses are not required and, as a result, simply draw attention to the sense of relief that emanates from David's inability to handle Oliver's Real presence. Instead of 'exchang[ing] with the Other the embarrassing idiosyncrasy of the obscene enjoyment', David's 'harmless' and 'well done' comments reveal a 'false obscene solidarity masking the underlying power relations – a paradigmatic case of the "postmodern exercise" of power' (Žižek, 2002: 13). Consequently, while David's political correctness is quickly re-established, such an exercise of power is also undermined through the concrete enactment of a politically correct performance that is performed in all its nonsensicality. Rather than laugh at the racist joke, then, we laugh at the comedy that is performed *in* David's politically correct presumption.

Furthermore, if we consider that in the first performance the other is absent; that is, Oliver plays no part, then it is clear that his appearance in the second performance serves to emphasise the contingency that emerges in the 'gap' between the first and second scenes. As previously noted, it is this 'contingent bit which dwells in the gap, which is produced by the very gap, and this imperceptible bit is the stuff that comedy puts to maximum use' (Dolar, 2005: 200). In other words, the Real is what emerges from the content of the first scene (the 'black man' and his accompanying 'cock') and its dis-continuous repetition in the second scene (a 'black man' finishing a joke about a 'black man's cock'). This is achieved in the tension – or, comic suspense – which is accomplished in Oliver's entrance. In recognising Oliver (and this is something that is most effectively made apparent when one watches the scene in question), David's reactions serve to heighten the scene's Real anxiety. It is through the scene's comedy that we can approach this anxiety.

More importantly, the asymmetrical 'gap' that is performed in scene two is not merely comical – in the sense that where we expect two, we get the same – but that such a 'gap' underscores the protraction of the joke into a comedy sequence, with the joke's inherent inconsistencies taking on a protracted significance. Again, we can turn to Zupančič to help trace this dynamic:

> If, then, the first step of the comic is this splitting divergence of the One – which produces the initial comic pleasure – what constitutes its second step? It consists simply in the comedy playing and constructing, from that point on, with this duality in a specific way: showing us the inner connections and mutual implications of the two elements of the duality. … Comedy is always a

> play with the inner ambiguity of the One. Comic duality is the inconsistency of the One (not simply its 'composition').
>
> *(2008: 122)*

This 'duality' is clearly reflected in the minimal difference between scenes one and two. In addition, while the above analysis has sought to map this inconsistency, with regards to the inherent contradictions in political correctness, it is also apparent that we cannot return to the joke's original racism. Indeed, 'when in comedy some (imaginary) Oneness or Unity splits in two, the sum of these two parts never again amounts to the inaugural One; there is a surplus that emerges in this split, and constantly disturbs the One' (Zupančič, 2008: 185). Accordingly, it is from this point onwards that both the joke and David's attempts to maintain a degree of political correctness are revealed to be 'split' and disturbed. That is, whereas in the first performance, the punchline (the 'black man's cock) serves as the Master-Signifier which retroactively determines the joke's sequence, it is in the second performance that, through a parallax shift, this Master-Signifier transfers from the 'significance' of the 'black man's cock' punchline (and the performance of this punchline) to a protracted comic sequence from which the *joke* itself and David's subsequent repetitions underscore the comedy of scenes three and four.

'...some of them can be a little sensitive': Self-estrangement and political correctness 'between the lines'

In the third scene, it becomes clear that someone has complained about David's racist joke. Both David and Gareth are called to a meeting with Jennifer (a partner of the Wernham Hogg firm and overseer of the Slough-Swindon merger) and Neil. In David's office, Jennifer and Neil reprimand David and Gareth for the inappropriateness of the joke. Clearly shocked that someone has complained about the joke, David immediately assumes that the complaint has come from Oliver, only to be told it was a female member of staff. While David protests that the joke cannot be racist, because Oliver found it funny, he is encouraged by Jennifer to repeat the joke in order to determine whether it is suitable for work. The joke is repeated and Jennifer asserts that it is offensive. She is immediately rebuked by David on the condition that the joke cannot be offensive because he doesn't 'say anything bad about black people', before stating, 'It's a compliment, if anything'. Exasperated, Jennifer reports that the joke's stereotype is an offensive myth. Gareth responds:

GARETH: I don't know Jennifer. I could show you a magazine where... literally *(Gareth puts his hands out in front of him measuring a foot-long gap between his outstretched forefingers)*

JENNIFER: *(Jennifer leans in, clearly dismayed)* Could you?

GARETH: Well, I haven't got it with me... but, when you're next in.

Gareth, while not understanding the sarcasm in Jennifer's remarks, continues to consider the suggestion. The camera cuts to Jennifer and Neil, both of whom look at David and Gareth in disbelief. Amidst the tension, David argues that he could change the joke by removing the reference to 'black' and, therefore, keep 'big cock'. Again, David is rebutted by Jennifer and she explains that such jokes should be kept outside the workplace. Clearly frustrated by the ongoing exchange, Jennifer finishes the meeting. Each character and the camera crew stand up and head to the door. Jennifer and Gareth leave the room but, before leaving, David, looking at the camera, grabs Neil by the arm in order to keep him in the room with the camera crew.

DAVID: She has a right to be careful, because some of them can be a little sensitive… you know, so…

NEIL: (*slightly confused by David's statement*) Sorry… who can?

David looks at the camera and shrugs his shoulders, clearly annoyed that Neil has questioned his remarks.

DAVID: (*slightly frustrated that he has to repeat himself*) Some… some people… can… take things the wrong way.

Neil nods ambivalently and goes to leave the room, before David speaks again…

DAVID: Oops, as an actress said to a Bishop (*David begins giggling, then stops abruptly, realising what he's said*)… And that's not a gay stereotype… the wrong way… I'm not saying that is the wrong way, I'm saying it's a way. Some women like it the wrong way, don't they (*David looks at the camera, when making the suggestion*)… and they're straight. (*Again, David stops abruptly, realising that he's said something else that may be taken the wrong way*) It doesn't matter if you're straight or gay, you know… A lot of people are… 1 in 10 apparently… that seems a bit high, doesn't it? But you know… you might be gay (*looking at Neil*)… if you are, good luck to ya, you know… just… just make sure its legal (*David looks at the camera*)… and be safe. OK.

David heads out the door alongside Neil. As the two men leave, David gives Neil a slow pat on the back, with the impression that the two men have made some form of connection.

In this scene, David continues to argue that the joke was inoffensive, primarily because Oliver didn't take offence and instead found it funny. What is more, we see the performance of the joke repeated for a third time – the same joke continued through its discontinuity. However, much like the previous two performances, while the content of the joke remains the same, we get a different response, this time reflected in Jennifer's reprimanding tone. Furthermore, in a continuation of the second performance, we see how David's responses reveal his true comic value as he exposes the underlying fantasy that structures the incongruity between himself and his politically correct image (Ladegaard, 2014). This fantasy is brought to bear in all its concrete materiality as David continues to object to the joke being racist and even suggests making changes to the joke, such as removing the 'black' reference. This is emphasised towards the end of scene where David refers to those 'sensitive' members of the staff who clearly can't take a joke. Neil's clarifications only serve to accentuate David's politically incorrect performance as he stumbles from awkward statement to awkward statement, each time clarifying his remarks with a look to the camera and a politically correct reply.

Again, much like scenes one and two, this third scene displays the repeated performance of the Royal Family joke. While Jennifer admonishes the joke's unsuitability for the workplace environment, David's attempts to re-signify the joke, by removing the reference to 'black', works to emphasise the joke's formal significance. In fact, this content-form relation is noted by Billig, who, while drawing upon the work of Critchley (2002), highlights how:

> one word changes a joke from being 'true' humour to the most bigoted humour. To use Freud's terminology, the 'joke-work' is identical. And if the joke is clever 'true' humour in the one form, why, with one different word, does it suddenly become reprehensibly unfunny? Any theory of racist humour must confront this problem.
>
> *(Billig, 2005: 26)*

This is especially pertinent when, as Billig (2005) notes, the 'joke-work' remains the same. In fact, despite David's suggestion that he remove the word 'black' from the joke's content, it is clear that the joke maintains a formal significance that serves only to sustain the 'problem' of racist humour.

If we consider that Billig's (2005) account draws attention to the importance of a particular word, and its subsequent removal, then what becomes apparent in this scene is how David's politically correct performance works to maintain a number of more obvious 'incorrect' remarks, which he excessively performs in an attempt to 'de-racialize' the joke's racist significance. David's reference to the 'little lady' in the second performance (a female member of staff who is in a wheelchair) and his later use of double-entendres ('as an actress said to a Bishop') and homosexual clarifications – again, quickly corrected when he adds that even women can like anal sex, as long as it's safe and legal – come together in the open acknowledgment that even Neil might be gay (and if he is, good luck to him). Rather than simply changing the particular context of a racist/offensive joke or merely replacing/removing the racist/offensive terminology that is used, David's performance highlights the excessive underside that frames the joke's content. What is most apparent is that throughout his various gaffes we are left laughing at David's continued desire to manage and regulate his behaviour with numerous politically correct assertions, supported with knowing looks at the camera. Accordingly:

> While this kind of comedy extracts laughter from the over-investment in social identities, the desire to *be* somebody, it is also always – and precisely at the point when a character identifies the most with his social role, when he or she *is* somebody – involved in disidentification, offering a glimpse of the

contingency of the social order in the exposure of the gap between the desiring subject and its ego-ideal.

(*Ladegaard, 2014: 117–118*)

This contingency is best exemplified when we consider how David's 'double-entendres' follow a form of 'self-censorship' that, while appeasing abstract notions of political correctness, obfuscate underlying concerns. Here, we can observe how 'glimpses' of the social order's contingency are often revealed in 'coded' forms. For example, while commenting upon the electoral campaigns of the US conservative politician Jesse Helms, Žižek highlights how Helms's:

> racist and sexist message is not publicly acknowledged (on the public level, it is sometimes even violently disavowed), but is instead articulated 'between the lines', in a series of double-entendres and coded allusions. The point is that this kind of self-censorship (not openly admitting one's own fundamental message) is necessary if, in the present ideological conditions, Helms's discourse is to remain operative: if it were to articulate directly, in a public way, its racist bias, this would render it unacceptable in the eyes of the predominant regime of the political discourse; if it were to effectively abandon the self-censored coded racist message, it would endanger the support of its targeted electoral body.
>
> (*2008b: 33*)

What Žižek's example draws attention to is the very ways in which racist and sexist messages can work within certain ideological conditions which openly disavow these messages in the first place. Though Helms's clearly racist concerns were masked through forms of self-censorship, it was their 'between the lines' articulation that allowed them to be performed and, subsequently, hidden.

To this extent, it is across scenes one to three that we can observe how David's adoption of certain 'double-entendres and coded allusions' serve to perform the inherent contingency of his performance and, specifically, the instability *within* political correctness. For example, in the first scene, David transgresses his political correctness through his ability to clarify the joke's political incorrectness (he asks Gareth: 'It's not racist, is it?'). Instead of challenging the joke's racism, such acknowledgment simply provides a space for it to be performed. This inversion falls apart in the second scene when David achieves his political correctness in all its absurdity: in this case, congratulating a black man for not objecting to a racist joke. In the third scene, we see political correctness neither resisted nor ignored, but performed through an endless stream of clarifications and (failed) self-censorship. What is significant, is how these various instances can be viewed as 'offering a glimpse of the contingency of the social order' (Ladegaard, 2014: 117–118) and, specifically, of the operation of 'maintaining' – at least in principle – the appearance of political correctness. To help subvert this appearance, we can return to a discussion of the comedy character.

As noted in Chapter Two, Zupančič's true and false comedy distinctions can be used to offer further clarification on the importance of the comedy character as a decidedly subversive form. Indeed, as evident in the above scenes, one key feature of *The Office* series was its mockumentary format; a format that provided various characters the opportunity to acknowledge and talk directly to the camera ('talking-head sequences'). Such acknowledgment is usually performed during moments of awkward tension. This is apparent in the first scene where Tim's exasperated expression is used to engage the audience in a sense of disbelief; a disbelief that is steered towards Gareth's unawareness that the joke he is telling relies upon a racial stereotype. In this third scene, however, David's glances play a prominent role, with David frequently glancing towards the camera throughout the scene. The effect of this is that we are subsequently included via this 'outside' observance, through which we are invited to monitor, observe and judge his behaviour.

In the case of Ricky Gervais (the actor), playing David Brent (the comic character), the 'gap' between actor/character is transposed into the comic character. It is 'David's' frequent glances to the camera that perform his self-estrangement and, as a consequence, expose the 'gap'. In doing so, the universal is redoubled via its concrete manifestation *in* the character David, so that it is through David's self-estrangement that the universal is concretised, or, in other words, it is through David that the limitations of the universal are laid bare in its own self-estrangement. This 'redoubling' is performed throughout the scene, with David glancing at the camera as he questions the joke's racism and when he awkwardly defends the joke. While such moments emphasise David's 'inability to conform to social consensus and our value systems', it is more a case that 'we rejoice at seeing him getting his comeuppance after regularly violating the limits of moral propriety' (Jacobi, 2016: 304). More importantly, it is not simply the case that David 'violates' these 'limits' and that it is *this* violation which is comical, but rather it is his own actions which perform the 'limit' to such a 'politically correct propriety'. As noted, it is the very limits of political correctness which are performatively 'redoubled' in the comedy character. Indeed:

> This is why, for Hegel, comedy is not simply a turn from the universal (from universal values of the beautiful, the just, the good, the moral …) towards the individual or the particular (as always and necessarily imperfect, limited and always slightly idiotic), but corresponds instead to the very speculative passage from the abstract universal to the concrete universal.
>
> *(Zupančič, 2008: 38)*

It is this 'speculative passage' which David's comic performance reveals. In other words, it is through 'the full assertion of universality' – in this case political correctness – that we get 'the immediate coincidence of universality with the character's/actor's singularity' (Žižek, 2006a: 107). Through David's concrete attempts to perform the universality of political correctness, the passage from abstract universal to concrete universal is performed through its own non-coincidence. The fact that David seeks to maintain his politically correct standard, despite his exceptions (his various faux pas), serves to highlight the very deadlock that renders immanent the universality of political correctness (Žižek, 2010). In doing so, David stands for the gap within political correctness and its own negation (Žižek, 2015).

'That is what I'm trying to achieve... that's the melting pot': The presumptuous authority of political correctness

After various cut-scenes, which depict David sitting alone in his office, it is clear that David remains upset by the fact that an unknown member of the team complained to Jennifer. Once Neil and Jennifer have left and the employees return to work, David makes an attempt to determine who spoke to Jennifer. After calling members of the new Swindon branch together, David asks for the members of staff who complained to reveal themselves. Upon the request, two female members of the Swindon branch raise their hands. While David points out that only 'two' members of staff complained, another Swindon colleague, who didn't originally raise his hand, explains that he also found the joke offensive, and this is followed by another member of staff who states that they too found the joke offensive. Notably, throughout this scene, it is white members of staff who have complained about the joke. Perplexed by this, David points to Oliver and, again, makes the suggestion that Oliver didn't find the joke offensive.

COLLEAGUE 4: Well what's he got to do with it?

DAVID: Well if he doesn't mind us laughing at him, what harm's been done?

COLLEAGUE 1: Well why is it that only black people should be offended by racism?

DAVID: Good point... first sensible thing you've said all day. Because I say, come one, come all, we're all the same, yeah. (*David looks at Oliver*) Let's ...

COLLEAGUE 1: So, is that why you've only got *one* black guy in the *whole* organisation?

DAVID: Wrong! Yeah... Indian fella in the warehouse and there used to be one Indian fella, used to work up here. Lovely chap, he left, didn't like it, up to him. You know... if I had my way, the place would be full of *them*... (*when David makes the comment 'them', he points to Oliver*). Wouldn't it Gareth?

GARETH: Well, yeah... half-and-half.

DAVID: Yeah. (*David turns to Oliver*) You are half-and-half aren't you?

OLIVER: I'm mixed-race... yes.

DAVID: That is my favourite, yeah. That is what I'm trying to achieve... that's the melting pot (*David brings his hands together and coalesces his fingers*)... please! So... there's your racist, for yah. So...

(*With a sense of proud smugness, David looks on at the Swindon colleagues who stand in front of him. It is clear that he feels that he has made his point and that he's not a racist. The camera cuts to the Swindon staff, who look back with shocked*

> *expressions. As the camera cuts to David, he gives the group a wink and walks off patting one of the employees on the back as he goes).*

In this fourth and final scene we see David continue to defend the joke, making a number of further gaffes and politically incorrect assertions along the way. However, what remains important to this scene is the fact that David believes he is remaining within the confines of a politically correct demeanor. In particular, the scene offers a unique take on the sense of grievance which underscores our accounts of racism. Without admonishing the joke's racist stereotype, due to the fact that it is now clear that Oliver was not the member of staff who complained, we instead see the scene provide a subversive account of such an 'obvious' conclusion. Indeed the portrayal of the black man taking offence is one that could very easily be declared as: 'playing the race card' (Lentin, 2018). Accordingly, the ambiguity surrounding Oliver's performance is what, for both David and the audience, presents Oliver as a 'true object of anxiety' (Žižek, 2005: 215). That is, while 'no longer prepared to play the role of victim', Oliver's actions resist 'the anonymous passive universality of a victim' (Žižek, 2005: 215), with his own actions being marked by a more general reluctance to engage with the debate between David and the members of staff.

If we consider that 'the fragile web of civility is the "social substance" of free independent individuals, it is their very mode of (inter)dependence' (Žižek, 2006b: xii), it is clear that this scene goes someway to commenting upon this civility as David's inappropriateness and the office's racial demographics are called into question. What becomes clear is how the 'position of enunciation' becomes a point of contention with various 'white' staff members complaining about the joke's racism. Though this could be interpreted as depicting a feigned-political correctness, with each white colleague feeling obliged to complain about the joke on behalf of Oliver, it is perhaps notable that each 'politically correct' complaint fails to achieve the same sense of admonition that David's own attempts to be 'politically correct' provide. Instead, David's various rebuttals remain naively tied to his own sense of political correctness as he seeks to congratulate the member of staff (Colleague 1) on their 'politically correct' statement as well as defend the office's employment of black people. Importantly, through David's 'politically correct' responses, we see a reassertion of racial difference, enacted through his various faux pas ('Indian fella'; 'them', when pointing to Oliver; 'half and half', a reference to 'mixed-ethnicity') and promulgated through the 'allowed transgression' that he believes Oliver's enjoyment of the joke provides.

Accordingly, though believing that he maintains a politically correct standard, Brent's numerous cringe-worthy statements reveal the inherent exceptions that underscore the universality of political correctness (yes, you can say that, but not *that*). As evident in both the third and fourth scenes, whenever Brent believes that he is making a politically correct statement he excessively goes too far which results in offending the exact groups he wishes to include. Rather than supporting political correctness as a universal notion, these instances reveal how it can be subverted through its own exceptions. Moreover, David's true comic value is made apparent via his ability to perform political correctness in all its abstract absurdity. In other words, David is able to perform and uphold his socio-symbolic status as the 'cool' office manager by naively retaining his politically correct persona. In doing so, 'He is not transformed by experience. Just the reverse: the "experience" in question is transformed by the triumph of his sheer presumptuousness, his belief in himself' (Kottman, 2008: 10). Here, 'Brent's knowing and studied attempt to *perform* political correctness' comically provides the concrete universal that renders PC's 'inauthenticity' (Westwood and Johnston, 2011: 796).

Across the four scenes, political correctness is no longer an abstract universal notion that seeks to manage and regulate cultural differences, but instead in the extended comic sequence we watch political correctness in all its concrete reality; a reality that is brought to bear via the very concrete materialisation of the incongruity which is inherent to political correctness. It is in this way that David's:

> struggle with political correctness is emblematic for our society. PC-language is often just rhetorical make-up, covering up the existing inequalities that persist. Like Brent, we go through the motions and watch our language, but this verbal correctness stands pale against the obvious inequalities and difference that continue to exist beneath the surface.
>
> *(Nys, 2008)*

In his 'politically correct' persona, then, David's over-identification with a politically correct performance underscores a number of contradictions, most notably the assumption that 'simply avoiding certain configurations of words is enough to prevent the offensive surplus – in its avoidance, it perpetuates the power of those configurations to guarantee that one is absolved from responsibility' (Yao, 2012: 3). Such liberation is reflected by the fact that he seems to interpret his racist joke as an 'allowed transgression'; a transgression that is conferred by Oliver stating that the joke is funny. This is exemplified when we consider 'how today's discourse on tolerance is always accompanied, at a deeper libidinal level, by a fundamentally intolerant kernel of repressed enjoyment' (Vighi and Feldner, 2007: 47) – a point reflected in Gareth's assertions in the third scene that he has magazines (clearly pornographic) that can help debunk 'the myth'.

Consequently, in scenes three and four, David continues to provide a number of politically incorrect faux pas, all of which excessively undermine his attempts to maintain his politically correct persona. It is in this sense that we are able to see how, through a concrete materialisation, the abstract absurdity of political correctness as a form of social regulation can be subversively undermined. Drawing from Zupančič (2008), Kottman explains that:

> Rather than signal a shift from the perspective of universal values to limited and imperfect individuals in their concrete materiality, comedy for Hegel lays bare the limitations and imperfections of the abstract universal itself. Comedy reveals the pitfalls to which our oldest values are exposed. Or, rather, comedy

> demonstrates that these values turn out to be no more and no less grand than their appearance on the world stage, in the lives and loves, the ups and downs, of individual selves.
>
> *(2008: 8)*

As a result, 'It is only at the peak of its abstraction, of full coincidence with itself, that the Universal becomes truly comical and truly concrete' (Hajdini, 2015: 203). David's failed attempts at self-censorship – in the end, his failure to say anything without clarifying it – reveals his comic self-estrangement. It is through his attempts to 'regulate' the joke (clarifying whether it is racist in scene one; highlighting its inappropriateness in scene two; stating that he'll change the reference to 'black' in scene three; and his continued defence of the joke in scene four) that David's political correctness is performed.

It is here that we can draw a fundamental connection between Zupančič's 'baron who slips on a banana peel' and David 'who slips on a racist joke'. In the former, what is:

> obvious [is] that the capital human weakness here … is precisely the baron's unshakeable belief in himself and his own importance: that is to say, his presumptuousness … *This* is the feature that makes him 'human,' not the fact that he falls into a muddy puddle or slips on a banana peel. … And, of course, we should not overlook the fact that what is really funny and makes us laugh most in our archetypal (imaginary) comedy is not simply that the baron falls into the puddle but, much more, that he *rises* from it and goes about his business as if nothing has happened. The puddle itself is thus not the site of the concrete reality (in which anybody turns out to be only human), but one of the props or devices through which the very concreteness or humanity of the concept itself – in our case, the concept of baronage or aristocracy – is processed, crystallized, and concretized.
>
> *(Zupančič, 2008: 29–30)*

In the case of David, his presumptuousness is reperformed in his own 'unshakeable belief' that he has told a funny joke. What David's responses concretely perform is the inherent limitations in the universality of political correctness as it 'is processed, crystallized, and concretized'. It is this 'unshakeable belief' which maintains the scenes' comic suspense.

Furthermore, what underscores David's presumptuousness is, much like the baron, his 'unshakeable belief' in his own political correctness. Just before we see David confront the staff, we are shown a number of close-ups of David, sitting at the desk in his office. Unbeknown to David, the camera, zooming-in through his office window, provides a close-up on David's face. The shot is notable for the sense of complexion that is evident in David's facial expressions, with the day's events clearly playing on his mind. While one could conclude that this serves to present David coming to terms with the fact that the joke may not have been the best joke to tell at an office 'welcome event', it is clear from his later actions that no sense of realisation has prevailed. Instead, what we get in this final scene is a comic reversal of Pippin's (2009) analysis of John Wayne's 'Ethan' in *The Searchers* (1956).

Set in the 'American West', *The Searchers* centres on the character of Ethan who is given the task of rescuing his niece Debbie (Natalie Wood) after she is abducted by Comanche Indians, whom she subsequently lives with for several years. Notably, 'Ethan's explicit intent throughout the film has been not to save her, but to kill her; in other words he was motivated by the racist idea that a white girl taken captive by the Indians deserves only to die' (Žižek, 2010: 119). Yet, upon encountering Debbie, Ethan has a sudden change of heart and doesn't kill her. In commenting upon this change, Pippin notes:

> What we need to discover here is that he [Ethan] did not know his own mind well, that he avowed principles that were partly confabulations and fantasy. We (and he) find out the depth and extent of his actual commitments only when he finally must act.
>
> *(2009: 240–241)*

Drawing attention to this analysis, Žižek highlights how 'One can thus say that, in the moment captured by this shot of his perplexed face, Ethan discovered himself as a neighbor, in the impenetrable abyss of his subjectivity' (2010: 120). In other words, when encountering Debbie's reluctance to leave her captors, Ethan is subject to realising his own strange behaviour – that he, just like the other, is strange and marked by a sense of self-understanding that posits the 'impenetrable abyss of his subjectivity' (Žižek, 2010: 120). This strange sense of self-understanding is what 'undermin[es] his identity as Ethan' (Žižek, 2010: 120) and which presents his self-estrangement from the community around him.

Certainly, whereas Ford's film is not a comedy, what Pippin's (2009) analysis reveals is a similar formal structure akin to the earlier cited example of the South African policeman calmly handing the black protestor her shoe (Žižek, 2002). What remains important when comparing Ethan and David is how, in the aforementioned scenes, David fails to portray the same sense of self-reflexivity that underscores Ethan's recognised strangeness. While Ethan's self-understanding echoes Lacan's alienation-separation distinction, via the fact that Ethan achieves a *separation* from his own fantasies (thus recognising his own lack), it is David's failure to 'separate' himself, which, though constituting his significance as a comedy character, ensures that the universal (political correctness) achieves self-consciousness in the character 'David Brent'. In other words, it is not that David *represents* political correctness – not in the same way that we can consider Ethan *representing* a pre-US Civil War 'frontier spirit' and his subsequent realisation that such a 'way of life' is coming to an end – but rather it is that David *is* political correctness. David embodies the lack at the heart of the universal's self-consciousness; which is to say that the universal is revealed in itself, through its own negativity and its own subversion. Importantly, this is not a subversion that 'mocks' political correctness, but, in contrast, is a subversion which openly performs its 'already present' limitations *in* David (Žižek, 2017: 342 [italics removed]). As a 'true comedy character', David's comedy performance is political correctness at work.

Further considerations

The comic subversion of David Brent: Lack and excess in the comedy character

In an analysis of David's comic value, Gray mentions the following 'talking head' scene, where David asserts:

> There are limits to my comedy. There are things that I will never laugh at, like the handicapped, because there's nothing funny about them, or any deformity. It's like when you see someone look at a little handicapped, and they go, 'Oh, look at him, he's not able-bodied, I am. I'm prejudiced.' Well, at least the little handicapped fella is ableminded. Unless he's not, it's difficult to tell with the wheelchair ones. So, just give generously to all of them.
>
> *(Gervais and Merchant, 2002: 115 cited in Gray, 2005: 159)*

Gray adds, 'If viewers are *not* embarrassed by this speech it is because it jams so many failures of discourse control into a small space that the very excess is pleasurable' (2005: 159). More to the point, when considered in light of McGowan's lack/excess dialectic, then it becomes clear that it is through David's lack of awareness that his excess is comically performed. Indeed, it would seem that David's excessive continuation in the description of handicapped individuals echoes his excessive transgressions in the above analysis.

As previously mentioned, David doesn't stop at making racial stereotypes but, over the course of each scene, resorts to a number of excessive descriptions regarding homosexual, disabled and 'mixed-race' individuals. These references are matched by his insistence that the joke cannot be racist because Oliver does not find it offensive. To this extent, without lack, that is, without the lack of awareness that David displays (most notably, not to tell racist jokes at work), we wouldn't have the excess which makes each scene comical. In fact, if we stick with David's lack of awareness, we would get a very different scene, involving David apologising for his remarks, or an altogether more worrying scene, where David simply ignores Oliver and continues with the joke. Instead, it is through David's capacity to embody lack and excess that his comedy is performed. Consequently, while 'the more excessive the affected person acts, the more this person's lack becomes evident' (McGowan, 2017: 45), in the case of David, it is his 'lack' of social awareness which overlays an excessive desire to be funny.

To this extent, we can align the character of David Brent alongside McGowan's analysis of Buster Keaton. As argued in Chapter Two, while 'Chaplin embodies exclusion, … Keaton exposes an internal excess within society' (McGowan, 2016: 602); an excess which draws attention to society's inherent contradictions. We can apply this to David's capacity to highlight the internal contradictions within political correctness and how, in his attempts to 'fit in' with the politically correct workplace, David finds himself out of place (McGowan, 2016). To return to McGowan's analysis of Keaton's 'excess', which locates his comedy at 'a point within the social order that reveals the order's failure and absence of self-identity' (McGowan, 2016: 603), it is:

> Keaton [who] creates a more radical comedy because it illustrates how the social order subverts itself rather than trying to subvert it from the outside. That is to say, the failure of the social order derives from its own contradictions, and Keaton's films direct our attention toward these contradictions.
>
> *(McGowan, 2016: 612)*

Certainly, Keaton's approach is not without its risks, as McGowan (2016) notes in Keaton's depiction of black savages in *The Navigator* (1924): 'The savages have a stereotypical look and act buffoonish throughout the encounter. Here, Keaton employs a standard Hollywood racist image without any irony' (McGowan, 2016: 612). The problem here is that it is Keaton's use of a stereotypical image which undermines his political intent. Accordingly, one could make the same criticism of the above scenes, where Gervais and Merchant deliberately draw upon a racial stereotype in order to induce a comic effect, yet, much like Keaton, such 'dismissal [… would] miss the elucidative value that Keaton's racism has for us' (McGowan, 2016: 613) and, by extension, the value of *The Office* as well. Here, McGowan notes that Keaton's:

> is a specific form of racism, not that of the Klan [Ku Klux Klan] or even the contemporary opponent of affirmative action who retreats from the fantasy of the racial other's seemingly strange enjoyment. Instead, it is a racism that fails to consider the difference between society's self-exclusion and those whom it excludes.
>
> *(2016: 613)*

To this end, it is society's inherent self-exclusion which Keaton's comedy accentuates. While 'this universal failure of belonging' is what results in 'societies hav[ing] recourse to racism, xenophobia, and other form of exclusion' (McGowan, 2016: 613), it is the obfuscation of society's inherent exclusion which results in such pervasive forms of exclusion. While this can be considered in relation to the previously mentioned spectacle and spectre distinctions (here, the spectre of race underlies the obfuscated exclusion that remains inherent to race's spectacle), in the case of *The Office*, it is through David's excessive attempts to 'include' that underlying contradictions in political correctness are performed. That is, in his attempts to be 'politically correct', David's excessive performance renders the internal contradictions of a politically correct rhetoric that can never achieve its universal aims. It is this lack within political correctness that 'produce[s] a potential self-undermining excess', which can reveal 'something uncontrollable, something inherently disturbing, even self-sabotaging, about humour' (Karlsen and Villadsen, 2015: 531). It is in this way that 'Managers who try to exploit humour as a tool for managerial control' will 'always be introducing an element of something ambiguous and uncontrollable into the organization' (Karlsen and Villadsen, 2015: 531).

It is through David's excess, then, that the inherent lack within political correctness is performed and, more importantly, how politically correct assertions can be subverted through their own excessive exceptions. Notably, David's failure is achieved through an excess of political correctness that performs the abstract embodiment of political correctness through his frantic attempts to maintain his politically correct persona. It is here that, 'As an embodiment of an abstract universal concept in a concrete individual, the comic hero introduces the moment of self-consciousness which the abstract universal lacks in itself' (Ladegaard, 2017: 182). It is important to remember that such a 'moment of self-consciousness' is closely tied to a 'comic hero' who reveals, in his own actions, the universal's absurdity (Roche, 2002). As a consequence, this is exposed when, in his desperate attempts to maintain a politically correct identity, David *is* the 'functionless concreteness' of political correctness (Hajdini, 2015: 204). As noted in McGowan's (2016) account of Keaton, this is certainly a risky gesture and it is a risk that both Gervais and Merchant echo in their use of the racial stereotype. Nonetheless, it is the way in which the stereotype and the joke are used which permits its subversive effect.

From joke to comedy sequence

In accordance with Zupančič's (2008) joke and comedy distinctions, what we see in the above scenes is a formal structure whereby the same joke is discontinuously performed over a protracted comic sequence. That is, it is clear that we are witnessing the telling of a joke – the Royal Family playing twenty-questions – and then seeing this joke played out over a protracted comic sequence. More importantly, the joke doesn't change, the punchline stays the same, but the surprising presence of Oliver retroactively redefines the preceding racist meaning. Certainly, this is not to suggest that the joke is no longer racist, but that, formally, the direction of the joke has changed from the racist punchline, to Brent's awkward inability to finish the joke. In other words, the repetition of the joke is parallaxically shifted into a comic sequence.

As noted in Chapter Two, a comic sequence works from an extended temporal structure, whereby the comic 'tension' is discontinuously repeated. Such discontinuity is marked by David's repeated attempts to defend the joke, with his assertions forming the underlying antagonism across the four scenes. Rather than simply telling a racist joke, what the above scenes achieve is a fundamental subversion of the joke's narrative. This occurs in two ways: 1) in the joke's inherent inconsistencies, which are brought to bear through the parallax that is achieved between scenes one and two; and, 2) in the discontinuity that is achieved across scenes one to four, which serve to embed the 'joke' within a protracted 'comic' sequence.

It is in extending this inconsistency through a comic sequence that the joke undergoes a comic subversion. In particular, with regards to the comic suspense which is established in scene two, we can return to Zupančič's contention that:

> As the word itself already indicates, suspense is a tension, an exciting and anguished expectation constituted and maintained by the fact that its crucial elements are not realized but remain 'in the air' as a possibility and/or a threat. … Comic suspense, … springs not from such a suspended realization but, rather, from an overrealization or a prerealization. What makes and inaugurates a comedy is that something like a hot potato immediately falls from the cataclysmic sphere which, in classic thrillers, hangs above the protagonists like a menacing cloud. The comic suspense is all in the question of *how the protagonists will deal with this 'hot potato,' how they will manage it, handle it, what they will do with it; where it will burn them; how far (and in what directions) they will go to avoid being burned; how it will catch up with them nevertheless.*
>
> *(2008: 92 [italics added])*

Here, we can draw attention to how the scene effectively achieves its comic suspense (it's 'hot potato') by leading one to question how David will 'manage' and 'handle' Oliver's entrance. In fact, in later scenes, we continue to observe the lengths in which David intends to go in order not to 'be burned' (how far will he go before he accepts the joke is racist?). To this end, it is through such 'comic suspense' (how will David deal with this situation?) that the performance of the joke is brought together via a minimal difference. That is, in both the first and second performances, we have the same joke told, with no difference in its 'content', but instead a minimal difference is identified in the joke's 'form' (its structured performance). To this extent, what becomes apparent in the second scene is that the 'newness' of the joke is achieved, not by anything *new* in the content of the joke, but by the failure of David to finish the joke and Oliver's subsequent finishing (Analisi, 2016). This emphasises how:

> The shift to be made in a properly dialectical analysis is thus from the condition of impossibility to the condition of possibility: what appears initially as the 'condition of impossibility', as an obstacle, becomes the enabling condition of what then transpires.
>
> *(Žižek, 2006b: xxv)*

When this is related to Oliver's appearance in the second scene, rather than obstructing the joke, Oliver's presence enables the continuation of the comic sequence. In fact, what is 'Crucial for the proper comic effect is not a difference where we expect sameness but, rather, *a sameness where we expect difference*' (Žižek, 2006a: 109 [italics added]). Indeed, we initially expect Oliver to object to the joke. Instead, however, the scene cleverly renders a certain similarity to the first performance. The joke is told, its content is the same and, to a certain extent, it is accepted as being funny. What is significant, however, is that the comedy of the scene emerges from having the same punchline retold, but this time by Oliver. In this way, the scene maintains its comic significance, but in a decidedly subverted form.

Therefore, it is not that the comic sequence 'confronts the Real', but rather repeats it (Zupančič, 2008). That is, it is through David's politically correct presumption that the comedy of each scene is concretely performed via the universal's ability to render those inherent antagonisms which it creates. We see this 'antagonism' performed in David's repeated attempts to defend the joke and his subsequent decline into further forms of offence. It is in this way that comedy can take on a subversive significance via its ability to 'ex-pose' the Real. Indeed, this is 'not the Real of what happened, but the structural Real (or impasse) the suppression of which constitutes the very coherence of our reality' (Zupančič, 2008: 58). It is 'this [which] is the real core of comedy' (Zupančič, 2008: 58) and which includes the 'other side' of what was known, but not acknowledged; the surprise of what was there, but not necessarily seen. Therefore, to conclude this analysis, a final consideration of the significance of the Real will be provided.

'A scene of extraordinary warmth': Making sense of David and Oliver's interaction

To help elucidate this final consideration, we can return briefly to the second scene. As noted, while David is left awkwardly responding to Oliver finishing the joke, there is a moment of subtle realisation between David (briefly, aware of the joke's racial significance) and Oliver (who, while looking at David, reassures him that the joke is 'good' and 'funny'). The moment is one marked by tension, shock and a certain 'comic' relief, but what is perhaps of greater significance is the way in which this tension permits a strange sense of warmth. This is depicted quite blatantly in David's forced realisation that he's telling an offensive racist joke (something he knows but has been willing to ignore) and Oliver's persistence to hear the joke. While David fails to acknowledge the (im)personal moment of Real human interaction – a failure that allows the tension of the comic suspense to be sustained throughout the proceeding scenes – it nonetheless depicts a certain moment whereby the symbolic racial differences that frame each scene are momentarily muted (in fact, this moment echoes the policemen-protestor exchange in the example from apartheid South Africa, see Chapter Four). The thinking behind this interaction stems in part from Žižek's (2018) analysis of the ending of Marvel

Studio's *Black Panther* (2018). In commenting on the ending of the film, Žižek directs attention to what he refers to as 'a scene of extraordinary warmth' (2018: 247). In this scene:

> the dying Killmonger sits down at the edge of a mountain precipice observing the beautiful Wakanda sunset, and T'Challa, who has just defeated him, silently sits at his side. There is no hatred here, just two basically good men with a different political view sharing their last moments after the battle is over. It's a scene unimaginable in a standard action movie that culminates in the vicious destruction of the enemy.
>
> *(Žižek, 2018: 247)*

It is this same sense of muted confrontation which is echoed in the brief exchange that David and Oliver share in scene two. Instead of being destroyed through examples of racial confrontation, what is significant in this moment is that there is some*thing* that is shared between the two men, be it a moment of 'extraordinary warmth', or a more open acknowledgment of the potential excessive idiosyncrasies which frame our social relations.

Accordingly, while the briefness of this 'moment' is quickly dissolved, what is comically rendered between David and Oliver is a certain depiction of the 'Thing' that is briefly shared, but which is subsequently lost in the proceeding scenes. One could venture that this shared 'Thing' is exactly what David seeks to explain in scene three and what he hopes to revive in scene four, with each attempt succumbing to further failure. However, the significance of the 'Thing' is that it provides a certain passage to the Real via an acknowledgment of that 'excessive' element that inherently constitutes the other. This is not a material 'Thing', but some*thing* in the other – that little bit of the Real – which we like but, nonetheless, struggle to put our finger on. It is this inexplainable yet incommensurable 'Thing' which is shared amongst a group of friends, who, when together, inexplicably share some*thing* that inevitably maintains the friendship. As a result, what we see depicted in this scene is what could be referred to as a moment of authentic interaction: an acknowledgment of that 'excessive' and potentially 'troubling' element – in this case David's hubris in telling a racist joke – which both performs and confronts the inherent obstacle that is brought to light when we share an obscene joke. It is the silent acknowledgment of this excessive quality, this prospective failure and this potential for miscommunication, which bears witness to the saliency of comedy's social efficacy.

Certainly, this in no way ignores the 'racist' significance of the joke, an ignorance that in many ways would let David 'off the hook' (as we've seen in the above analysis, David is more than capable of digging his own hole), nor does it subsume David and Oliver's interactions in a fantasy depiction of cross-racial harmony. Instead, it directs our focus to the inherent tensions that are imminently captured in the everyday faux pas and personal gaffes that frame our social interactions. Bearing in mind that in our day-to-day lives we cannot live a life akin to a sitcom script, there remains something significant in drawing attention to those moments of miscommunication and misunderstanding. Indeed, it is this acknowledgment that can help permit a more considered connection with the strangeness of the other and, more importantly, *ourselves*.

References

Analisi, S. 2016. Comedy, repetition and racial stereotypes on television. *Cinergie*, 9, 103–116.

Bebber, B. 2014. *Till Death Us Do Part*: Political satire and social realism in the 1960s and 1970s. *Historical Journal of Film, Radio and Television*, 34 (2), 253–274.

Bergmann, R. and Højlund, H. 2019. Fiery soul fantasies in a project-based welfare setting: The case of project school sports. *Critical Policy Studies*, 13 (3), 261–279.

Billig, M. 2005. Comic racism and violence. In: S. Lockyer and M. Pickering, eds. *Beyond a Joke: The Limits of Humour*. Basingstoke: Palgrave Macmillan, 25–44.

Black Panther. 2018. Film. Walt Disney Studios Motion Pictures.

Boakye, J. 2019. Smooth, angry, cool, powerful: How we talk about blackness [online]. *The Guardian*. Available from: www.theguardian.com/books/2019/apr/13/smooth-angry-cool-powerful-how-we-talk-about-blackness [Accessed 20 January 2020].

Brabazon, T. 2005. 'What have you ever done on the telly?' *The Office*, (post) reality television and (post) work. *International Journal of Cultural Studies*, 8 (1), 101–117.

Cauley, K. 2019. Word: Woke [online]. *Believer Mag*. Available from: https://believermag.com/word-woke/ [Accessed 1 March 2019].

Chow, B. 2014. The tickling object: On Žižek and comedy. In: B. Chow and A. Mangold, eds. *Žižek and Performance*. Basingstoke: Palgrave Macmillan, 224–252.

Critchley, S. 2002. *On Humour*. London: Routledge.

De Jongste, H. 2017. Culture and incongruity in *The Office* (UK). *Language & Communication*, 55, 88–89.

Delay, T. 2014. Excess: The obscene supplement in Slavoj Žižek's religion and politics. *International Journal of Žižek Studies*, 8 (2), 1–20.

Dolar, M. 2005. Comedy and its double. In R. Pfaller, ed. *Schluss mit der Komödie!/Stop That Comedy!*Vienna: Sonderzahl, 181–210.

Dolar, M. 2017. The comic mimesis. *Critical Inquiry*, 43, 570–589.

Flisfeder, M. 2012. *The Symbolic, The Sublime, and Slavoj Žižek's Theory of Film*. New York, NY: Palgrave Macmillan.

Gherovici, P. and Steinkoler, M. 2016. Introduction. In: P. Gherovici and M. Steinkoler, eds. *Lacan, Psychoanalysis, and Comedy*. New York, NY: Cambridge University Press, 1–22.

Gilroy, P. 2004. *After Empire: Melancholia or Convivial Culture?* Abingdon: Routledge.

Goncalo, J. A., Chatman, J. A., Duguid, M. M. and Kennedy, J. A. 2015. Creativity from constraint? How the political correctness norm influences creativity in mixed-sex work groups. *Administrative Science Quarterly*, 60 (1), 1–30.

Gray, F. 2005. Privacy, embarrassment and social power: British sitcom. In: S. Lockyer and M. Pickering, eds. *Beyond a Joke: The Limits of Humour*. Basingstoke: Palgrave Macmillan, 146–161.

Hajdini, S. 2015. The comedy of the great depression: On Chaplin's *Modern Times*. *Crisis and Critique*, 2 (1), 195–215.

Heller, A. 2005. *Immortal Comedy: The Comic Phenomenon in Art, Literature, and Life*. Lanham, MD: Lexington Books.

Hsiao, L.-C. 2010. Color (un)conscious: Psychoanalysis, resistance, and the specter/spectacle of race. *Concentric: Literary and Cultural Studies*, 36 (1), 159–187.

Jacobi, P. 2016. Life is stationary: Mockumentary and embarrassment in *The Office*. In: J. Kamm and B. Neumann, eds. *British TV Comedies: Cultural Concepts, Contexts and Controversies*. Basingstoke: Palgrave Macmillan, 295–310.

Kamm, J. and Neumann, B. 2016. Introduction: The aesthetics and politics of British TV comedy. In: J. Kamm and B. Neumann, eds. *British TV Comedies: Cultural Concepts, Contexts and Controversies*. Basingstoke: Palgrave Macmillan, 1–22.

Karlsen, M. P. and Villadsen, K. 2015. Laughing for real? Humour, management power and subversion. *Ephemera: Theory & Politics in Organization*, 15 (3), 513–535.

Kilborn, R. 2003. *Staging the Real: Factual TV Programming in the Age of Big Brother*. Manchester: Manchester University Press.

Kingsbury, P. 2017. Uneasiness in culture, or negotiating the sublime distances towards the big Other. *Geography Compass*, 11 (6), 1–11.

Kottman, P. A. 2008. Slipping on banana peels, tumbling into wells: Philosophy and comedy. *Diacritics*, 38 (4), 3–14.

Kunkle, S. 2012. Embracing the paradox: Žižek's illogical logic. *International Journal of Žižek Studies*, 2 (4). Available from: http://zizekstudies.org/index.php/IJZS/issue/view/10 [Accessed 1 March 2019].

Ladegaard, J. 2014. Laughing matters: Four Marxist takes on film comedy. In: E. Mazierska and L. Kristensen, eds. *Marx at the Movies: Revisiting History, Theory and Practice*. Basingstoke: Palgrave Macmillan, 102–122.

Ladegaard, J. 2017. The comedy of terrors: Ideology and comedy in Marlowe's *Doctor Faustus*. *Textual Practice*, 31 (1), 179–195.

Lentin, A. 2018. Beyond denial: 'Not racism' as racist violence. *Continuum*, 32 (4), 400–414.

McGowan, T. 2014. The barriers to a critical comedy. *Crisis and Critique*, 1 (3), 201–221.

McGowan, T. 2015. *Psychoanalytic Film Theory and the Rules of the Game*. New York, NY: Bloomsbury.

McGowan, T. 2016. The location of silent comedy: Charlie Chaplin's outsider and Buster Keaton's insider. *Quarterly Review of Film and Video*, 33 (7), 602–619.

McGowan, T. 2017. *Only a Joke Can Save Us: A Theory of Comedy*. Evanston, IL: Northwestern University Press.

McNeil, D. 2010. *Sex and Race in the Black Atlantic: Mulatto Devils and Multiracial Messiahs*. New York, NY: London.

Murray, D. I. 2018. Political correctness at work is worth the effort [online]. *Forbes*. Available from: www.forbes.com/sites/forbestechcouncil/2018/11/16/political-correctness-at-work-is-worth-the-effort/#5adb76953d81 [Accessed 1 March 2019].

Nys, T. 2008. Look at the ears! The problem of natural kinds. In: J. J. Wisnewski, ed. *The Office and Philosophy: Scene from the Unexamined Life* [ebook]. New York, NY: John Wiley & Sons.

Pippin, R. B. 2009. What is a Western? Politics and self-knowledge in John Ford's *The Searchers*. *Critical Inquiry*, 35, 223–246.

Roche, M. W. 2002. Hegel's theory of comedy in the context of Hegelian and modern reflections on comedy. *Revue Internationale De Philosophie*, 3 (221), 411–430.

Schwind, K. H. 2014. 'Chilled-out entertainers': Multi-layered sitcom performances in the British and American version of *The Office*. *Comedy Studies*, 5 (1), 20–32.

Soper, K. 2009. The pathetic carnival in the cubicles: *The Office* as meditation on the misuses and collapse of traditional comedy. *Studies in American Humor*, 3 (19), 83–103.

Swyngedouw, E. 2015. Depoliticized environments and the promises of the Anthropocene. In: R. L. Bryant, ed. *The International Handbook of Political Ecology*. Cheltenham: Edward Elgar Publishing, 131–148.

The Navigator. 1924. Film. Metro-Goldwyn.

The Office. 2001–2003. TV Series. BBC Two/One.

The Office. 2002. Series 2, Episode 1, 'Merger'. BBC Two. 30 September.

The Searchers. 1956. Film. Warner Bros.

Tyler, M. and Cohen, L. 2008. Management in/as comic relief: Queer theory and gender performativity in *The Office*. *Gender, Work and Organization*, 15 (2), 113–132.

Vighi, F. and Feldner, H. 2007. *Žižek: Beyond Foucault*. Basingstoke: Palgrave Macmillan.

Vogt, E. 2007. Exception in Žižek's thought. *Diacritics*, 37 (2–3), 61–77.

Wallace, R. 2018. *Mockumentary Comedy: Performing Authenticity*. Cham, Switzerland: Palgrave Macmillan.

Westwood, R. and Johnston, A. 2011. Reclaiming authentic selves: Control, resistive humour and identity work in the office. *Organization*, 19 (6), 787–808.

Yao, D. 2012. Learning to tickle: How to transmit knowledge as if re-telling a joke. *The International Journal of Žižek Studies*, 6 (2), 1–12.

Žižek, S. 2001. *The Fright of Real Tears: Krzysztof Kieslowski between Theory and Post-Theory*. London: British Film Institute.

Žižek, S. 2002. The only good neighbor is a dead neighbor. *Identities: Journal for Politics, Gender and Culture*, 2 (2), 9–31.

Žižek, S. 2005. *The Metastases of Enjoyment: Six Essays on Women and Causality*. London: Verso.

Žižek, S. 2006a. *The Parallax View*. Cambridge, MA: MIT Press.

Žižek, S. 2006b. Preface to the paperback edition: The big other between violence and civility. In: R. Butler and S. Stephens, eds. *Slavoj Žižek: The Universal Exception*. London: Continuum, vii–xxxii.

Žižek, S. 2006c. *How to Read Lacan*. London: Granta Books.

Žižek, S. 2008a. *The Sublime Object of Ideology*. London: Verso.

Žižek, S. 2008b. *The Plague of Fantasies*. London: Verso.

Žižek, S. 2010. *Living in the End Times*. London: Verso.

Žižek, S. 2012. *Less Than Nothing: Hegel and the Shadow of Dialectical Materialism*. London: Verso.

Žižek, S. 2015. *Absolute Recoil: Towards a New Foundation of Dialectical Materialism*. London: Verso.

Žižek, S. 2017. *In Defense of Lost Causes*. London: Verso.

Žižek, S. 2018. *Like a Thief in Broad Daylight: Power in the Era of Post-Humanity*. London: Allen Lane.

Zupančič, A. 2003. *The Shortest Shadow: Nietzsche's Philosophy of the Two*. Cambridge, MA: MIT Press.

Zupančič, A. 2008. *The Odd One In: On Comedy*. Cambridge, MA: MIT Press.

Zupančič, A. 2016. Power in the closet (and its coming out). In: P. Gherovici and M. Steinkoler, eds. *Lacan, Psychoanalysis, and Comedy*. New York, NY: Cambridge University Press, 219–234.

CONCLUSION

Comedy: Unpredictable, complicated and frustrating

The purpose of this book has been to critically consider the subversive potential of comedy. Indeed, this remains an important sub-topic within comedy studies, one in which the effects of comedy, humour and the telling of jokes bear opposing aims. That is, while on the one hand, examples of comedy can bring relief, dissolve tension and offer the opportunity for a 'break' from the norm, on the other, such forms of subversion can just as easily be used to fund, maintain and uphold hegemonic powers. For the latter, laughter, comedy and humour prove to be a mere safety-valve that all the while continues to ensure the status quo.

Set against this predicament, this book has examined comedy as a decidedly unpredictable, complicated and, at times, frustrating phenomenon. It has been noted how examples of comedy can prove conducive for producing moments of incongruity, which can reveal to the subject both a banal but also a profound sense of incoherence or disjuncture. To help elucidate upon this incongruity, the work of both Critchley (2002) and Heller (2005) was considered in order to discuss the extent to which comedy can elucidate the subject's constitution as well as shed light on our existential condition. Consequently, while for Critchley, subversion occurs from the anti-nihilism that this incongruity creates; for Heller, it emerges from the sense of alienation that is achieved when we notice something that was not previously seen. In both instances, however, the subject remains beholden to an understanding of comedy that is figured around the distance between the ego and superego (Critchley's 'Super-Ego II') or from the unbridgeable abyss that is formed between our genetic and social a priori (Heller).

Yet, whether such incongruity can be perceived as 'subversive' is problematised when one considers that the incongruity in question can be used for both reactionary and conservative ends, and, as the above has considered, from a distance that externalises the subject. Accordingly, while comedy can help critique and even support transgressive forms, challenging the status quo and holding powerful individuals and groups to account, at the same time it can serve to ridicule less powerful groups, undermining those who seek to challenge dominant discourses and, as a consequence, work to support social hierarchies.

Today, this is reflected in a propensity for comedies that focus heavily on cynicism, satire and irony. These forms of comedy reflect 'inherent transgressions', which permit the apparent subversion of ideology through forms of cynical distance. For most politicians and their critics, examples of satire and a malignant cynicism towards 'the system' end up culminating in forms of protest that remain beholden to 'Trump Baby balloons' and to a media ecosystem that both expects and incorporates such reaction. As noted in Chapter Two, such forms of cynicism can be allied with Zupančič's 'false' and 'true' comedy distinctions, with examples of false comedy maintaining a certain impotency when challenging those in power. This is reflected in the distance that false comedy maintains *between* the universal and the concrete, with the universal kept largely intact. In fact, when false comedy seeks to reveal the comedy of humanity, it simply replaces social hierarchy with abstract authority (Pound, 2010, 2015; Zupančič, 2008). Nowhere is this more apparent than in the case of political correctness.

Political correctness and comedy's subversion

In order to examine comedy's subversive potential, this book has considered how such subversion can be applied to the hegemonic power of political correctness. Certainly, as detailed in Chapter One, the relation between comedy and political correctness is one that can be located in the emergence and success of Alternative Comedy in the UK and, more widely, to a neoliberal consensus that has served to privilege the autonomy of the individual and a politicisation of one's identity. Here, it was noted that our current (neo)liberal predicaments posit a constellation that, while drawing upon discourses pertaining to multiculturalism, cultural diversity and tolerance, all encapsulated within a wider identity politics, such discourses ultimately pay too much attention to cultural displays of 'difference' (culturalisation of politics), ignoring structural forms of inequality that expound these differences. Central to this critique was the importance of the other in both encouraging forms of political correctness, while also supporting racist fantasies that admonish the other's otherness. In both instances, the formal structure remains the same: examples of political correctness and a desire to promote multiculturalism work from a universality that both supports and maintains the privileged position of the multicultural, cosmopolitan subject. What remains ignored and/or kept at a distance is exactly *that* which makes the other, 'other'.

The significance of political correctness is not simply achieved via its regulated dictates and desire for 'tolerance', but rather from its contravening tendencies to evoke both passion and derision. Writing in 1994, Sarah Dunant noted that one of the remarkable achievements of political correctness was its ability to 'offen[d] both the right and a good deal of the left at the same time' (1994: xi). Today, these antagonisms remain. Much of this can be tied to the various ways in which political correctness can stand for positive values, such as compassion and decency, as well as serving to buttress, or at least draw attention to, obvious forms of racism, sexism, homophobia, etc. It is for this reason that, as Quirk asserts, 'many comedians are deeply and unapologetically committed to practicing political correctness in their own work, and ready to recognise and defend it as best practice within their profession' (2018: 60). Certainly, in the context of racism, the approach that is presented in this book is not one that believes political correctness causes racism. Rather, it is the extent to which examples of racism remain an effect of the very regulations that political correctness propagates in its attempts to manage, contain and frame the other. Again, it is in this context that political correctness achieves its universal position, formed from the fact that political correctness requires 'racism' and the 'racist other' in order to maintain its privileged universal status.

To this end, it is not enough that we simply call for more political correctness, nor should we simply oppose it. As noted by Daly in his work on subversion:

> Subversion is not simply a neutral practice; rather it is something that takes place in a historically structured way. With today's multiculturalist ethos we get all kinds of subversions which, although they do challenge existing authorities and do de-naturalize a whole range of social/sexual relations, do not manage to threaten the underlying principles of the socio-economic order itself – on the contrary, such subversions often serve as a way of preserving the very dynamism of that order.
>
> *(2010: 21)*

For Daly, then, 'the more radical question is whether forms of subversion can be developed that are capable of subverting the very logics of existing subversion' (2010: 6). In explaining his 'subversion of subversion', Daly outlines:

> the development of forms of subversion that do not condone existing logics of subversion but which seek rather to undermine and repudiate the latter and to thereby open up new spaces of political possibility and creativity. It would mean not only breaking with the implicit grammar and interdictions of political discourse (the veiled agreements over the 'need' for low corporate taxation, for re-capitalizing global markets, for continuing with providing incentives for financiers-investors and so on), but also more direct, and even violent, forms of confrontation as well. Both are ultimately aspects of the same undertaking: the de-identification with 'due process' and the existing horizons of possibility and political choice.
>
> *(2010: 15)*

This book has elaborated on this process by considering how comedy can afford such a path, offering neither a complete withdrawal from forms of confrontation (as seen in Critchley and Heller's incongruent distance) nor a simple hyper-active resistance to forms of inequality (as seen in multicultural discourses). Instead, as detailed in Chapter Four, attention has been given to exploring how comedy can induce a parallax shift in our capacity to approach topics such as racism. By exploring comedy's ability to expose the inherent 'gap' or inconsistencies of the symbolic order/big Other, this approach has considered the various ways in which certain universal notions can be concretely performed *through* comedy. That is, in a process akin to Daly's (2010) 'subversion of subversion', the efforts of this book have sought to ground such a development in the failed possibilities that comedy can expose.

In order to meet this aim, it has been argued that specific attention should be paid to examining comedy's 'form' in 'the mode of the comic processing itself' (Zupančič, 2008: 30). Such an approach steers away from merely acknowledging the racist, sexist or homophobic content of certain jokes or comedy sequences, towards an exploration of the formal structure of those instances where mis-communication, faux pas and failure form part of the comic mode. As Chow details in relation to stand-up comedy:

> It is well known that stand-up often misfires: the room doesn't unite in laughter, it splits, divides, the fault line often directly separating the performer from the audience. These 'misfires', when the joke misses its target, … point us to another politics of comedy, less frequently considered by comedians and scholars.
>
> *(2014: 225)*

Indeed, it has been the conviction of this study that such 'misfiring' proves constitutive of both the comic sequence and human interaction in general. It is in the act of comically performing these misfires, both unintentionally, as in the case of Chow's (2014) stand-up example, and in the deliberate performance of such a misfire, as in the case of *The Office*, that a more subversive realtering of the socio-symbolic field can be achieved (Žižek, 1998a). To this extent, this study echoes Kamm and Neumann's claim that:

> the specific achievement of TV comedy might well be to teasingly tackle conflicts and social challenges that seem irresolvable at the time of enactment, thus not so much showing a way out of cultural predicaments, but rather allowing to assess them from a different, transgressive perspective.
>
> *(2016: 7)*

It is this perspective which has been considered in the analysis of *The Office* and, in particular, its performance of a 'black man's cock' joke. What has remained central to this analysis, and what proved crucial in the selection of the 'Merger' episode, was the extent to which the comic performance sought to deliberately and unapologetically perform a racist joke and, in so doing, draw attention to both the spectacle and spectre of race.

Race, racism and political correctness: A subversive performance

In combining psychoanalytic approaches to race and racism with Hsiao's (2010) spectre and spectacle distinctions, this analysis has highlighted how the efforts of political correctness, while drawing attention to race's spectacle – through racial/ethnic equality initiatives and multicultural agendas (spectacles which simply reassert the artificiality of racial difference) – ultimately ignore the spectral significance of race as a category of in-visibility. It is this spectacle which keeps the spectre at a distance, encouraging post-racial declarations which ignore ongoing forms of racism and racial inequality. What this spectre avers is the Real of racism, that which is disavowed, but which nonetheless proves an effect-cause of racial difference as it is performed across a variety of symbolic and imaginary constructions.

Here, the comic performance of a 'black man's cock' joke, and its extended comic sequence in the 'Merger' episode, was selected due to its direct subversion of the spectacle of 'blackness' through a performance that deliberately enacted a racist trope. This does not ignore the spectacle of race, but, in the character of Oliver, renders the spectre of race visible via the comic sequence. Nor is this visibility achieved through a form of cynical distance – it is not an ironic performance that deliberately uses racism to merely transgress what is believed to be an inherently transgressive example – instead, the multiple failures of the proceeding scenes and the inherent failure of David to maintain his politically correct status, prove to be a decidedly awkward and, indeed, frustratingly comic experience. As a result, the impasses that David's excess presents prove indicative of the Real (McGowan, 2017). Here, the inefficiency of political correctness is laid bare, not in its open denouncement nor in its reassertion, but through deliberately suspending its efficiency and failing to offer some path out of David's ongoing predicament. We can see this in the following ways.

First, through a repetition of the Real, we are, over the course of the four scenes, repeatedly subject to the joke's performance and to the continual failure of David to acknowledge his politically correct presumptions and the effect this is having. It is in this way that the joke's racism is used as a means of navigating the symbolic rules and conventions that structure human interaction and, in particular, to those forms of exclusion that exist within the socio-symbolic order, in this case, *within* political correctness itself. The novelty here is not the enjoyment of repeating the racist joke, but the novelty of the repetition itself. Equally, this repetition is not used to create something 'new'. This would signify a 'change in perspective' on behalf of David, who subsequently undergoes a process of realisation, from which he leaves the episode a 'changed man'. As scene four reveals, there is no change in David's perception of the joke, instead, the repetition of the joke and David's excessive attempts to continually *deflect* its racism serve to expose the effects of the Real through a comic performance that allows the inconsistency – the gap – at the heart of both the subject and the big Other to be performed.

Second, it is through the comic sequence that we observe a certain redoubling that, in the confines of the symbolic authority afforded by political correctness, reveals how the ambiguities *within* political correctness can be mediated *through* the big Other. That is, in scene one, we witness the false appearance of David's political correctness, with the joke's racist significance being acknowledged but maintained. In scene's two to four, however, we see the falsity of this appearance openly performed in various instances that radically require the joke to be told and re-told. It is with each re-telling that the sequence excessively and reflexively performs the inherent failure of political correctness, with each instance failing to curb the racism which it is required to prohibit. As a result, neither David nor Oliver act in defiance of the big Other nor do they oppose the symbolic mandates prescribed by political correctness, but instead the performance of the comic sequence ensures that it is through David's attempts to be 'politically correct' that what is usually prohibited – the telling of a racist joke – is both performed and enacted under the aegis of the big Other (see Chapter Four). This is continued in the third scene, when Jennifer helps to continue the comic sequence by asking David to repeat the joke. To this extent, it is through the very authority which is tasked with curtailing, preventing and dispelling forms of racism (being an office manager) that we observe the open performance of a racist joke. In this way both the joke and its performance are subversively re-articulated.

Third, the comedy sequence approaches, but also *uses*, the potential misfires that underscore human interaction and which serve as a constitutive feature of David's interactions with Oliver and his colleagues. Rather than precluding any form of interaction that seeks to manage or regulate examples of racism, the sequence opens a space where the antagonisms within the socio-symbolic order are laid bare. This works against the ideological operation of political correctness, where, instead of approaching racism, it deliberately masks or occludes its existence by ignoring any direct encounter with the *possibility* of racism.

Therefore, rather than proclaiming or demonstrating a fantasy of political correctness, the comic 'moment marks the intrusion of a radical openness in which every ideal support of our existence is suspended' (Žižek, 2012: 9), but also performed. It is in this sense that 'the very kernel of our being can be watched and performed only as comedy' (Zupančič, 2008: 182). Moreover, Zupančič's 'true comedy', defined 'as the expression of the universal in the concrete' (Berlant and Ngai, 2017: 234) is, in the case of political correctness, 'a universal which is no longer (re)presented as being in action, but *is* in action' (Zupančič, 2008: 27). By way of highlighting comedy's Real subversion, the following and final discussion will serve to conclude Zupančič's (2008) analysis of comedy and the concrete universal with the possibility of critiquing future examples of political correctness.

The Real 'ex-posed': The concrete universal, parallax and excess

As detailed in the above conclusions, the purpose of this study has been to expose that intimate space which is shared, and in the case of *The Office* performed, when we tell a joke or when we watch a comic performance. In part, it is in these performances that the ontological constitution of the symbolic order/big Other is exposed as being grounded in a fundamental 'gap'. This 'gap' has been reflected in the various instances where the inconsistency of the symbolic order/big Other is identified in the concrete universal. As a result, comedy reveals those instances where our social norms, values and politically correct standards prove illusive and impotent. This is an approach that steers towards antagonism, but which is not intended to be antagonistic. Instead, our relation to antagonism bears witness to the Real, a traumatic presence that undermines our social interactions, but which can also draw attention to that which gets 'too close' (Žižek, 1998b). It is this 'closeness' which is performed in comedy and which is reflected in the sense of awkwardness we feel when a joke or comedy sequence reveals something Real (when a joke gets 'too close'). Comedy's subversion emanates not from ignoring this tension, but from repeating and returning to this tension via the Real. As a result:

> the Real 'ex-posed' by comedy is usually not the Real of what happened, but the structural Real (or impasse) the suppression of which constitutes the very coherence of our reality. By ignoring the Real of what happened, comedy succeeds in displaying the crack in the midst of our most familiar realities. And *this* is the real core of comedy.
>
> *(Zupančič, 2008: 58)*

It is in ex-posing the Real that the 'crack' within our reality can be performatively demonstrated through comedy. Here, the incomplete ontological constitution of material reality is exposed through its own ex-sistence. It is in accordance with this ontological incompleteness that the inherent inconsistencies of the symbolic order (the gap within any signifying system, 'the missing signifier'), the big Other ('the big Other does not exist') and the subject (the relation of the subject to the Real/the divided subject) have been conceived. Central to this consideration, however, has been envisaging how such incompleteness can, in the case of comedy, be provided a subversive significance. Notably, this has been approached via the contention that comedy's subversion does not occur from a reactionary position but, instead, emerges from *within* the discourses and universal assumptions which both structure and orientate our socio-symbolic and imaginary constructions. In other words, from the 'split' or 'gap' which constitutes these abstract constructions, and which is made visible in their concrete manifestation (Daly, 2010; Žižek, 2006a). More to the point, it is in acknowledging this 'gap' that one can steer clear of those inherent transgressions that always-already draw upon subversive elements in order to maintain the status quo. As noted in Chapter One, it is this un-subversive subversion which has underscored postmodernism's political impotency and its culturalisation of politics. Under postmodernism, ideology is *post*-ideological, and it is in this way that ideology occurs through forms of cynical distance that maintain our relation to the ideological field. This is reflected in examples of comedy that draw upon irony, satire and cynicism.

In contrast, this study has delivered its own 'traversal' via the subversive significance of Zupančič's (2008) concrete universal and Žižek's (2006a) parallax view. When considered together, it has been argued that both terms can be used to examine those instances where the modal logic of a particular situation is undermined from within this modality itself (Daly, 2010). Importantly, while such an approach seeks neither to 'cure' nor 'banish' racism, it instead presents an alteration in the relational structures that produce racism. In other words, it seeks to examine those formal structures which constitute racism's recurrence across different socio-historical contexts. To help elucidate this, we can return to the general use of stereotypes in both society and comedy. Indeed, if we consider that the use of stereotypes remains embedded in the societies, cultures, traditions and histories of the groups that use them, then it is perhaps of greater concern that their possible adoption remains a fundamental feature of any society or group that contains individuals who can be delineated based upon their 'race', religion, gender, sexuality and/or (dis)ability. What remains significant, therefore, is how directly confronting these stereotypes serves only to maintain the hegemonic position of the particular stereotype that is being admonished. That is, it transfers it to a position of universal significance – the moot point – from which it continues to hold a certain standard. Certainly, this is not to ignore the inaccuracy or the impact of a particular stereotype; instead, what it calls for is a consideration of how these stereotypes, and their already established subversions, are subverted. It is this process of subversion which is enacted in *The Office* and which bears witness to the comic impasses that arise in examples of political correctness.

As detailed in Chapter Five's analysis, it was argued that political correctness finds itself facing its 'unbearable' concrete antagonism in the 'Merger' episode: a black man who finds a joke about a racial stereotype concerning black men funny. To this end, we don't see a criticism of or resistance to political correctness through its 'content' (the racist joke), as evident in the various ways in which David's telling of the joke is admonished by the staff and his subsequent rebuttals, but instead in David's concrete responses: his patronising 'harmless' and 'well done!'; his concern that the joke is a compliment; and his assertion that 'mixed-race' is his 'favourite'. In this sense, it is not that David is an ignorant, right-leaning racist, but rather a confused liberal, desperately performing a politically correct rhetoric that comically reveals the inherent inconsistencies in political correctness itself. More importantly, this critique is not levelled from a position *outside* of political correctness. That is, the comedy performed does not seek to make fun of or satirise the politically correct individual. To do so would present a form of critique that remains grounded in a position that is *separated from* political correctness, echoing the criticisms that have been levelled at Critchley and Heller. Rather, what the episode performs is the failure and inconsistency of political correctness when it is *in action*. It is, in other words, in the inherent excessiveness of political correctness – its regulated management of human interaction; its ability to maintain the other at a 'safe' distance; its capacity to approach cultural differences through spectacle and artificiality – that its slip-ups, misfires and inconsistencies are laid bare. Accordingly, while Gilroy asserts that 'Brent's weaknesses, in particular his vanity and absolute lack of principle, make him into a representative character who, incidentally, captures all the inconsistencies and shallowness of the New Labour project' (2004: 151), it is the contention of this book that the 'inconsistencies' and 'shallowness' of political correctness are not necessarily 'represented', but instead are performed *in* the character of David Brent. In part, this is achieved through David's ability to 'include' Oliver's presence in the joke. Such 'inclusion' highlights the pretense of the universal, which seeks to include that which remains its 'included exception'. Instead, such 'Inclusion does not eliminate failure but excessively reproduces it' (McGowan, 2016: 611), providing an 'excessive engagement that turns the agent into a singular universality' (Žižek, 2010: 125) via the concrete universal. In other words, political correctness 'enters into dialectical tension with its own particular content' (Žižek, 2010: 336). In short, this presents an attempt to maintain, ex-pose and re-approach our relations to such tension (the Real), through forms of anxiety that deliberately require a new way of looking at things.

Over the course of this study, and in accordance with Zupančič's concrete universal, this new way of looking at things has been supplemented with the short-circuiting that Žižek's parallax view prescribes. Central to both notions is the extent to which they can 're-align' our perspective on reality, drawing attention to what was previously ignored or obscured. As noted, Zupančič's concrete universal does not ignore or eradicate the universal, but rather through a parallax view can expose the shift in perspective that reveals the inherent contradictions and impasses that emerge from performing this universal in action. Through a comic parallax shift, we can observe how 'the universal is on the side of undermining the universal' (Zupančič, 2008: 28). Here, the Real of racism and the spectre of race are brought to bear via that point of tension, antagonism or exclusion that neither generates nor explicitly undermines the universal, but which exposes its inherent 'gap'. This application of the concrete universal posits the scenes' true comedy, repeating the Real via a form of reflexive mobilisation that critically exposes the inconsistencies in political correctness.

Political correctness: In principle, yes; in practice, no

A key part of this book has been to explore the assertion that political correctness works from a position of abstract universality – indeed, that it is a 'mute medium' from which all cultures, identities, sexualities, ethnicities etc., can come together under some universal whole (Žižek, 2017). A fight for every culture, but a fight that fails to ever truly acknowledge, or appreciate, the Real differences and inherent antagonisms which structure such a 'fight' in the first place. In contrast, this book has served to examine the effectiveness of political correctness when conceived as an 'actual universality [which] "appears" (actualizes itself) as the experience of negativity, of the inadequacy-to-itself' (Žižek, 2012: 361 [italics removed]). Following Zupančič, it is this 'negativity' and 'inadequacy-to-itself' that comedy performs. What becomes evident from this approach, however, is the extent to which examples of political correctness can, to a certain extent, be maintained in order to 'hold on' to that experience of negativity and inadequacy which such a comic rendering can provide. That is, to what extent can examples of political correctness be used to preserve a critical understanding of the 'potential' universality which constitutes society's 'impossibility', and, by extension, how can it shed light on the various antagonisms and stumbling blocks that underscore our social relations? In short, how can political correctness remain comically subversive?

In answer to these final questions, we can consider how our approach to political correctness can be allied with Žižek's (2010) reflections on the 'death penalty'. Indeed, Žižek grounds his example on 'a wonderful Jewish story about an anti-death-penalty Talmud specialist who, embarrassed by the fact that the death penalty is ordained by God himself, proposed a delightfully practical solution' (2010: 20). He explains:

> one should not directly overturn the divine injunction, that would have been blasphemous; but one should treat it as God's slip of tongue, his moment of madness, and invent a complex network of sub-regulations and conditions which while leaving the possibility of a death penalty intact, ensure that this possibility will never be realised.
>
> *(Žižek, 2010: 20)*

Žižek's adoption of this story proves constitutive of his approach to the concrete universal, revealing a subversive significance. Indeed, as Žižek notes:

> The beauty of this procedure is that it turns around the standard trick of prohibiting something in principle (torture, for instance), but then slipping in enough qualifications ('except in specified extreme circumstances ...') to ensure it can be done whenever one really wants to do it.
>
> *(2010: 20)*

More to the point, 'one accepts the final catastrophe – the obscenity of people killing their neighbours as a form of justice – as inevitable, written into our destiny, and then one engages in postponing it for as long as possible, hopefully indefinitely' (Žižek, 2012: 982).[1] What we see from this example is a deliberate rendering of the dictum: in principle, yes; in practice, no.

If we consider cases of torture such as the violation of human rights by the US Army and CIA at Abu Ghraib prison (Iraq), then we can see that, despite their disavowal of the practice of torture (in principle, no), ultimately, forms of torture were maintained under 'exceptional circumstances' (in practice, yes). In the case of the Talmud specialist, however, we experience the obverse – in principle, yes (torture is allowed), but in practice, no (the complex array of sub-regulations that prevent the act from occurring). As a result, it is in this latter example that the failure to achieve the principle is continually performed through its failed practice. Indeed, this same approach can be applied to political correctness and, more importantly, can be given a comic significance.

As argued throughout this book, the intention has never been to openly call for more racism; instead, it has, through the form of comedy, sought to trace a path that, while not ignoring racism (the Real), seeks to obtain a position where its effects are distrusted, played with and, in short, made fun of. In other words, one can comically perform the essential ineffectiveness of a practice that, in principle, is maintained, but which ultimately remains beholden to the failure of its realisation. Furthermore, it is comedy's ability to perform PC's sub-regulations as well as its incessant attempts to manage and dictate the correct form of human interaction, which is subsequently enacted in its practiced 'no'. Significantly, this is not an attempt to reassert further regulation, but an endeavour to accept the 'inevitable' obscenity that comedy can arouse in order to comically (and indefinitely) subvert the regulated way in which political correctness seeks, in practice, to manage human interaction. In short, it is to view political correctness *as a comic form* that, when applied, comically fails to meet its desired objectives: a universal practice that continually looks for exceptions to the rule (a universalised exception).

To this extent, what comedy can expose is the tensions that inevitably surround the telling of a joke or the performance of a 'risky' comic sequence. This is certainly not intended to fetishise the 'risk' involved. Indeed, as Flisfeder (2019) asserts, if a fetish is what hides the lack in signification, then the approach undertaken in this book is that 'race' is an inherently lacking symbolic-imaginary signification (see Chapter Three). Accordingly, it is in performing and drawing attention to this lack that 'the precious "middle ground" of civility, which mediates between uncontrolled private fantasies and the strictly regulated forms of intersubjective behaviour', can be upheld (Žižek, 2006b: xii). That is to say, it is this 'middle ground' in human and social interaction which bears witness to the 'contingent, self-reflective individuals that subjects must come to accept' in order to 'affirm the commonality which binds them' (Dews, 1995: 22). In the case of comedy, this can help mobilise such idiosyncrasies (our shared sense of strangeness) as a way of retaining our anxiety to the Real. Here, Žižek asserts:

> Politeness (manners, gallantry) is more than just obeying external legality and less than pure moral activity. It is the ambiguously imprecise domain of what one is not strictly obliged to do (if one doesn't do it, one doesn't break any laws), but what one is nonetheless expected to do. We are dealing here with implicit unspoken regulations, with questions of tact, with something towards which subjects have as a rule a non-reflected relationship, something that is part of our spontaneous sensitivity, a thick texture of customs and expectations woven into our inherited substance of mores … Therein resides the self-destructive deadlock of Political Correctness: it tries to explicitly formulate, legalize even, the stuff of manners.
>
> *(2018: 167)*

The capacity of political correctness to penalise this behaviour is its inherent weakness and one that, through the adoption of the concrete universal and parallax view, can expose the comedy at its heart. In other words, it is in comically performing and exposing this 'self-destructive' deadlock at the heart of political correctness that a process of subversion can be maintained. The key here is to remain within sight of the 'inevitable' failure which underscores this principle. Therefore, though in principle, 'yes', one should not go out of their way to mock or deride certain individuals or groups; in practice, our response to political correctness should be 'no'. One should comically and indefinitely postpone or subvert the various ways in which this principle is enacted and pursued. It is in the process of continually guaranteeing such practice that political correctness can be subversively administered *through its failure*. It is in comically performing this failure that comedy's Real subversion can be achieved.

Note

1 Žižek (2012) draws upon Dupuy's 'enlightened catastrophism' to help elaborate upon this example.

References

Berlant, L. and Ngai, S. 2017. Comedy has issues. *Critical Inquiry*, 43, 233–249.
Chow, B. 2014. The tickling object: On Žižek and comedy. In: B. Chow and A. Mangold, eds. *Žižek and Performance*. Basingstoke: Palgrave Macmillan, 224–252.
Critchley, S. 2002. *On Humour*. London: Routledge.
Daly, G. 2010. Causes for concern: Žižek's politics of loving terror. *The International Journal of Žižek Studies*, 4 (2), 1–23.
Dews, P. 1995. The tremor of reflection: Slavoj Žižek's Lacanian dialectics. *Radical Philosophy*, 72, 17–29.
Dunant, S. 1994. Introduction: What's in a word? In: S. Dunant, ed. *The War of the Words: The Political Correctness Debate*. London: Virago Press, vii–xv.
Flisfeder, M. 2019. Postmodern Marxism today: Jameson, Žižek, and the demise of symbolic efficiency. *The International Journal of Žižek Studies*, 13 (1), 23–56.
Gilroy, P. 2004. *After Empire: Melancholia or Convivial Culture?* Abingdon: Routledge.
Heller, A. 2005. *Immortal Comedy: The Comic Phenomenon in Art, Literature, and Life*. Lanham, MD: Lexington Books.
Hsiao, L.-C. 2010. Color (un)conscious: Psychoanalysis, resistance, and the specter/spectacle of race. *Concentric: Literary and Cultural Studies*, 36 (1), 159–187.
Kamm, J. and Neumann, B. 2016. Introduction: The aesthetics and politics of British TV comedy. In: J. Kamm and B. Neumann, eds. *British TV Comedies: Cultural Concepts, Contexts and Controversies*. Basingstoke: Palgrave Macmillan, 1–22.
McGowan, T. 2016. The location of silent comedy: Charlie Chaplin's outsider and Buster Keaton's insider. *Quarterly Review of Film and Video*, 33 (7), 602–619.
McGowan, T. 2017. *Only a Joke Can Save Us: A Theory of Comedy*. Evanston, IL: Northwestern University Press.
Pound, M. 2010. Comic subjectivity: Žižek and Zupančič's spiritual work of art. *The International Journal of Žižek Studies*, 4 (4), 1–17.
Pound, M. 2015. Political theology and comedy: Žižek through rose tinted glasses. *Crisis and Critique*, 2 (1), 171–191.
Quirk, S. 2018. *The Politics of British Stand-Up Comedy: The New Alternative*. Gewerbestrasse, Switzerland: Palgrave Macmillan.

Žižek, S. 1998a. *Tarrying with the Negative: Kant, Hegel, and the Critique of Ideology*. Durham, NC: Duke University Press.

Žižek, S. 1998b. Love thy neighbour? No, thanks! In: C. Lane, ed. *The Psychoanalysis of Race*. New York, NY: Columbia University Press, 154–175.

Žižek, S. 2006a. *The Parallax View*. Cambridge, MA: MIT Press.

Žižek, S. 2006b. Preface to the paperback edition: The big Other between violence and civility. In: R. Butler and S. Stephens, eds. *Slavoj Žižek: The Universal Exception*. London: Continuum, vii–xxxii.

Žižek, S. 2010. *Living in the End Times*. London: Verso.

Žižek, S. 2012. *Less Than Nothing: Hegel and the Shadow of Dialectical Materialism*. London: Verso.

Žižek, S. 2017. *Against the Double Blackmail: Refugees, Terror and Other Troubles with the Neighbour*. London: Penguin.

Žižek, S. 2018. *Like a Thief in Broad Daylight: Power in the Era of Post-Humanity*. London: Allen Lane.

Zupančič, A. 2008. *The Odd One In: On Comedy*. Cambridge, MA: MIT Press.

INDEX

For Product Safety Concerns and Information please contact our EU representative GPSR@taylorandfrancis.com
Taylor & Francis Verlag GmbH, Kaufingerstraße 24, 80331 München, Germany

www.ingramcontent.com/pod-product-compliance
Lightning Source LLC
LaVergne TN
LVHW010649300926
849161LV00005B/1077
* 9 7 8 0 3 6 7 5 0 8 9 5 1 *